About the Author:

Brent Q. Hafen received his Ph.D. from the University of Southern Illinois. A former associate editor of *Health Education,* Dr. Hafen has held the position of Professor of Health Science at Brigham Young University, and is the author of several major health education texts.

$17.95

C0-BEH-470

NUTRITION,
FOOD,
AND WEIGHT
CONTROL

NUTRITION, FOOD, AND WEIGHT CONTROL

Expanded Edition

Brent Q. Hafen
Brigham Young University

with contributions from
Laren R. Robison
Brenda Peterson
Katherine G. Elliott
Roberta Setzer

ALLYN AND BACON, INC.
Boston, London, Sydney, Toronto

Library of Congress Cataloging in Publication Data

Hafen, Brent Q
    Nutrition, food, and weight control.

    Bibliography: p.
    Includes index.
    1. Nutrition.   2. Obesity.   3. Reducing
diets.   I. Title.
QP141.H186 1980b   613.2'5   80–15207
ISBN 0–205–06825–1

Series Editor: Hiram Howard

Printed in the United States of America

Contents

Preface   vii

Preface

Although the United States has perhaps the safest, most adequate, and most nutritious food supply in the world, inadequate nutrition is one of our nation's major health problems. Many Americans have poor eating habits, which may lead to malnutrition, overweight, obesity, or increased risk for various diseases.

Even though weight control is a concern of almost half of the adult population, many people have fallacious concepts about appropriate ways to lose weight. A plethora of information and misinformation on nutrition and weight control makes it difficult for the typical layperson (or the professional who is not directly involved in the area of nutrition) to determine what is accurate scientifically. Recent studies show evidence of confusion over vitamins and minerals, fats, trace elements, vegetarianism, fiber, sugar, and fad diets.

Nutrition, Food, and Weight Control represents a gleaning from the research and writings of many prominent experts in the field of nutrition and weight control. It covers both popular and traditional concerns. Not only does the book consider what we do know about nutrition; it also suggests ways of applying that knowledge for the purpose of improving health.

This book is intended as a practical reference for health educators, home economists, nurse practitioners, and any other professionals who are educating or advising others on practical nutritional matters. Unit 1 covers traditional areas of nutritional concern, while Unit 2 delves into such popular concerns as fiber, sugar, food additives, vegetarianism, and nutrition and disease. Unit 3 is devoted to obesity and weight control—what obesity is, what causes it, how to control it, and evaluations of various diets and methods that are supposed to control weight. The Appendixes provide reference material for individual nutritional evaluation or teaching purposes. A glossary has supplementary definitions for those terms printed in boldface type throughout the book.

In terms of money and human suffering, one can well argue that every dollar and hour spent on nutritional instruction may save tens of dollars and hours in medical care, because improvements in nutrition seem to have a direct effect on the level of health. Although there is sufficient nutritional information available for those who know how to seek it out, there are few books that adequately cover both traditional nutritional topics and contemporary concerns in easy-to-understand language. It is the hope of the author that the information provided herein may fill that need.

B.Q.H.

NUTRITION, FOOD, AND WEIGHT CONTROL

UNIT 1

BASIC NUTRIENTS

1

Agriculture: Food and People

From our earliest beginnings the most valuable commodity has been food; the most important practice, agriculture. Too often food production and food availability are taken for granted, especially in the United States and other developed nations, because, for the most part, food abundance and variety have continued without interruption. The real value of food seems to become apparent to most people only during shortage.

In reference to the world community, however, Jonathan Swift is still right: "Whoever could make two ears of corn or two blades of grass to grow upon a spot where only one grew before would deserve better of mankind and do more essential service to their country than the whole race of politicians put together."[1] And certainly two of Malthus's observations in 1798 are as true today as they were when he made them: First, that food is necessary to the existence of man. Second, that the passion between the sexes is necessary and will remain necessarily in its present state.[2]

It is safe to assume that, at least in the immediate future, population will continue to grow, and food production and availability will continue to be a primary focus of world attention and concern.

A second dimension of the food picture sometimes hidden by the necessity of making more ears of corn or blades of grass grow is that of quality.

Historically, a focus on quantity (yield) has always preceded concern with quality. The simple expediency of "you got to eat to think, you got to eat to work," makes this so. Research on quality requires a tremendous investment in time, effort, and finances. Fortunately, in the United States, where one farmer feeds himself or herself and fifty-six other people, the burden of food production is lifted, allowing fifty-six people to follow other pursuits. Therefore, research can be done. Unfortunately, at the present time in the United States less than 2 percent of the federal research budget is allocated for agricultural research. This is an interesting situation in a nation producing over 80 percent of the world's exportable food.

It is important that people understand food—its source, its supply, and its quality. The consumer, especially in large cities, is far removed from the site of food production, and there is little that identifies items on a supermarket shelf with the forms in which they were produced. Therefore, in the developed nations,

This chapter was prepared by Dr. Laren R. Robison, Chairman, Department of Agronomy and Horticulture, Brigham Young University.

especially in the United States where less than 4 percent of the population are farmers, food at the farm level is not understood.

There is a constant barrage of food-related literature which places us on the brink of disaster due to the lack of land, crop yield barriers, adverse weather, lack of water, etc. It suggests we are unknowingly being poisoned by agricultural chemicals, and that use of "organic" food-producing methods would somehow increase the quality of food. The literature would have us further believe that proteins, vitamins, and minerals are removed during processing from food which is then wrapped, distributed to the supermarkets, and sold to the naive consumer. Such reports from consumer activist groups and "food faddists" leave most consumers uncertain of what to believe.

LAND AVAILABLE

The argument that the world is running out of agricultural land dates back to Malthus. Neo-Malthusians in recent years have taken the same posture and are recycling his conclusions. The arguments sound plausible but miss some important points.

First, it is true that the greater part of the land available and suitable for crop production is not deep Iowa farm soil. It is mostly raw land (pastures, grassland, and forests) and needs the hand of a farmer to put it into production. However, there is a great deal of difference between not having any land and having land that needs development. All of the farmland being used today has gone through that development cycle. No one would argue that the economic returns must exceed the investment, and capital must be made available for pioneers. For this to become a national policy, however, would merely require that new priorities be set.

Second, the amount of land devoted to grain is increasing at about 1 percent per year worldwide and more than double that in parts of Latin America and Africa. Most authorities would agree that the amount of potentially arable land in the world is from 3.0 to 3.2 billion hectares (7.4 to 7.9 billion acres).[3] This is roughly twice the amount of land that is currently under cultivation and about three times what is actually being harvested. In the United States in 1969, there was estimated to be approximately 472 million acres of cropland being used for crops, soil improvement, and pasture. By 1974, almost all of the readily available cropland had been returned to crop production; however, an additional 266 million acres of land not classed as cropland could produce crops if needed. So even in the United States we are using only about 64 percent of the potentially available land. Thus, the food supply–available land situation is not so bleak either in the world or in the United States.

CROP YIELDS

As the most easily developed arable land has yielded to population pressure, and as the necessity for more food has exceeded land development, there has been a transition from "area" to "yield" agriculture; that is, obtaining more kilograms from the same hectare. This started primarily in the developed countries, because yield agriculture requires tremendous financial input into research, programs, and facilities. When this transition spread from developed to less developed countries, and yield increases occurred, especially in wheat and rice, the term "green revolution" was coined.

Plants provide almost 95 percent of the world's food supply either directly or indirectly.[4] Nutritionists have long maintained that a healthy diet includes carbohydrates and fats for energy, combined with a proper balance of other nutrients—vitamins, minerals, proteins, and water, provided by daily servings from the "Four Basic Food Groups." A cursory review of these groups indicates a relatively higher proportion of animal products, most of which are readily available only in developed nations. The world runs on grains, and plants are a poor person's meat. Plants provide directly 88 percent of the calories and 80 percent of the protein eaten by people.

The world's principal food crops, in approximate order of importance, are (1) cereal grains, (2) seed legumes, (3) root and tuber crops, (4) sugar crops, and (5) tropical crops. A listing of these important food crops is given below.

IMPORTANT MAJOR FOOD CROPS

Cereal Grains	Seed Legumes	Root and Tuber Crops	Sugar Crops	Tropical Crops
Rice	Field Beans	Potatoes	Sugar Cane	Bananas
Wheat	Peanuts	Sweet Potatoes	Sugar Beets	Coconut
Corn	Chick Peas	Casava		
Barley	Pigeon Peas			
Sorghum	Soybeans			
Millet	Mung Beans			
Oats	Broad Beans			
Rye				

A secondary but extremely important source of food is the fruit and vegetable crops. One of the great untapped sources of food, which could play a tremendous role in supplying vitamins, minerals, and carbohydrates, is small garden plots. Research on garden plots of different sizes has indicated that a significant amount of food can be produced in a small area of land.

Garden Size (sq. ft.)	Pounds of Fresh Vegetables Produced
5 × 5	59
10 × 10	184
15 × 25	403
20 × 20	485
50 × 50	1,847

Brigham Young University, Agronomy & Horticulture Dept., 1977–78.

This research was conducted in the temperate zone. Tropical and semitropical yields would be larger due to the longer growing period.

The potential for production increases is tremendous. Clifton Cox of Armour Food Company suggests that all the following yield increases could be obtained simultaneously using present technology.

Commodity	*% Increase*
Grain Sorghum	94
Barley	68
Corn	66
Soybeans	42
Oats	29
Wheat	20

Most impressive, however, are those statistics which indicate something that has been accomplished, rather than estimates of the future. The past history of American agriculture is perhaps the best example. Even though acreage has been reduced by government "set aside programs," yields and total pounds of any given crop in any given year continue to climb. Record yields of crops are compared to average production and 1985 estimated yields in Table 1-1.

Table 1-1. Yields from Some Major Food Crops in the United States

	Average Yield Bushels Per Acre 1979	**Record Yields**	**Expected Yields by 1985**
Barley	50	212	80
Corn	109	352	150
Oats	54	296	80
Potatoes	272 cwt	875 cwt	400 cwt
Rice	101	—	130
Sorghum	63	320	80
Soybeans	32	110	40
Wheat	34	216	50

Modified from "Food Production: Technology and the Resource Base," Wittwer, S. H., *Science*, Vol. 188, pp. 579–584, Table, 9 May 1975, copyright by the American Association for the Advancement of Science.

A similar story can be told of rice and wheat in Mexico, India, Pakistan, the Philippines, and other developing nations. Improvements in yield have been effected through a number of means — breeding techniques, fertilizer, irrigation, and pest management.

Breeding Techniques   Standard breeding techniques have accomplished much in the past and will continue to be the principal means of improvement in the foreseeable future. A good example is the change in plant architecture of rice. Because the flag leaf on new varieties does not droop below the panicle (head), the leaves can function more efficiently in capturing sunlight from photosynthesis, thus providing the needed carbohydrates for improved rice production. Hybrid corn is perhaps the stellar achievement in American agricultural research. A 352.64-bushel record yield in 1977 certainly points the way to the future. Equally significant for developing nations is the initial development and utilization of high-yielding varieties of rice and wheat. These varieties now account for approximately 26 percent of the rice and 50 percent of the wheat acreage in Asia and the near East. The People's Republic of China announced the development of a spring wheat reported to yield over 100 bushels per acre even under adverse conditions. Of course, a major objective of crop breeding programs now is the development of varieties with higher protein content and improved amino acid balance, particularly the amino acid lysine. (See section on Food Quality.)

In the future, the technique of isolation could revolutionize agriculture and be a major avenue for building new species, improving yield, and improving nutritional quality. This technique isolates different cell protoplasts, fuses them, and subsequently regenerates them.

Fertilizer

Fertilizer is probably the single most important industrial input into agricultural productivity. Improving the efficiency of fertilizer uptake and use by plants is already a major goal of industry and university agricultural scientists. It is estimated that only 50 percent of the nitrogen and less than 35 percent of the phosphorus and potassium applied as fertilizer in the United States is being recovered by crops.[5] The remainder is lost to the environment. If these losses could be alleviated, tremendous increases in crop production could be expected. This would be especially true in the warm, tropical areas of the world, where losses are the highest.

Some of the innovations in the process of development or trial utilization are slow-released nitrogen fertilizers, improved methods of placement and application, new formulations of fertilizer for foliage application, and new fertilizer sources.

Irrigation

No factor affecting plant life is so clearly defined as water. Moisture determines the productive capacity of a crop, because all of the vital processes of plant cells take place in water. Agriculture worldwide suffers from a deficit of water.

Indeed, the development of irrigation is a primary target of most nations, developed or developing, because optimal use of crop resources comes from land that is irrigated. The utilization of tube wells in Asia, the redirection and utilization of entire rivers in Pakistan, the development of a superb trickle irrigation technique in Israel, the development of new water application techniques, and the breeding of crop varieties with greater water use efficiency will result in substantial improvements in crop productivity. It is estimated that approximately 30 percent of the food produced for mankind occurs on the 12 to 15 percent of land that is irrigated.[6] Thus, tremendous improvement in food production could come about through this one crop management tool.

Pest Management

It has been said that agriculture is a controversy with nature. Agriculture is interested in only a relatively few species of plants produced in mass plantings and, more often than not, as a monoculture. This has been encouraged by product demand and needs. Simply stated, farmers grow what will return to them the greatest financial incentive. This kind of agriculture, monoculture, encourages the development of associated plant pests—weeds, insects, disease, etc.

The question with pesticides, those chemicals used to mitigate pests, is not so much what the future will hold in terms of new products, technology, or uses, but what will happen to food supplies if environmental groups and federal regulatory agencies continue to stifle use in the name of conservation. It is estimated that crop yields in the United States would be reduced by 50 percent and food prices would rise four- or fivefold in the absence of pesticides.[7] This is already happening in some of the developing nations of the world. Worldwide losses from pests amount to approximately 30 percent of the total world harvest. Pesticides are at present the principal agent of control, simply because there are few alternatives available. Biological control is a possibility for the future, but is not very effective as yet. Meanwhile, pesticides are being developed which will be target specific. Researchers are also placing more emphasis on pest management, which integrates various control methods and places less emphasis on a single system such as pesticides.

Much could be written about each of the previous topics, and many examples given to show research programs and applications. Other research which will affect food supplies in the future will concern plant growth regulators, tillage systems, controlled environments (greenhouses), nutrient film and hydroponic techniques, new foods, and multiple cropping. While population increase will be a major focus of concern in the world, it will come at a time when the technology and capability to produce an adequate food supply will also be available.

FOOD QUALITY

Food quality can be measured in many different ways and is affected by every step in the production cycle from the seed to the table. The quality of the food we eat is largely determined by the harvesting and processing technology used and the way meals are prepared in the home. One aspect, however, which is more subtle and which only now is beginning to be revealed, is the effect on quality of specific varieties of species and management and production practices. (The same holds true for animal species and their management.)

The energy and nutritive value of food crops depends upon their chemical composition. All crops are different in their composition; furthermore, even though two species of plants may have similar nutrient content as determined chemically, they may act quite differently biologically. The differences are far more closely related to the genetic endowment of the plants than to their production. If plants are well nourished during their period of growth, they will provide high-quality food characteristic of their species.

Since plants provide 90 percent of the world food supply either directly or indirectly, the question to ask is "Is it possible to create 'supernutritious' plants so that at least the major nutritional needs of the people are satisfied?" For instance, is it possible to develop varieties of crops where the protein content could be raised and the amino acid balance changed to make them more nearly equivalent to the quality of animal protein?

Progress today on raising grain protein levels and increasing the level of critically deficient amino acids has been remarkable. A major research objective is the improvement of protein content and/or quality in plants, primarily because there is no better or cheaper way to improve protein needs of people, especially in the developing nations. In the United States and other developed nations, animal products will still continue to be the major source of protein. Even here, however, improved crops will improve animal production. The biological value of protein (for both human and animal consumption) in corn, rice, and wheat has been improved through the identification and use of breeding materials with increased lysine content. Rice, wheat, and barley selections with higher protein content have been identified, and some varieties are in commercial production. Rice selections with 2 percent higher protein than commercial varieties have been developed. "Lancota," a new hard, red winter wheat variety, has a yield equal to that of other released varieties but with 1 or 2 percent better protein, and "hyproly" barley has been used successfully as a parent in breeding programs to increase lysine content in several new barley selections which will become available soon. Not only is there a great deal of genetic potential to be tapped even in those crops where research has been already done, but much could be and is being done with many of the other grain crops, including sorghum, millet, and triticale.

In the case of sorghum, high lysine selections have been identified, and progress toward commercial production is moving rapidly. Triticale, a manmade cereal combining the characteristics of wheat and rye, has potential for becoming a major grain crop. The yield and protein of several selections of triticale are equivalent to those of wheat, and the amino acid balance is superior. Seed legumes are undergoing a similar change to improve their protein digestibility and nutritional value. Continued research in converting legumes to packaged, textured vegetable proteins will make them more acceptable to the consumer as meat substitutes.

Root and tuber crops are also undergoing the same development. Researchers at the International Potato Institute in Lima, Peru, have discovered potatoes with quite different characteristics than those commonly known—they have found potatoes with significant amounts of protein and high vitamin A. The same is true of sweet potatoes, which serve as an important source of energy in Africa, Asia, and South America. Research on the Latin American cassava indicates its future importance for food production. The Mayaguez Institute of Tropical Agriculture in Puerto Rico has also catalogued a large number of tropical plants which could be developed into food.

SUMMARY

There is good evidence that the world food problem, from the standpoint of diet, is not so much protein deficiency as caloric inadequacy. In other words, if caloric intake were increased, in many instances proteins would be adequate because the body would then assimilate them from the food source.

Food supplies in the United States are adequate at the present time and for the foreseeable future. Generally, food quality in the United States is the best in the world. Indeed, malnutrition in the United States is far more a matter of improper food choice and lack of nutritional education than a matter of inadequate food availability.

NOTES

1. Jonathan Swift, *Gulliver's Travels* (London: Oxford University Press, 1938), p. 158.
2. T. R. Malthus, *An Essay on the Principle of Population* (London: Ward, Lock, and Co., 1890), p. 448.
3. *World Food and Nutrition Study* (Washington: National Academy of Sciences, 1975), p. 65.
4. Marilyn Chou et al., *World Food Prospects and Agriculture Potential* (New York: Praeger Publishers, Inc., 1977).
5. "Food and Agriculture," *Scientific American,* September 1976.
6. Chou, *World Food Prospects.*
7. *Facts from Our Environment,* Potash Institute of North America, 1972.

2

Those Necessary Nutrients

In this land of plenty, millions of Americans aren't eating wisely. Not because they haven't enough to eat, but because they eat too much of the wrong things or too little of the right things. Food is what you eat, nutrition is how your body uses food. And if you are not eating foods to meet your bodily needs, you may be suffering from poor nutrition.[1]

Few people have a basic understanding of nutrition. Literally, "you are what you eat." Protein, carbohydrates, fats, vitamins, minerals, and water are all essential to nourish the body.

Not all foods contain the same nutrients and not all nutrients serve the same purpose in the body. The important thing is to remember that no one food does everything and all foods have something to offer. A variety of different types of food will provide all the nutrients most of us need. This chapter will discuss the nutrients protein, carbohydrates, fats, and water, while vitamins and minerals will be discussed in Chapters 3 and 4.

PROTEINS

What Are Proteins?

Next to water, proteins are the most abundant substance in body cells. They perform almost endless functions in the body. Jean Mayer states, "They are the most complex substances known to man." In fact, one scientist has called them "the noblest piece of architecture invented by nature."[2]

For some reason, proteins have taken on somewhat of a supernatural quality among many misinformed consumers. Claims such as the following abound: "Proteins are body builders and muscle makers," "They are excellent diet foods, as they contain no calories and burn up fat." Actually, these claims are groundless. Proteins are, in fact, vital to life and growth, but they are not a wonder food.

Perhaps the best way to explain proteins is by explaining about Gutenberg's invention in 1454.

Back in 1454, Johann Gutenberg, a citizen of Strasbourg, invented moveable type . . . what was so special was that instead of having to make each letter individually in each word of each sentence, as you would carve your name on a tree, Gutenberg made molds from which he could produce dozens of copies of each letter. These could be dropped into place to print anything of any length: short poems and long ones, plays, novels, histories, recipes, encyclopedias, newspapers, magazines and so on.[3]

Proteins work on the same principle. Proteins are the sentences. The letters are the twenty **amino acids,** comparable to the twenty-six letters in the American alphabet. A writer can produce innumerable words by joining the twenty-six letters in various combinations. From the twenty amino acids, millions of proteins can be formed.

Functions of Proteins

As stated earlier, proteins are vital to life. Thus they received their title from the Greek word meaning "of first rank."[4] Since each cell type requires a different kind of protein, thousands of them exist in the body.

Proteins account for the tough, fibrous nature of hair, nails, and ligaments, and for the structure of muscles. They are a part of **hemoglobin**, which transports oxygen in the blood; of **insulin**, which regulates blood sugar; and of the enzymes necessary for digestion of food.

Proteins (actually amino acids) are required by the body for building and maintaining body tissues, and are part of deoxyribonucleic acid (DNA), which controls the genetic code and thus all hereditary characteristics in body cells. The greatest amounts of proteins are needed when the body is building new tissues rapidly, such as during infancy, pregnancy, or when a mother is nursing a child. Extra protein also is needed when excessive destruction or loss of body protein has occurred from **hemorrhage**, burns, surgery, infections, or other causes. Contrary to popular belief, except for the small amount of protein needed for developing muscles during conditioning, people engaged in sports and other strenuous physical activities do not need increased protein, provided their diets supply enough calories from carbohydrates and fats to meet their energy needs.

Proteins are needed for building the thousands of enzymes which control the speed of chemical reactions in the body, and for making hormones such as thyroxine, which regulates **metabolism** (metabolism is a term for the chemical processes occurring in the body). Proteins also are needed to form antibodies, which combine with foreign proteins that enter the body, producing an **immunity** response that helps ward off harmful infections. They also help regulate the water balance and the acid-base balance in the body.

Proteins, like carbohydrates and fats, can be burned to supply energy. When the diet does not supply enough **calories** from the other two nutrients, proteins are used for energy, even at the expense of building body protein.

Some protein is needed regularly in the diet because the body has little protein reserve. If more protein is eaten than is required for the nitrogen needs of the body, it is used for calories or is converted to body fat. (Nitrogen is used for maintenance of existing tissues and other essential nitrogen-containing compounds in the body, such as amino acids.) Thus, one can become fat from eating excess calories in the form of protein just as much as from too many calories from carbohydrates or fats.

Contrary to popular belief, growth cannot be stimulated by ingesting large amounts of protein unless a protein deficiency is present. The body has its blueprint for growth and development already made up as a result of inheritance. The best method of stimulating muscle growth is through physical activity: "If you work a muscle under load it will increase in size."[5]

Types of Proteins

To be used in the body, protein in food must be broken down by digestion into amino acids and absorbed into the blood. The efficient building of body tissues requires a well-balanced mixture of amino acids. Some nonessential amino acids can be made by the human body, but several must be provided preformed from foods, and therefore are known as the essential amino acids.

There are eight essential amino acids that adults who have achieved their full growth require in their diet. These are:

isoleucine	phenylalanine
leucine	threonine
lysine	tryptophane
methionine	valine

Arginine and histidine, two additional amino acids that the body produces in small amounts, are needed in larger quantities for growth or for any situation that requires building. Thus it is proper to say that for any growing individuals there are ten essential amino acids.

The rest of the amino acids are:

alanine	glycine
asparagine	hydroxyproline
(from aspartic acid)	proline
aspartic acid	serine
cysteine	thyroxine (and
cystine	triiodothyronine)
glutamic acid	tyrosine
glutamine	
(from glutamic acid)	

The various essential amino acids are required in different amounts by the human body. Food proteins providing all of the essential amino acids in the proportions needed by humans are called "complete" or high quality. If a protein low in an essential amino acid is too unbalanced, it will not support either growth or maintenance. When combined, two proteins with different amino acids may complement one another and provide protein of high biological value.

Because animal body composition is similar to that of humans, animal products are closer to the balance of amino acids required by humans than plant foods. Meat, fish, poultry, milk, cheese, and eggs are all sources of high-quality protein. Vegetable proteins are usually low in one or more of the essential amino acids. **Legumes** (peas and beans) contain larger amounts of and better quality protein than other plant sources.

Even though animal protein (meat) is one of the best sources of amino acids, it is felt by some nutritionists that we consume too much animal protein in the United States.[6] A discussion of some of the problems inherent in a high intake of animal protein will be discussed in Chapter 12, and in the section on fats in this chapter.

Table 2-1 gives the comparative quality—not the quantity—of proteins in our foods.

Table 2-1.

Group 1 (Superior)	Human milk, eggs
Group 2 (Excellent)	Cow's milk, cheese, meat, fish, oats, rye, rice, sweet potatoes, spinach
Group 3 (Satisfactory)	Wheat germ, flour, peas, potatoes, lentils, cottonseed meal, sunflower seeds, millet, soy flour
Group 4 (Useful)	White flour, almonds, Brazil nuts, cashews, peanuts, barley flour

From "Protein The Master Builder," by Jean Mayer, *Family Health Magazine*, August 1974, pp. 38–39, 58. Reprinted with permission of *Family Health Magazine,* August 1974 © . All rights reserved.

Protein in the Diet

How much protein do you need? Every balanced diet needs adequate protein in order to replace body tissues. For most adults, 70 grams of good-quality protein a day is more than enough. The amounts of protein recommended by the Food and Nutrition Board, National Academy of Sciences-National Research Council, for individuals of different ages are given in Table 2-2. However, the recommended amount of protein is sufficient only if it contains the various essential amino acids. A hundred grams of gelatin protein would satisfy the total amount required, but it would not sustain life because gelatin lacks some important essential amino acids.

Table 2-2.

Children	1–3 years	23 grams
	4–6	30
	7–10	36
Males	11–14	44 grams
	15–22	54
	over 22	56
Females	11–14	44 grams
	15–18	48
	over 18	46
	pregnant	+30
	lactating	+20

From Food and Nutrition Board, National Academy of Sciences, *Recommended Dietary Allowances,* eighth revised edition, National Research Council, Washington D.C., 1974.

Generally, a combination of animal and vegetable protein is the best means of obtaining sufficient amounts of protein daily. It is possible, however, to maintain good health without eating meat at all. Certain combinations of vegetable proteins will supply the essential amino acids. Some vital animal proteins, such as vitamin B_{12}, must be taken as supplements for a healthy vegetarian diet.[7]

No doubt there are some in the United States who have protein intake levels below the recommended allowance because of a combination of interrelated social, economic, cultural, and health factors. However, most take in amounts of protein well above the recommended allowance, and therefore are not in need of protein supplements.[8]

CARBOHYDRATES

All carbohydrates are made of the chemical elements carbon, hydrogen, and oxygen. The hydrogen and oxygen are always in the same proportion as in water—H_2O. The name itself indicates the combination—carbo (carbon) hydrate (water). Figure 2-1 shows some carbohydrate chains. Note the presence of the chemical elements carbon, hydrogen, and oxygen.

What Are Carbohydrates?

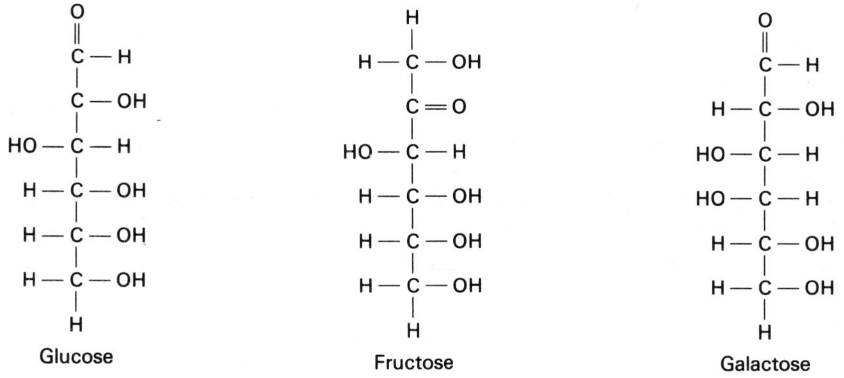

Figure 2-1. Some Chemical Examples of Carbohydrates

The carbohydrates which provide nourishment in our foods are the various sugars and starches. Glucose, the simplest unit of six carbon atoms, is the main carbohydrate. A chain of **glucose** units is a **starch**. Two other common building blocks aid glucose in forming the various carbohydrates. These are fructose, found in the carbohydrates of fruit, and galactose, found only in milk. These three building blocks, called single sugars, are all formed by hooking the same number of carbon and water units together in different ways.

In plants, two glucose blocks are often connected together, forming maltose. This combination is called a disaccharide or double sugar. Add more glucose units to this union and a starch is formed. In the body, several units of glucose form what is called **glycogen**, or animal starch. This is stored in the liver and the muscles as a ready source of energy. When glucose is needed by the body, glycogen is simply broken down into individual units of glucose.

Sucrose, or table sugar, is perhaps the most common of the disaccharides. It is formed from one unit of glucose and one of fructose. Milk sugar is formed by combining one unit of glucose and one of galactose. It is, therefore, another disaccharide.

Functions of Carbohydrates

The major function of carbohydrates in the diet is to provide energy for the work of the body. They also allow the body to manufacture some of the B-complex vitamins and form part of the structure of many biological compounds. In addition, carbohydrates add flavor to our food.

Types of Carbohydrates

On nutrition labels, the grams per serving of several types of digestable carbohydrates are listed. The best known of these are starch, glucose, sucrose, and lactose.

Starch is the most important carbohydrate food source. Since plants store energy for future use (including nourishment of embryo plants) in starch form, the seeds of plants such as the cereal grains, legumes, and potatoes are the richest sources of starch. Cereals contain principally starch, but important vitamins and minerals are also present in the outer layer and germ of the grain or kernel. Refinement, as in milling white flour, removes much of the outer layer and the germ. Enrichment of white bread and flour restores three of the B vitamins that are lost in processing and adds iron.

Starchy foods are not very flavorful if eaten raw. Cooking swells the starch granules, breaks them open, makes them taste better, and allows them to be more easily digested. In some vegetables, such as corn and peas, a sweet taste is present while the plant is immature. This disappears as the plant ripens and the sugar content changes to starch. In some fruits, such as bananas, the unripened fruit contains starch, which changes to sugar on ripening.

It takes longer to break down a large starch molecule than a sugar. This may be an advantage, since this slower process supplies needed energy material constantly over a longer period of time. Simple sugars are ready for absorption almost immediately, and that immediate absorption may place demands on the metabolic processes of the body, as they attempt to cope with an oversupply of glucose in the blood. Thus some nutritionists think it is better to take much of our fuel and energy foods in the form of the large starch molecules rather than in the very quickly and easily digested sugars.

Many other people feel that starches are the least desirable of the carbohydrates because of their calories. However, the first and most basic need of the body is for calories as fuel and energy sources. And eating unrefined starches also helps supply needed vitamins, minerals, **fiber**, and small amounts of protein.

Through digestion, the body changes the starch in foods to glucose, which can be used as a source of energy by all of the tissues in the body. If the body receives more glucose than it can use as energy, small amounts can be stored as glycogen (sometimes called animal starch) in the liver and muscle tissues, but excess carbohydrates are rapidly converted to fat. However, since one can become overweight by consuming excess calories of any type, one should not think of carbohydrates as any more fattening than protein or fat.

Sucrose (common table sugar) is mostly produced from sugar cane and sugar beets; the sugars from the two sources are identical chemically. Refined sugar is an unusual food in that it is pure carbohydrate; therefore, it is only a source of calories, and contains no vitamins, minerals, protein, or fat. Almost all other food sources contain some combination of essential nutrients.

The United States per capita consumption of sugar at present is over 100 pounds a year, a substantial increase over the consumption prior to this century.

The increase is related to our increased consumption of soft drinks, cakes and other bakery products, candies, syrup, jams and jellies, and other manufactured products which have a high sugar content. Many of these foods contribute calories without providing much in the way of other nutrients. These calorie-rich foods should not be consumed at the expense of foods which provide essential vitamins, minerals, and protein, and it should be remembered that an excess of calories from any source leads to obesity.

Lactose, or milk sugar, is produced by mammals to serve as an energy source for the young. The enzyme lactase must be present to digest lactose. Some people are lacking in this enzyme after early childhood and may find it difficult or impossible to digest milk. Infants and post-weaning children can also have milk sensitivity or intolerance caused by a congenital deficiency of lactase.

Carbohydrates in the Diet

Carbohydrates are economical to produce in abundance—a characteristic that helps a majority of the people in the world to survive. In the United States and Canada, carbohydrates provide 40 to 50 percent of the total food energy, while the entire population of the world obtains about 70 percent of its energy from carbohydrates. The cereal grains (such as wheat, rice, corn, and oats), potatoes, many fruits, vegetables, peas, beans, taro, cassava (tapioca), and sugar cane and sugar beets are major world sources of carbohydrates. Many processed foods are rich in carbohydrates, including breads and other baked goods, jams and jellies, molasses, noodles, spaghetti, and dried fruits.

Of the two basic carbohydrate energy-providers, starch and sugar, starch has been the main energy source in the United States. However, carbohydrates are less predominant in the American diet today. There are several apparent reasons for this decreasing consumption. A key factor may be the rise in real income, permitting a movement away from a diet high in greens, beans, and whole grains, a diet that had been enforced by economics.

In addition, there is relatively little advertising of fruits, vegetables, and whole grains. This point was raised by Dr. Joan Gussow of Columbia University:

> No amount of information about the nutritive or non-nutritive qualities of the foods advertised will compensate for the total imbalance in the nature of the foods advertised on television. The nature of the foods advertised is largely highly processed foods, many of them snack foods, highly sugared, highly salted . . . We should have advertising of fruits and vegetables. They should be public service announcements selling people on those components of the diet which, in fact, they are not currently being sold on—dairy products, beans and rice and grains, and other forms of protein foods . . . And all these foods don't get sold because they do not have a high enough mark-up.[9]

FATS

What Are Fats?

The term **"fat"** produces many reactions. For the average consumer it means body fat and has unpleasant connotations. However, scientists will tell us that fat as a nutrient is essential and good for the body. Many other terms also come to mind when discussing fats. Nouns like glyceride and lipid and adjectives like saturated, unsaturated, and polyunsaturated are among them. But what do they mean?

Fats are composed essentially of fatty acids and glycerol. Each fatty acid is made up of carbon atoms joined like links on a chain. The carbon chains vary in length, with most edible fats containing between four and twenty carbons. Because typical fats or oils consist of three fatty acids linked to a glycerol molecule, they are called **triglycerides**.

Each carbon atom has hydrogen atoms attached as the charms might be on a bracelet. When each carbon atom in the chain has attached to it as many hydrogen atoms as it can hold (two), it is called a **saturated fatty acid**; when a hydrogen atom is missing from two neighboring carbons, a double bond forms between the carbon atoms and the fatty acid is called unsaturated. For example, a monounsaturated fat is a fatty acid that contains one such double bond. A fatty acid that contains more than one such double bond in the chain is called polyunsaturated. The **polyunsaturated fatty acid** called **linoleic acid** is of particular nutritional importance because the body cannot manufacture it; hence, it is an essential fatty acid and must be supplied in the food one eats.

Unsaturated fatty acids and fatty acids composed of shorter chains have lower melting points and are liquids (oils) at room temperature. All food fats, animal or vegetable, contain a mixture of saturated, polyunsaturated, and monounsaturated fatty acids. Generally, animal fats are more saturated than the liquid vegetable oils.

Within the category of liquid vegetable oils there is still considerable variation. For instance, coconut oil is more highly saturated than the others; it is a liquid because it has short carbon chains. Oils such as safflower, corn, cottonseed, peanut, and soybean are especially rich in linoleic acid, and thus the labels on products containing these oils often state "high in polyunsaturates" or "high in polyunsaturated fatty acids." When oils have **"hydrogenated"** on the label, hydrogen has been added to make the product more solid. Margarine is an example of an oil processed this way. As a result, the vegetable oils are less unsaturated.[10]

Function of Fats   The fats in our foods serve a variety of functions. Some fat is essential in the diet to provide linoleic acid, which is necessary for proper growth and a healthy skin. However, only a small amount of linoleic acid is required to meet this need—about 1 to 2 percent of an individual's total daily calories. Fats also carry fat-soluble vitamins into the body and aid in their absorption. In addition, fats serve as a concentrated source of energy, and because they slow digestion and the emptying of the stomach, they delay the onset of hunger. Fats also contribute to our enjoyment of foods, because they add flavor and improve the texture.

Fats are called a concentrated source of energy because they have an energy value more than twice that of carbohydrates or proteins; that is, one gram of fat provides nine calories, while one gram of protein or carbohydrate provides only four calories. This means that foods rich in fats add much to the caloric content of the diet; those calories in excess of body needs create fat deposits in the body. Fat deposits may be good or bad; some fat in the tissues helps to cushion the body organs and to prevent heat loss through the body's surface. Too much fat deposited, of course, leads to being overweight. By some estimates, as much as half of the U.S. population is overweight to some degree, and many nutritionists feel that this is the greatest nutritional problem in our country.

A reduction in fat-rich foods is a sensible way to limit calories in the diet in order to reduce or control weight. In judging the amount of fat in one's diet, it is very easy to underestimate the total. Most people think about only the visible fats— butter, margarine, lard, cooking and salad oils. But much of the fat in the diet comes from less visible sources—the small fat particles and streaks in meat from well-fed animals; the varied amounts in nuts, meats, and poultry; the fat added in the cooking of foods; and the fat contained in many processed foods.   *Fats in the Diet*

Table 2-3 gives the fat content of several representative types of foods.

Table 2-3

Percent Fat	Food
90–100	Salad and cooking oil and fats, lard
80–90	Butter, margarine
70–80	Mayonnaise, pecans, macadamia nuts
50–70	Walnuts, dried unsweetened coconut meat, almonds, bacon, baking chocolate
30–50	Broiled choice T-bone and porterhouse steaks, spareribs, broiled pork chop, goose, cheddar and cream cheeses, potato chips, french dressing, chocolate candy
20–30	Choice beef pot roast, broiled choice lamb chop, frankfurters, ground beef, chocolate chip cookies
10–20	Broiled choice round steak, broiled veal chop, roast turkey, eggs, avocado, olives, chocolate cake with icing, french-fried potatoes, ice cream, apple pie
1–10	Pork and beans, broiled cod, halibut, haddock, and many other fish, broiled chicken, crabmeat, cottage cheese, beef liver, milk, creamed soups, sherbet, most breakfast cereals
Less than 1	Baked potato, most vegetables and fruits, egg whites, chicken consommé

From *Fats in Food and Diet,* U.S. Department of Agriculture, Bulletin No. 361, p. 5.

In recent years, consumers have read and heard much about the amount of fat they eat as well as about the kind of fat they eat (saturated vs. unsaturated or polyunsaturated). Most of the controversy involves the relationship of dietary fats and cholesterol to **atherosclerosis**, a disease in which **cholesterol** and other fatty substances are deposited on the inner walls of arteries.

Cholesterol is a normal constituent of blood and tissues and is found in every animal cell. Some of the cholesterol in human blood and tissues is synthesized by the body, and some is supplied by diet. The amount supplied by diet varies greatly depending on the kinds and amounts of foods included.

The amount of cholesterol in the diet is positively related to the amount of cholesterol in the blood. Ordinary diets are likely to supply 600 to 900 milligrams of cholesterol daily. A low-cholesterol diet usually provides about 300 milligrams of cholesterol daily. Such a small amount is difficult to achieve in the usual American diet and may well be lower than is necessary for a healthy individual on a well-balanced diet.

There is evidence not only that fat and saturated fat tend to increase serum cholesterol levels but that direct consumption of cholesterol does so as well. A high level of blood cholesterol has been identified as one of several risk factors in the development of atherosclerosis and coronary heart disease. Some evidence has indicated that saturated fats in the diet tend to cause an increase in cholesterol levels, while polyunsaturated fats tend to result in decreased levels. However, many factors other than diet are involved, and these will be discussed in Chapter 12.[11]

Since the beginning of the century, the amount of nutrient fat available per person per day has risen from about 125 to 156 grams. Nutrient fat is easier to obtain now because of more plentiful food sources. This increase is equivalent to about 2½ tablespoons of butter or regular margarine; or a little more than 2 table-spoons a day of vegetable oil; or about 24 pounds a year in nutrient fat.

Discussing the sources of the increase, a Department of Agriculture report says:

> The same foods did not always account for the increase in fat throughout the 60-year period, but for most years salad and cooking oils were the chief contributors. Following salad and cooking oils, dairy products and shortening shared equally in the contribution to the gain in nutrient fat during the first 15 years. However, in the last seven years, meat provided the largest increase in fat, followed by salad and cooking oils and then by shortening.[12]

It is not unusual for fat to supply 45 to 50 percent of the total calories in an American diet. In a nationwide survey, fat supplied an average of 45 percent of the total calories in the diets of young and middle-aged men.[13] The higher fat consumption trends have been underway in other nations as well.

One of the principal reasons for reducing the consumption of fat is to make a place in the diet for complex carbohydrates (starches), which generally carry higher levels of micronutrients than fat without the health complications of fat (to be discussed in Chapter 12).

There is no specific definition of moderation, but for most of us it means using less fat than we are in the habit of using. This applies especially to the fat we add to food during preparation and at the table.

Some advocates of moderation believe that 38 to 40 percent of the total calories from fat is a reasonable goal. In most diets this reduction can be achieved by simply cutting down on the amount of visible or separable fat used.[14]

Governmental and professional groups in the United States and eight other nations have recommended decreases in total fat consumption to ranges from 25 to 35 percent of total calorie consumption.[15]

The following excerpt from a presentation by the American Heart Association to the Federal Trade Commission relates consumption goals to commonly used food measures:

> A relatively small number of foods do contribute a major proportion of the cholesterol and saturated fat in the American diet. For example, in our

1972 report, the Inter-Society Commission for Heart Disease Resources recommended the reduction of dietary cholesterol to less than 300 mg. per day. We noted that the average American daily cholesterol intake was approximately 600 mg. per day. A single egg yolk, however, contains 250 mg. cholesterol by itself, nearly the daily allowance. We further recommended an intake of less than 20 percent of total calories to be obtained from saturated fat. Assuming a caloric intake of 2,500 calories per day, the average American should take in no more than 250 calories or less than 27 grams of saturated fat per day. One cup of whole milk contains 5 grams saturated fat. One cup of ice cream contains 8 grams; six ounces of ham approximately 8 grams. These are very substantial portions of the maximum recommended allowance for a day. Therefore the contribution of individual foods to the cholesterol and saturated fat intake in the diet can be highly significant.[16]

With respect to overall fat consumption, one should select more foods that derive 30 percent or less of their calories from fat. Tables 2-4 and 2-5 give, respectively, the fat and cholesterol content of selected foods. Since high levels of fat, saturated fat, and cholesterol most often enter our diets in the process of acquisition of protein, particularly through red meat, more of our protein needs should be satisfied from fish, poultry, and vegetable sources.[17]

It is important to remember, however, that fat is an important constituent of the diet and is important to health in many ways. A diet too restricted in fat lacks flavor and satiate value; a greater volume of food is needed to satisfy the appetite and meet energy needs. Fats are also the chief sources of essential fatty acids, as well as carriers of some essential vitamins, namely A, D, E, and K. Too little fat can result in a diet that is deficient in these nutrients.

However, many nutrients are important in fat utilization, including calcium, magnesium, chromium, zinc, vanadium, niacin, biotin, pantothenic acid, vitamin B_6, and vitamin E. The specific action and quantitative requirement for some of these are not completely understood. For example, when the proportion of fat as polyunsaturated oils increases in the diet, the requirement for vitamin E increases.

An individual's utilization of fats is affected by many other factors, such as the endocrine system (thyroid, adrenal, pituitary, ovarian, pancreatic, and other glands); aging, which slows down physiological processes so that enzyme mechanisms are unable to keep up with our usual patterns of eating; and diseases, which may interfere with the absorption and metabolism of fat.

WATER

Water is a most important nutrient. It stands next to air in importance to life. You can get along for days, even weeks, without food, but only a few days without water.

Water is necessary for all the processes of digestion. Nutrients are dissolved in water so they may pass through the intestinal wall and into the bloodstream for use throughout the body. Water carries waste out of the body and also helps to regulate body temperature.

The body's most obvious source of water is the water a person drinks, but some is produced by the body's burning of food for energy. Coffee and tea are mostly water, as are fruit juices and milk. Soup is a water source, as are many fruits and vegetables. Even meat can be up to 80 percent water.

Table 2-4. Fat Content and Major Fatty Acid Composition of Selected Foods (in Decreasing Order of Total Saturated Fatty Acid Content within Each Group of Similar Foods)

[In percent]

Food	Total fat	Fatty acids Total saturated	Total monounsaturated	Total polyunsaturated
Animal fats:				
Chicken	100.0	32.5	45.4	17.6
Lard	100.0	39.6	44.3	11.8
Beef tallow	100.0	48.2	42.3	4.2
Avocado	15.0	2.0	9.0	2.0
Beef products:				
T-bone steak (cooked, broiled—56 percent lean, 44 percent fat)	43.2	18.0	21.1	1.6
Chuck, 5th rib (cooked or braised—69 percent lean, 31 percent fat)	36.7	15.3	17.5	1.5
Brisket (cooked, braised, or pot roasted—69 percent lean; 31 percent fat)	34.8	14.6	16.7	1.4
Wedge and round-bone sirloin steak (cooked or broiled—66 percent lean; 34 percent fat)	32.0	13.3	15.6	1.2
Rump (cooked or roasted—75 percent lean; 25 percent fat)	27.3	11.4	13.1	1.2
Round steak (cooked or broiled—82 percent lean; 18 percent fat)	14.9	6.3	6.9	.7
Cereals and grains:				
Wheat germ	10.9	1.9	1.6	6.6
Oats (puffed, without added ingredients)	5.5	1.0	1.9	2.2
Oats (puffed, with added nutrients, sugar covered)	3.4	.6	1.2	1.4
Barley (whole grain)	2.8	.5	.3	1.3
Domestic buckwheat (dark flour)	2.5	.5	.8	.9
Cornmeal, white or yellow (whole-ground, unbolted)	3.9	.5	.9	2.0
Shredded wheat breakfast cereal	2.5	.4	.4	1.3
Wheat (whole grain, Hard Red Spring)	2.7	.4	.3	1.3
Wheat flakes breakfast cereal	2.4	.4	.3	1.2
Rye (whole grain)	2.2	.3	.2	1.1
Wheat meal breakfast cereal	1.4	.3	.1	.7
Wheat flour, all purpose	1.4	.2	.1	.6
Rice (cooked brown)	.8	.2	.2	.3
Bulgur from Hard Red Winter wheat	1.5	.2	.2	.7
Oatmeal or rolled oats, cooked	1.0	.2	.4	.4
Rye flour	1.4	.2	.1	.6
Cornstarch	.6	.1	.1	.3
Rice (cooked white)	.2	.1	.1	.1
Farina (enriched, regular, cooked)	.2			.1
Corn grits, cooked	.1			.1
Dairy products:				
Nondairy coffee whitener (powder)	35.6	32.6	1.0	
Cream cheese	33.8	21.2	9.4	1.2
Cheddar cheese	32.8	20.2	9.8	.9
Light whipping cream	32.4	20.2	9.6	.9
Muenster cheese	29.8	19.0	8.7	.7
American pasteurized cheese	28.9	18.0	8.5	1.0
Swiss cheese	27.6	17.6	7.7	1.0
Mozzarella cheese	19.4	11.8	5.9	.7
Ricotta cheese (from whole milk)	14.6	9.3	4.1	.4
Vanilla ice cream	12.3	7.7	3.6	.5
Half and half cream	11.7	7.3	3.4	.4
Chocolate chip ice cream	11.0	6.3	2.6	.4
Canned condensed milk (sweetened)	8.7	5.5	2.4	.3
Ice cream sandwich	8.2	4.7	2.6	.5
Cottage cheese (creamed)	4.0	2.6	1.1	.1
Yogurt (from whole milk)	3.4	2.2	.9	.1
Cottage cheese (uncreamed)	.4	.2	.1	
Eggs:				
Fried in margarine	15.9	4.2	7.2	1.9
Scrambled in margarine	12.6	3.7	5.5	1.4
Fresh or frozen	11.3	3.4	4.5	1.4
Fish:				
Eel, American	18.3	4.0	9.0	2.7
Herring, Atlantic	16.4	2.9	9.2	2.4
Mackerel, Atlantic	9.8	2.4	3.6	2.4
Tuna, albacore (canned, light)	6.8	2.3	1.7	1.8
Tuna, albacore (white meat)	8.0	2.1	2.1	3.0
Salmon, sockeye	8.9	1.8	1.5	4.7
Salmon, Atlantic	5.8	1.8	2.7	.5
Carp	6.2	1.3	2.7	1.4
Rainbow trout (United States)	4.5	1.0	1.5	1.4
Striped bass	2.1	.5	.6	.7
Ocean perch	2.5	.4	1.0	.7
Red snapper	1.2	.2	.2	.4
Tuna, skipjack (canned, light)	.8	.2	.2	.2
Halibut, Atlantic	1.1	.2	.2	.4
Cod, Atlantic	.7	.1	.1	.3
Haddock	.7	.1	.1	.2

Food	Fatty acids			
	Total fat	Total saturated	Total monoun-saturated	Total polyun-saturated
Fowl:				
Chicken (broiler/fryer, cooked or roasted dark meat)	9.7	2.7	3.2	2.4
Turkey (cooked or roasted dark meat)	5.3	1.6	1.4	1.5
Chicken (broiler/fryer, cocked or roasted light meat)	3.5	1.0	.9	.9
Turkey (cooked or roasted light meat)	2.6	.7	.6	.7
Lamb and veal:				
Shoulder of lamb (cooked or roasted, 74 percent lean; 26 percent fat)	26.9	12.6	11.0	1.6
Leg of lamb (cooked or roasted, 83 percent lean; 17 percent fat)	21.2	9.6	8.5	1.2
Veal foreshank (cooked or stewed, 86 percent lean; 14 percent fat)	10.4	4.4	4.2	.7
Nuts:				
Coconut	35.5	31.2	2.2	.7
Brazil nut	68.2	17.4	22.5	25.4
Peanut butter	52.0	10.0	24.0	15.0
Peanut	49.7	9.4	22.9	15.0
Cashew	45.6	9.2	26.4	7.4
Walnut, English	63.4	6.9	9.9	41.8
Pecan	71.4	6.1	43.1	17.9
Walnut, black	59.6	5.1	10.8	40.8
Almond	53.9	4.3	36.8	10.1
Pork products:				
Bacon	49.0	18.1	22.8	5.4
Sausage, cooked	32.5	11.7	15.1	3.9
Deviled ham, canned	32.3	11.3	15.2	3.5
Liverwurst, braunschweiger, liver sausage	32.5	11.0	15.5	4.1
Bologna	27.5	10.6	13.3	2.1
Pork loin (cooked or roasted, 82 percent lean; 18 percent fat)	28.1	9.8	13.1	3.1
Ham (cooked or roasted, 84 percent lean; 16 percent fat)	22.1	7.8	10.4	2.4
Fresh ham (cooked or roasted, 82 percent lean; 18 percent fat)	20.2	7.1	9.5	2.2
Canadian bacon (cooked and drained)	17.5	5.9	7.9	1.8
Chopped ham luncheon meat	17.4	5.7	8.3	2.2
Canned ham	11.3	4.0	5.3	1.2
Salad and cooking oils:				
Coconut	100.0	86.0	6.0	2.0
Palm	100.0	47.9	38.4	9.3
Cottonseed	100.0	26.1	18.9	50.7
Peanut	100.0	17.0	47.0	31.0
Sesame	100.0	15.2	40.0	40.5
Soybean, hydrogenated	100.0	15.0	23.1	57.6
Olive	100.0	14.2	72.5	9.0
Corn	100.0	12.7	24.7	58.2
Sunflower	100.0	10.2	20.9	63.8
Safflower	100.0	9.4	12.5	73.8
Shellfish:				
Eastern oyster	2.1	.5	.2	.6
Pacific oyster	2.3	.5	.4	.9
Ark shell claim	1.5	.4	.3	.3
Blue crab	1.6	.3	.3	.6
Alaska king crab	1.6	.2	.3	.6
Shrimp	1.2	.2	.2	.5
Scallop	.9	.1		.4
Soups:				
Cream of mushroom (diluted with equal parts of water)	3.9	1.1	.7	.8
Cream of celery (diluted with equal parts of water)	2.3	.6	.5	1.0
Beef with vegetables (diluted with equal parts of water)	.8	.3	.3	
Chicken noodle (diluted with equal parts of water)	1.0	.3	.4	.2
Minestrone (diluted with equal parts of water)	1.1	.2	.3	.5
Vegetable (diluted with equal parts of water)	.9	.2	.3	.4
Clam chowder, Manhattan style (diluted with equal parts of water)	.9	.2	.2	.5
Table spreads:				
Butter	80.1	49.8	23.1	3.0
Margarine (hydrogenated soybean oil, stick)	80.1	14.9	46.5	14.4
Margarine (corn oil, tub)	80.3	14.2	30.4	31.9
Margarine (corn oil, stick)	80.0	14.0	38.7	23.3
Margarine (safflower oil, tub)	81.7	13.4	16.1	48.4
Vegetable fats (household shortening)	100.0	25.0	44.0	26.0

From Consumer and Food Economics Institute, U.S. Department of Agriculture, Agricultural Research Service, Hyattsville, Maryland. "Comprehensive Evaluation of Fatty Acids in Foods," *Journal of The American Dietetic Association,* May 1975; July 1975; August 1975; October 1975; March 1976; April 1976; July 1976; September 1976; November 1976; January 1977; unpublished data on shellfish and margarine.

Table 2-5. Cholesterol Content of Common Measures of Selected Foods (in Ascending Order)

Food	Amount	Cholesterol
		Milligrams
Milk — skim, fluid or reconstituted dry	1 cup	5
Cottage cheese, uncreamed	½ cup	7
Lard	1 tablespoon	12
Cream, light table	1 fluid ounce	20
Cottage cheese, creamed	½ cup	24
Cream, half and half	¼ cup	26
Ice cream, regular, approximately ten percent fat	½ cup	27
Cheese, cheddar	1 ounce	28
Milk, whole	1 cup	34
Butter	1 tablespoon	35
Oysters, salmon	3 ounces, cooked	40
Clams, halibut, tuna	3 ounces, cooked	55
Chicken, turkey, light meat	3 ounces, cooked	67
Beef, pork, lobster, chicken, turkey, dark meat	3 ounces, cooked	75
Lamb, veal, crab	3 ounces, cooked	85
Shrimp	3 ounces, cooked	130
Heart, beef	3 ounces, cooked	230
Egg	1 yolk or 1 egg	250
Liver, beef, calf, hog, lamb	3 ounces, cooked	370
Kidney	3 ounces, cooked	680
Brains	3 ounces, raw	more than 1700

From "Cholesterol Content of Foods," R.M. Feeley, P.E. Criner, and B.K. Watt. Reprinted from the *Journal of the American Dietetic Association* 61:134, 1972.

Water in the Diet   Water is essential for life. If you are not drinking enough, you may tire easily and find it hard to concentrate. Many people drink less water than is optimum for the best functioning of the body. The shipwrecked sailor who goes without water for much more than forty-eight hours will die.

Your need for liquids depends on your size and weight. As a general guide, adults should drink between one and a half and two quarts of fluid a day. Children, of course, need proportionately less. Water, which makes up more than half your body weight, is constantly being lost and must be replaced. Not all this water is lost through urination. It is also lost through perspiration and unseen and unfelt evaporation through the skin. Some water comes from your lungs; you can see this moisture by breathing on a mirror.

It is very important that you drink enough. If you drink too little, the salts and minerals excreted by your kidneys may not be flushed completely from your system. These minerals are the building blocks for kidney stones. Also, many doctors believe that bacteria, which cause infections, can grow more easily when urine flow is low. However, very large amounts of urine may weaken certain protective mechanisms that suppress the growth of bacteria.

It also is very important to spread out drinking over the waking hours. If all fluids are drunk in a two-hour period, the kidneys will excrete the excess quickly and the body will not benefit. Miners and other workers who do not have a handy water supply often think that they can drink a lot of water before work and not need any more until the end of the day. Not only is this untrue, it also is dangerous. If one operates on this theory, by the end of the day the urine will be very concentrated—a favorable breeding ground for both kidney stones and urinary tract infections.

You don't have to waterlog yourself to replenish your body's water supply. Fruit juice and coffee supply water to the body, as does tea, milk, or other beverages. In fact, 85 percent of the average person's total fluid intake represents fluids other than water. But if you miss a coffee break or develop a sudden dislike for Coke, then you should replace it with water. Coffee sometimes causes diuresis, the medical term for increased urination. If coffee goes "straight through you," then your body is not gaining water from this source.

Retired persons and persons who live alone frequently do not drink enough, simply because a cup of coffee is no fun when it is not accompanied by conversation. One way to be sure to drink an adequate amount is to follow a schedule until it becomes habit. Drink with meals; take time in mid-morning and mid-afternoon to drink water, juice, or a soft drink; and have something to drink in the evening while watching television or reading a book.

During exercise or hard work, fluids lost through excess sweating must be replaced. If you eat a great deal, additional fluids are needed to get rid of the extra salt and minerals in the food and to replace fluids that are lost when that food is metabolized.

When you are not eating because of an upset stomach, a diet, or for any other reason, you need to drink more to replace the pint of water that comes from most normal daily food intake. During a fever, fluid intake should be increased to compensate for greater loss of water through the skin. When you eat extra salt, extra fluid is needed to excrete the salt in the urine.[18]

CALORIES AND ENERGY

The body needs energy for metabolic processes to support physical activities, growth, and lactation, and to maintain body temperature. A **calorie** has been described as "a measuring unit for the energy or heat that foods supply to the body."[19] The most accurate way of describing a calorie is "a calorie (kilocalorie) is the amount of heat needed to raise the temperature of one liter of water by one degree centigrade."[20]

Most people believe that calories are equivalent to fat, and therefore they spend most of their lives counting calories. A calorie is merely a unit of measure. The human body is like the combustion engine; it must have a ready supply of energy or it will stop. The heart, lungs, and other organs require this continual supply even when the body is in a state of rest. The number of calories utilized to keep the body functioning while in a state of rest is called the basal metabolic rate (BMR). The BMR can be influenced by such factors as age, body size, climate, lactation, pregnancy, and health status.

The more one exercises, the more energy must be produced. The energy comes from the breakdown of protein, fat, and carbohydrates when they combine with oxygen in the body. We need enough calories to keep the body functioning while in a state of rest plus enough to support any type of physical activity being performed.

Fuel values differ in the various nutrients. Protein measures out to 4.00 calories for a gram; fats, 8.90 for a gram; and carbohydrates, 4.00.[21] The nutrients vitamins, minerals, and water have no caloric value.

Calories are seldom worried about except when an imbalance is evident. Too few calories and the body cries out with hunger and disease. Too many calories and the body bulges out with pounds of embarrassment.

Calories must be balanced with activity, or malnutrition of one type or the other will prevail. For a more thorough discussion concerning basal metabolism, energy, and caloric needs, see Unit III.

SUMMARY

The nutrients in food are necessary to support growth, to repair constantly wearing tissues, and to supply energy for physical activity. The basic nutrient substances contained in foods are proteins, carbohydrates, and fats. Water is also important nutrient substance which aids in all body regulatory processes. Unless the diet supplies all the elements required for normal life processes, the human body cannot operate at peak efficiency for very long. If an essential nutrient is missing from the diet over very long periods of time, deficiency diseases may develop.

Each nutrient contained in food serves an important purpose in the body. Proteins are required by the body mainly for building and maintaining tissues. The major function of carbohydrates is to provide energy for body work. Fats serve a number of purposes, including aiding in the transport and absorption of fat-soluble vitamins, providing energy, and adding flavor to and improving texture of foods. Water is required in abundance by the body for all processes of digestion and for transport of nutrients, chemical substances, and waste products. Water also helps to regulate body temperature. No one nutrient is superior to another, and all are needed in the diet in appropriate proportions.

Proteins, carbohydrates, and fats all provide energy units for the body to use. Fat, the most concentrated source of food energy, supplies nine calories per gram; protein and carbohydrate each supply four calories per gram. A calorie is not a nutrient itself; rather, it is a unit of energy measurement. A calorie (sometimes called kilocalorie) is the amount of heat needed to raise the temperature of one liter of water by one degree centigrade. The body requires sufficient energy each day to maintain metabolic processes; to support physical activities, growth, and lactation; and to maintain body temperature.

In the United States today an abundance of good foods is available everywhere and within the economic reach of most people. A variety of different types of foods will provide all of the nutrients most of us need. No one food does everything, and all foods have something to offer.

NOTES

1. Pamphlet "Food Is More Than Something to Eat," U.S. Department of Agriculture and Health, Education, and Welfare in cooperation with the Grocery Manufacturers of America and the Advertising Council.
2. Jean Mayer, "The ABC's of Proteins," *Family Health,* May 1973, pp. 24-25.
3. Ibid.
4. Ibid.
5. "Proteins Part I," *The Health Letter,* Vol. III, No. 5, 1974.
6. Mark Hegstead, "Protein Needs and Possible Modifications of the American Diet," *Journal of the American Dietetic Association,* April 1976.
7. Jean Mayer, "Protein: The Master Builder," *Family Health,* August 1974, pp. 38-39, 58.
8. Joginder Chopra et al., "Protein in the U.S.," *Journal of the American Dietetic Association,* Vol. 72, March 1978, pp. 253-257.
9. Select Committee on Nutrition and Human Needs, U.S. Senate, *Dietary Goals for the United States* (Washington, D.C.: U.S. Government Printing Office, 1977), pp. 17-18.
10. Edward Damon, "A Primer on Four Nutrients: Proteins, Carbohydrates, Fats, and Fiber," *FDA Consumer,* February 1975, pp. 5-13.
11. Ibid.
12. Select Committee, *Dietary Goals,* pp. 17-18.
13. U.S. Department of Agriculture, *Fats in Food and Diet,* Bulletin No. 361.
14. Ibid.
15. Select Committee, *Dietary Goals,* pp. 17-18.
16. Ibid, pp. 37, 40, 41.
17. Ibid.
18. Adapted from: "Fluids: How Much Should I Drink?" by the National Kidney Foundation.
19. Jean Mayer, "Calories Still Count," *Family Health,* October 1974, pp. 42, 58, 60.
20. Ibid.
21. Ibid.

3

Vitamins: Myths and Miracles

The vitamin, because of its vast use in the United States, has appropriately been dubbed "The Great American Placebo."[1] **Vitamins** are devoured on a "just in case" basis, without consideration of possible ill effects. In 1972, the *Statistical Abstract of the United States* stated the vitamin production of 1970 as 23 million pounds. "Somebody with a bend for unusual arithmetic figured out that a vitamin pill is dropped down the gullet once every 0.214 seconds. That is pretty close to perpetual motion."[2]

Parents are even buying them freely for their children. TV shows sing out, "Yabba dabba doo, Yabba dabba doo, Flintstone vitamins are good for you . . ." One small boy in Kansas has now forgotten that song. After swallowing 40 children's vitamins at once, he spent two days in intensive care at the hospital with vitamin A and iron poisoning.[3] This case was added to the statistics of FDA's National Clearinghouse for Poison Control Centers. They reveal 4,000 cases of vitamin poisonings reported each year, with some 3,200 involving children.[4]

In recent years, numerous miracles have been ascribed to vitamins. If you have a cold, take vitamin C; sex life lagging, go buy some E. Everything from that tired rundown feeling to schizophrenia can supposedly be cured by the downing of this vitamin or that.

Many people will swear to you that vitamins provide added energy. They obviously do not know much about nutrition or the human body. Some vitamins (B expecially) do aid in the conversion of food into usable energy. However, in amounts greater than the Recommended Daily Allowances, they provide nothing of value. Only those with a rare, medically diagnosed, vitamin deficiency would benefit from an amount greater than the RDA levels.[5]

The fact is that most people get the proper amount of nutrients from the foods they eat. Rare indeed is the American who does not. Someone has stated, "The irony of all this is simply that Americans who have the best overall diet of any country in the world, and therefore the least need for diet supplements, are the world's greatest overusers of vitamin pills."[6]

Vitamin tablets do not produce miracles or make us healthy. Although a deficiency would make one ill, an excess of vitamins does not make one any healthier. The best guarantee for a healthy life is a well-balanced diet of the four basic foods.

What is the truth about vitamins? With so many reports of pro and con, one finds it difficult to wade through the bog of controversy presently engulfing the consumer.

VITAMINS—HISTORICALLY SPEAKING

In the early 1900s, it was believed that three compounds were needed in the diet to ward off beriberi, pellagra, and scurvy. They were presumed to be from a class of chemical compounds called amines, and were named for the Latin, *vita,* which means life. Later it was discovered that not all of the substances were amines, so the "e" was dropped, making our present day "vitamin."

In former years, the chemical makeup of vitamins was unknown, so they were identified by letters (A, B, C, D, E, etc.). Later, what was considered one vitamin turned out to be many, so numbers were added (B_1, B_2, B_6, etc.). When some vitamins proved unnecessary, they were omitted from the list. Thus, we find gaps in the numbers. Chemical names were assigned as the makeup of each vitamin was discovered. Now these names are frequently used to eliminate confusion.

Vitamins are measured in small amounts. The terms used are **IU** or International Units (which refers to the measurable amount of activity), milligrams, and micrograms.

The Food and Drug Administration presently holds the guillotine on safe and unsafe vitamin usage. Their aim is to protect the consumer from the proven hazards of dangerous amounts of nutrients. They also ensure that the consumer is better served through "accurate labeling, modest promotion, and rational formulation of vitamins and mineral products."[7]

To accomplish this task, the FDA set forth a method for designating daily vitamin allowances. In 1940, the Food and Nutrition Board of the National Research Council published the first edition of *Recommended Daily Allowances* **(RDA).**[8] Revised numerous times since then, these allowances will ensure an adequate intake of vitamins for most people. See Table 3-1.

It is important to understand that the RDA are not expressions of minimal nutrient requirements. "The Recommended Dietary Allowances are the levels of intake of essential nutrients considered, in the judgment of the members of the Food and Nutrition Board on the basis of available scientific knowledge, to be adequate to meet the known nutritional needs of practically all healthy persons."[9] The RDA were derived by increasing the average estimated daily requirements. While this increase ensures that almost everyone following the guidelines will have an adequate intake of nutrients, it probably inflates the amounts necessary for most people. The latest revision of the National Research Council RDA was in 1974. However, the United States RDA which are commonly used as a guide were derived from the National Research Council 1968 RDA, which are considerably above the actual nutrient requirements of the average person.

Now you may ask, "Just what are vitamins?" Dr. Joseph R. Dipalma, M.D., stated they are "organic chemical substances that serve as precursors of certain cofactors essential to the vital metabolic processes of the body. Except for a limited amount of vitamin D, they cannot be synthesized in the body but must be obtained from food. When one or more of them is lacking in the diet, a deficiency disease results."[10]

Vitamins fall into two groups: **fat-soluble** or water-soluble.

Table 3-1. Food and Nutrition Board, National Academy of Sciences–National Research Council Recommended Daily Dietary Allowances,[a] Revised 1974

	Age	Weight		Height		Energy	Protein	Fat-Soluble Vitamins			
								Vita-min A Activity		Vita-min D	Vita-min E Activity[e]
	(years)	(kg)	(lbs)	(cm)	(in)	(kcal)[b]	(g)	(RE)[c]	(IU)	(IU)	(IU)
Infants	0.0–0.5	6	14	60	24	kg × 117	kg × 2.2	420[d]	1,400	400	4
	0.5–1.0	9	20	71	28	kg × 108	kg × 2.0	400	2,000	400	5
Children	1–3	13	28	86	34	1,300	23	400	2,000	400	7
	4–6	20	44	110	44	1,800	30	500	2,500	400	9
	7–10	30	66	135	54	2,400	36	700	3,300	400	10
Males	11–14	44	97	158	63	2,800	44	1,000	5,000	400	12
	15–18	61	134	172	69	3,000	54	1,000	5,000	400	15
	19–22	67	147	172	69	3,000	54	1,000	5,000	400	15
	23–50	70	154	172	69	2,700	56	1,000	5,000		15
	51+	70	154	172	69	2,400	56	1,000	5,000		15
Females	11–14	44	97	155	62	2,400	44	800	4,000	400	12
	15–18	54	119	162	65	2,100	48	800	4,000	400	12
	19–22	58	128	162	65	2,100	46	800	4,000	400	12
	23–50	58	128	162	65	2,000	46	800	4,000		12
	51+	58	128	162	65	1,800	46	800	4,000		12
Pregnant						+300	+30	1,000	5,000	400	15
Lactating						+500	+20	1,200	6,000	400	15

[a] The allowances are intended to provide for individual variations among most normal persons as they live in the United States under usual environmental stresses. Diets should be based on a variety of common foods in order to provide other nutrients for which human requirements have been less well defined. See text for more detailed discussion of allowances and of nutrients not tabulated. See Table I (p. 6) for weights and heights by individual year of age.

[b] Kilojoules (kJ) = 4.2 × kcal.

[c] Retinol equivalents.

[d] Assumed to be all as retinol in milk during the first six months of life. All subsequent intakes are assumed to be half as retinol and half as β-carotene when calculated from international

FAT-SOLUBLE VITAMINS

Vitamins A, D, E, and K are soluble in oil; therefore digestion of these vitamins requires the presence of adequate amounts of digestible fat and bile salts in the intestinal tract. Once they are absorbed into the body, very little of the fat-soluble vitamins is lost by way of the kidneys. These vitamins can be stored in considerable amounts in body fat, muscles, and liver. Fat-soluble vitamins play an important part in the maintenance of good health, and adequate amounts of these vitamins are readily available from a well-balanced diet.

Vitamin A–Retinol Vitamin A is a pale yellow organic compound composed of carbon, hydrogen, and oxygen. Since it is stored in the body, there is rarely a deficiency. It is found in all animals. Green and yellow vegetables and yellow fruits are the best source of **carotene,** which the body then converts into vitamin A.

Water-Soluble Vitamins							Minerals					
Ascorbic Acid (mg)	Folacin[f] (μg)	Niacin[g] (mg)	Riboflavin (mg)	Thiamin (mg)	Vitamin B$_6$ (mg)	Vitamin B$_{12}$ (μg)	Calcium (mg)	Phosphorus (mg)	Iodine (μg)	Iron (mg)	Magnesium (mg)	Zinc (mg)
35	50	5	0.4	0.3	0.3	0.3	360	240	35	10	60	3
35	50	8	0.6	0.5	0.4	0.3	540	400	45	15	70	5
40	100	9	0.8	0.7	0.6	1.0	800	800	60	15	150	10
40	200	12	1.1	0.9	0.9	1.5	800	800	80	10	200	10
40	300	16	1.2	1.2	1.2	2.0	800	800	110	10	250	10
45	400	18	1.5	1.4	1.6	3.0	1,200	1,200	130	18	350	15
45	400	20	1.8	1.5	2.0	3.0	1,200	1,200	150	18	400	15
45	400	20	1.8	1.5	2.0	3.0	800	800	140	10	350	15
45	400	18	1.6	1.4	2.0	3.0	800	800	130	10	350	15
45	400	16	1.5	1.2	2.0	3.0	800	800	110	10	350	15
45	400	16	1.3	1.2	1.6	3.0	1,200	1,200	115	18	300	15
45	400	14	1.4	1.1	2.0	3.0	1,200	1,200	115	18	300	15
45	400	14	1.4	1.1	2.0	3.0	800	800	100	18	300	15
45	400	13	1.2	1.0	2.0	3.0	800	800	100	18	300	15
45	400	12	1.1	1.0	2.0	3.0	800	800	80	10	300	15
60	800	+2	+0.3	+0.3	2.5	4.0	1,200	1,200	125	18+[h]	450	20
80	600	+4	+0.5	+0.3	2.5	4.0	1,200	1,200	150	18	450	25

units. As retinol equivalents, three fourths are as retinol and one fourth as β-carotene.

[e] Total vitamin E activity, estimated to be 80 percent as α-tocopherol and 20 percent other tocopherols. See text for variation in allowances.

[f] The folacin allowances refer to dietary sources as determined by *Lactobacillus casei* assay. Pure forms of folacin may be effective in doses less than one fourth of the recommended dietary allowance.

[g] Although allowances are expressed as niacin, it is recognized that on the average 1 mg of niacin is derived from each 60 mg of dietary tryptophan.

[h] This increased requirement cannot be met by ordinary diets; therefore, the use of supplemental iron is recommended.

This vitamin is necessary for cell growth, reproduction, and healthy skin and respiratory tissues. It also keeps the outer layers of the skin from hardening, becoming dry and itchy, and thus more susceptible to infection. Acne, a condition unrelated to vitamin A deficiency, does not improve when the vitamin is taken orally. However, many dermatologists prescribe topical application of retinoic acid in solutions and creams to cause a mild drying and flaking of the skin and thereby a gradual removal of scar tissue.[11]

A deficiency of A has been shown to cause night blindness and xerophthalmia, a condition of the eye in which the tear glands dry up and the cornea may become ulcerated.[12]

An overdose of A can be perilous, because of its **toxicity**. Such symptoms as headaches, nausea, and irritability may occur from a buildup. Other more severe ailments include growth retardation in children, enlargement of the liver and spleen, loss of hair, rheumatic pain, and disturbance of the menstrual cycle. Occasionally in children, and young people who have taken large doses of vitamin A, an intracranial pressure builds up that resembles a brain tumor. This oftentimes causes unnecessary surgery to be performed.

Toxic reactions from overuse of vitamin A are most common in adolescents who are attempting to cure acne and in infants and young children whose mothers are overly enthusiastic about keeping their children healthy. Toxic symptoms from vitamin A may include skin rash, loss of hair, irritability, loss of appetite, or other of the previously discussed conditions.

Parents need to know that not only is more than the recommended daily intake dangerous, but for the normal child eating a normal diet, no supplement of vitamin A is necessary.[13] If you must take a supplement, do not exceed 5,000 IU per day.[14]

Vitamin D—Calciferol

Vitamin D is used in the absorption of calcium and phosphorus in bone formation. A lack of it causes rickets. Early signs are skeleton deformation: bowed legs, deformed spine, "pot belly" appearance, and stunted growth. Adults suffering from a deficiency of vitamin D can develop osteomalacia, a softening of the bones that may ultimately result in bone deformation.

Vitamin D is often called the "sunshine vitamin" because it is naturally formed in the body by a reaction to the sun's rays; it is mostly needed by children and by older people who lack exposure to sunlight. This is how the reaction occurs:

> Human skin contains a substance called 7-Dehydrocholesterol, located just beneath the corneum, the outermost layer of the skin. Infants' skin contains twice the adult concentration of the substance and regardless of race, the corneum of infants is thinner and less heavily pigmented than that of adults of similar coloring. When radiation from the sun is present, the 7-Dehydrocholesterol undergoes a series of conversions, the end result of which—though not a single substance—can, for all practical purposes, be called "Vitamin D."[15]

Other sources of this vitamin are fish, eggs, and fortified milk.

The daily dietary requirements for D are very small, because it is stored in the body like vitamin A. However, infants and children need a supplement of about 400 units of vitamin D per day. This is why all prepared milks and milk formulas in the United States are fortified with about 400 IU of vitamins per quart.[16]

An excess of D causes nausea, weight loss, weakness, and excessive urination. More severe symptoms include hypertension and calcification of soft tissues.

Concerning excess vitamin D intake, the Food and Nutrition Board of the National Academy of Sciences has stated:

> An excess intake of vitamin D can result in serious toxicity. Vitamin D is stored in the fatty tissues of the body and is present in the circulating plasma. Because vitamin D promotes absorption of calcium from the intestine, a large excess of stored vitamin D can cause excessive quantities of calcium in the blood (hypercalcemia) persisting for months after intake of vitamin D has been discontinued. Chronic hypercalcemia causes calcification of soft tissues with particularly serious injury to the kidney; associated general symptoms are weakness, lethargy, anorexia, and constipation.[17]

Excessive amounts of vitamin D are hazardous, and only individuals with diseases affecting vitamin D absorption or metabolism require more than 400 IU daily.[18]

Vitamin E is possibly the most mysterious of all vitamins; it is the hardest to research because it is virtually impossible to find a deficiency of it in humans. The amount of vitamin E needed by most people appears to be satisfied by the average well-balanced diet, even though some vitamin E is lost in food processing. It is found in plant materials, vegetable oil, eggs, whole grains, liver, fruits, and vegetables.

Vitamin E—the Tocopherols

Vitamin E acts as an antioxidant, helping to prevent oxygen from destroying other substances, such as vitamin A. In premature infants with a rare form of anemia, it has been effective as a cure. All other reports and wild claims of its healing powers have not been scientifically proven. In fact, one researcher states:

> Vitamin E is one of those embarrassing vitamins that have been identified, isolated and synthesized by physiologists and biochemists and then handed to the medical profession with the suggestion that a use should be found for it, without any satisfactory evidence that human beings are ever deficient in it or even that it is a necessary nutrient for man.[19]

Yet there are some who recommend vitamin E in large doses to cure a variety of disorders such as circulatory, reproductive, and nervous system diseases, acne, sexual impotence, muscular dystrophy, and diaper rash, as well as disorders of aging and those caused by air pollution.

The Committee on Nutritional Misinformation of the National Research Council states the following:

> Misleading claims that vitamin E supplementation of the ordinary diet will cure or prevent human ailments such as sterility, lack of virility, abnormal termination of pregnancy, heart disease, muscular weakness, cancer, ulcers, skin disorders, and burns are not backed by sound experimentation or clinical observations. Some of these claims are based upon deficiency symptoms observed in other species. Careful studies over a period of many years attempting to relate these symptoms to vitamin E deficiency in human beings have been unproductive. The wide distribution of vitamin E in vegetable oils, cereal grains, and animal fats makes a deficiency in humans very unlikely. Premature infants or individuals with impaired absorption of fats may require supplemental vitamin E, but they should, in any event, be under the care of a physician.[20]

All successful research involving the use of vitamin E as a cure for sterility has concerned mice and other animals. Vitamin E deficiency causes tissue swelling and brain damage in chickens, and faulty development of the placenta and destruction of the fetus in female rats, mice, hamsters, and guinea pigs, but experiments on humans have failed.[21]

Thus, we do need vitamin E, but, until proven otherwise, only in moderate amounts. If you do take supplemental vitamin E, do not exceed 100 IU per day. Self-medication of vitamin E can certainly be hazardous in that it may delay appropriate diagnosis and cure of an ailment. There is much controversy about whether or not there are other hazards of high-dose vitamin E supplementation:

> Reports of severe liver damage, urine problems, high levels of cholesterol formation in the blood, bleeding in heart patients on blood-thinning drugs, extreme weakness and fatigue, all have been associated with vitamin E dosages far beyond the recommended daily allowances—from 300 to 800 International Units daily. Yet vitamin E is not considered one of the potentially toxic vitamins, taken in large amounts.[22]

Vitamin K   Vitamin K is essential for the clotting of blood; therefore, it gets its name from the "koagulation factor," a Danish term coined by a Danish scientist named Dam in 1929.

Good sources for vitamin K are spinach, liver, kale, cauliflower, egg yolk, and dairy products. A deficiency causes hemorrhaging and liver injury. However, since most vitamin K is produced by bacteria in a person's colon, a deficiency is usually not the result of poor nutrition but rather is caused by a reduction of the intestinal flora. Such a reduction is often brought about by drugs.

This vitamin is adequately supplied by human and cow milk and thus no supplementation is necessary except to prevent hemorrhaging when individuals are in a diseased state or giving birth. Ingestion of large quantities of vitamin K supplements can result in red blood cell destruction.

WATER-SOLUBLE VITAMINS

Found in foods having a high proportion of water, each of the water-soluble vitamins performs one or more exclusive functions in body maintenance.

The most important vitamins in this category are vitamin C (**ascorbic acid**) and the B-complex group, including pantothenic acid, niacin (nicotinic acid), and **folic acid** (folacin). In general, they function as coenzymes in the processing of carbohydrates, protein, and fat in the body.

Water-soluble vitamins are required in extra amounts at certain times. For instance, additional amounts of water-soluble vitamins usually are needed during very cold weather, because low temperatures cause the vitamins to be heavily excreted in the urine. On the other hand, perspiration resulting from heavy-duty work in high temperatures also can deplete the body's supply of the vitamins and make supplementation necessary.

Excess quantities of these vitamins are not stored in the body. Quantities beyond the body's needs are removed in the urine. The required amounts must be obtained daily from food or other sources.

Thiamine—   Thiamine belongs to the B-vitamin complex. It was discovered in 1892 by Eijkman
Vitamin B$_1$ of Java. It comes in the form of colorless crystals and has a yeast-like smell and a salty taste. It is sold in the form of thiamine hydrochloride.

Thiamine is required for normal digestion. It is one of the keys to the release of energy during the metabolism of carbohydrates and it is essential for the orderly breakdown of **pyruvic acid**. Its other functions include aiding in growth, fertility, lactation, and the normal function of nerve tissues. It does not provide usable energy, but it aids in cellular energy production.

Beriberi is the most common result of a lack of B_1. Many minor problems may also arise. Some of these are fatigue, anorexia, constipation, labored breathing, weariness, nausea, tiredness of the calf, spastic colon, and depression.

Thiamine is found in abundant quantities in brewer's yeast, pork, beans, peas, nuts, and enriched and whole-grain breads and cereals. A significant increase in dietary carbohydrate increases the thiamine requirement. Thiamine deficiency is infrequent and supplementation is not necessary.

It should be noted here that thiamine works in conjunction with other B-complex vitamins, and must be accompanied by them. A self-prescribed dosage of one or the other vitamins from this complex would unavoidably cause a deficiency of others in the group.

A second danger with self-prescribed vitamin B is overdose. Many of the B vitamins interact with other drugs, so taking B vitamins without medical supervision can be fatal. Riboflavin can decrease the beneficial activity of tetracycline being taken for an infection. Pyridoxine can interfere with the action of Levodopa, a drug widely prescribed for the treatment of Parkinson's disease. Folic acid can lessen the effects of diphenylhydantoin, an antiepileptic medication. Large doses of the B-complex group as a whole can increase bloodclotting time, thus posing a critical threat of hemorrhage to someone who regularly takes an anticoagulant or has any disorder that might tend to cause bleeding episodes.

Riboflavin—
Vitamin B_2

Riboflavin helps the body obtain energy from carbohydrate and protein substances and enhances the building of body tissues. A deficiency causes sores and cracks on the lips and dimness of vision. This vitamin is found in abundant quantities in leafy vegetables, cheese, eggs, milk, lean meat, and enriched and whole-grain breads and cereals.

The need for vitamin B_2 increases as the intake of protein increases. A well-balanced diet is a sufficient source of riboflavin.

Pyridoxine—
Vitamin B_6

The functions of pyridoxine involve the breaking down, production, and supply of proteins as needed by the body cells. On a smaller scale it also helps process carbohydrates and fats.

Pyridoxine is found in a variety of foods including legumes, potatoes, wheat, corn, yeast, bananas, liver, kidney, and other meats. Milk and eggs are fair sources.

Infants with a genetically caused metabolic disorder who are suffering convulsions will respond to therapeutic doses of B_6 to correct the dietary lack. Aside from such a rare deficiency, milder forms of the vitamin shortage in the body can cause symptoms such as mouth soreness, dizziness, nausea, and weight loss. It is possible that deficiency of the vitamin may also reduce immunological protection.[23]

Large doses of the vitamin have been given effectively to treat vomiting during pregnancy. In addition, patients taking antidepressants and women using oral contraceptives often require vitamin B_6 supplementation. Healthy persons eating a balanced diet have no need of vitamin B_6 supplementation.

Cyanocobalamin—
Vitamin B_{12}

In 1926, Minot and Murphy discovered that Addison's Anemia could be controlled by ingestion of whole liver. In 1948, this same treatment cured another form of **anemia,** and a lack of B_{12} was named as the cause of this ailment.[24] This vitamin is necessary for the normal development of red blood cells and the function of all cells, especially those in the bone marrow, nervous system, and intestines. Along with anemia, a deficiency of this vitamin can cause a degeneration of the spinal cord, the symptoms of which often do not appear until after the damage is irreparable.

The only known sources of cyancobalamin are from the animal kingdom; it is not supplied by plants. Strict vegetarians, therefore, may suffer a deficiency of this vitamin and should consider supplementation. Good food sources include eggs, dairy products, liver, kidney, lean meats, and seafoods.

Periods of rapid growth in children, conditions causing abnormal blood loss (surgery, occult hemorrhage, menstruation), and added demands of the body during pregnancy and lactation may indicate the need for vitamin B_{12} supplementation.

Niacin—Nicotinic
Acid, Nicotinamide

The needle-like crystals of niacin in its pure form are said to be bitter tasting. Both forms of the vitamin—niacin (nicotinic acid) and niacinamide (nicotinamide)—have the same effects and functions. They are not related to the substance nicotine, found in tobacco.

Niacin, as part of two coenzymes, functions mainly in body cells to convert proteins and fats to provide energy when needed (proteins and fats can provide energy when carbohydrates are not available).

Pellagra is the disease associated with niacin deficiency. Because the functions of niacin and riboflavin are interrelated, their deficiency symptoms are similar. General or early signs of pellagra include weakness, loss of appetite, headache, and backache. The later stages of the disease include scaly **dermatitis,** swollen and reddened tongue (glossitis), diarrhea, confusion, and disorientation.

Tryptophane, an essential amino acid or protein-building material, is converted to niacin in the body (approximately 60 mg of tryptophane provide 1 mg of niacin). Therefore diets furnishing adequate amounts of protein will supply tryptophane for conversion to niacin. Because of the tryptophane they contain, beans, peas, peanuts, meat, poultry, fish, milk, and eggs are good sources of niacin. Enriched grain products also make an important contribution. In wheat, corn, and rye bran, a bound form of niacin occurs that cannot be utilized by humans. Corn and rice are naturally poor in niacin because they contain very little tryptophane.[25]

Pantothenic Acid

Pantothenic comes from the Greek word "pantothen," which means "in every corner," and reflects the fact that pantothenic is found in all forms of living things. The body has the ability to make significant amounts of pantothenic acid from the bacteria present in the intestines. Pantothenic acid plays an important role in the production of energy from carbohydrates, fat, and proteins. It is also involved in the formation of certain fat and protein compounds, as well as hormones.

The wide distribution of this vitamin among living things, coupled with the fact that it can be produced by the body, makes deficiency a rarity. The effects of a deficiency in animals or human beings have not been clearly demonstrated.

The best sources of pantothenic acid are yeast, kidney, heart, liver, egg yolk, and salmon. Other foods such as whole grains, legumes, peanuts, broccoli, sweet potatoes, cheese, and milk make a good contribution.[26]

Biotin

Biotin has also been called the "anti-egg white injury" factor, since a substance in egg white, avidin, has been shown to be responsible for the eczema and paralysis seen in rats fed an abundance of raw egg white. Raw egg white combines with biotin and prevents it from being utilized by the body. The symptoms can be corrected by giving sufficient biotin in the diet. Avidin is also made harmless by the heating of egg whites.

In combination with certain enzymes in the body, biotin plays an important role in the production of fat and protein substances (fatty acids, amino acids, and purines, one of the building blocks for nucleic acids, respectively). It is also involved in carbohydrate breakdown. A deficiency of biotin in human beings is rare and has been known to occur only when large amounts of raw egg whites are eaten. In a particular experiment, volunteers were fed a diet with adequate calories but low in biotin and containing approximately sixty egg whites for a period of about ten weeks. In the third or fourth week, these persons developed deficiency symptoms that included lassitude, dermatitis, muscle pain, anorexia, hyperesthesia (increased sensitivity of the skin or the senses), and anemia.[27]

Excellent food sources include liver and other organ meats, mushrooms, peanuts, egg yolk, legumes. Milk, other vegetables, fruits, and cereal grains contain lesser amounts in general. In addition, bacteria in the intestine seem to be capable of making biotin.

Folacin (Folic Acid)

Folacin is not present in its active form in nature, but is converted by the body. Folacin has an essential part in the production of vital protein substances such as nucleoproteins (substances found in all living cells and necessary for growth and development) and the protein portion of hemoglobin (in red blood cells) called heme.

A diet consistently lacking in folacin will lead to a type of anemia in which the red blood cells are produced in fewer numbers and are abnormally enlarged. (This is quite different from the anemia caused by a deficiency of vitamin B_{12}). This particular effect of folacin deficiency is understandable, since the vitamin functions in the making of red blood cells' hemoglobin. Inflammation of the tongue (glossitis) and gastrointestinal problems such as diarrhea may occur in some persons.

Since the vitamin is found in green leaves, its name was taken from the latin word "folium," meaning leaf. Excellent sources of folacin are deep-green leafy vegetables, liver, kidney, and yeast. Meats, fish, eggs, nuts, legumes, and whole grains are also considered good sources.

Vitamin C– Ascorbic Acid

James Link, Ship's Surgeon of the H.M.S. *Salisbury,* and "the Father of Nautical Medicine," discovered in 1747 that if the men aboard his ships ingested citrus fruit, they did not suffer the malady of scurvy. Later, in 1933, Waugh and King at the University of Pittsburgh and Suentgyolggi in Hungary identified the anti-scurvy factor as ascorbic acid. Because it saved sailors from scurvy, vitamin C has been credited with having done as much as Lord Nelson to break the power of Napoleon.

Today vitamin C is noted for its help in holding body cells together, strengthening blood vessels, and healing wounds. It aids in the production of amino acids, protects vitamins A and E from being naturally broken down, and prevents the breakdown of fat for energy once energy needs have been met. Vitamin C also helps tooth and bone formation and aids in resistance to infection.

The best sources of vitamin C are of course citrus fruits. Other good sources include berries, melons, green leafy vegetables, potatoes, and tomatoes.

Vitamin C for the prevention of colds is perhaps the hottest topic at present. There are some very highly esteemed advocates on both sides of the fence. Dr. Linus Pauling, winner of two Nobel prizes, came out with a book lauding the curative powers of vitamin C against the common cold.

But Jean Mayer, well-known nutrition expert, wrote concerning Dr. Pauling's report,

> We just do not know what the supersaturation of ascorbic acid does. I find it remarkable that some people who are most nervous about what they call untested chemicals in their food nevertheless dose themselves daily with a substance that is needed (and well understood) at the required levels but is actually an "untested chemical" when you take it in huge doses.[28]

Clinical observations and experimentation have not supported claims that daily vitamin C supplementation, in doses ranging from 500 mg to a full gram or more, will provide a cure for physical and mental stress or lessen the chance of vascular disease. No tests have conclusively proved that vitamin C can stay the cold either. However, some studies have shown that an increase of daily intake may reduce the frequency and severity of colds.

But even assuming the body's need for vitamin C increases during times of infection, inflammation, surgery, and maybe when an individual is smoking or taking oral contraceptives, the RDA is still usually sufficient. Any person eating a balanced diet with plenty of fresh fruits and vegetables consumes far more than the RDA in a typical day.

An overdose of vitamin C can cause kidney stones or severe diarrhea. In addition, it can harm diabetics by making accurate testing of diabetes impossible—because it is water-soluble and is passed off in the urine, it gives a false indication of sugar level. While many persons may be able to tolerate large doses of vitamin C for prolonged periods, others may be at risk.

> If a person chooses to experiment with higher doses, say in the thousands of mg. per day, they should bear in mind the fact that the potential for undesirable side-effects increases with dose and duration; if a person has been on high doses for more than one or two weeks, the body will have become used to the high dose and will need to be "weaned" off slowly to avoid a rebound fall in blood level.[29]

PSEUDOVITAMINS

Lipoic Acid   Lipoic acid (also thioctic acid and protogen) is not a true vitamin, but rather a substance capable of being dissolved in fat, and thus it is called a fatty acid. It is mentioned after B-complex vitamins because of its close relationship, in function, to thiamine (B_1). With thiamine, lipoic acid participates in the processing of carbohydrates to produce energy. The food sources of lipoic acid include yeast and liver.

PABA is one of the forms of folacin (folic acid), but it is not considered a vitamin. It is worthy of mention because certain minute organisms require it for growth, and because it is involved in the formation of folic acid.

Para-Aminobenzoic Acid (PABA)

Inositol is stored particularly in muscle, red blood cells, and brain and eye tissue. However, its role in human nutrition has not been identified. Human beings apparently make this substance from intestinal bacteria. Fruits, legumes, grains, nuts, meat, and milk contain varying amounts of inositol.

Inositol

It is debatable whether the two compounds choline and betaine should be classified as vitamins. They are components of body cells rather than enzyme helpers. Choline, which is manufactured by the body, prevents accumulation of fat in the liver and is involved indirectly in normal nerve functions. Betaine is made from choline and also has a role in the prevention of "fatty livers." Neither dietary requirements nor deficiency problems have been established. Choline is found in many foods, including egg yolk, legumes, whole-grain cereals, and organ meats. Very little occurs in fruit and vetetables in general.

Choline and Betaine

Laetrile, also known as "vitamin B_{17}," a drug derived from pulverized apricot pits, has been widely promoted for the prevention, treatment, and cure of cancer. Its major component is amygdalin. The laetriles are recognized as a family of chemical compounds. The FDA has ruled that they are not, however, essential nutritional components, since they do not promote any physiological process vital to the existence of living organisms.

Laetrile— Vitamin B_{17}?

Furthermore, there is no evidence that a disease state is produced or alleviated by the exclusion from or addition to the diet of the laetriles. The FDA reasons that if there were a vitamin B_{17} (as the product Laetrile is claimed to be), and if cancer were a vitamin B_{17} deficiency disease, then every animal deprived of the vitamin would succumb to cancer, while no animal given sufficient amounts of the substance would be afflicted. This follows the same reasoning that no person given adequate amounts of vitamin C ever has scurvy.[30] Thus, the FDA has concluded that Laetrile or amygdalin, or nitroloside is neither an essential nutrient nor a vitamin.

In fact, the Commissioner of Food and Drugs has issued the following warning on laetrile and has requested that it be publicized as much as possible.

> Whether sold as a drug (amygdalin) or as a "vitamin" (B_{17}), Laetrile is worthless in the prevention, treatment or cure of cancer. The substance has no therapeutic or nutritional value. Laetrile can be fatal for cancer patients who delay or give up regular medical treatment and take Laetrile instead.[31]

Laetrile contains cyanide and can cause poisoning and death when large quantities are taken by mouth. One infant died of cyanide poisoning after swallowing fewer than five Laetrile tablets. At least sixteen other deaths have been documented from ingestion of Laetrile ingredients (apricot and similar fruit pits). Laetrile is especially hazardous if the injection form is taken by mouth. This can cause sudden death.[32]

Laetrile is not routinely subject to Food and Drug Administration inspection for quality and purity the way all other drugs are. Analysis has shown some Laetrile to contain toxic contaminants—ampules of Laetrile for injection have been found with mold and other adulterants which can be dangerous when injected.

Those who persist in the use of Laetrile or its ingredients should:

1. Be prepared to deal promptly with acute cyanide poisoning if the oral product is used. Vigorous medical treatment must be started immediately or death can result.
2. Watch for early sumptoms of chronic cyanide poisoning, including weakness in the arms and legs and disorders of the nervous system.
3. Keep the drug out of reach of children.
4. Those who choose to use Laetrile should secure it from medically approved sources.

THE "NATURAL" CRAZE

This is a generation of nature lovers, and everything is geared to "getting back to nature," even vitamins. A vitamin that would cost one dollar in its "synthetic" form costs five dollars "natural."

Two fallacies are behind this "natural" vitamin craze: (1) Natural vitamins are superior to those synthesized by man; (2) Vitamin products sold as "natural" do not contain synthetic ingredients.

Chemists tell us that each vitamin, in order to be called such, must have a particular molecular structure. This remains the same whether the vitamin is synthesized in a laboratory or extracted from an animal or plant. For example, to be called vitamin A, a substance, no matter what its source, has to have a specific molecular arrangement. The body cannot tell the difference between a vitamin from an animal or plant and the same vitamin from a laboratory.

An investigator discovered some interesting things while visiting two manufacturers of "natural" vitamins:

> Their Rose Hips Vitamin C Tablets are made from natural rose hips combined with chemical ascorbic acid, the same vitamin C used in standard pharmaceutical tablets. Natural rose hips contain only about two percent vitamin C, and we were told that if no vitamin C were added, the tablet "would have to be as big as a golf ball."[33]

In any case, all vitamins, "natural" or synthetic, must contain a certain number of binding additives, such as ethyl cellulose, polysorbate 80 (a synthetic emulsifier), gum acacia, etc. It comes back to the same old story — if you want natural vitamin C, go buy an orange. Your pocketbook will appreciate it.

VITAMIN CURES

One of the greatest debates of all time is now in session. On one side are those who are convinced that vitamin therapy is a cure for everything from athlete's foot to cancer and mental retardation. On the opposite side are those who wait for experimental proof.

Research so far has provided no convincing evidence of unique health benefits occurring from the excessive consumption of any one nutrient. Dr. Jukes makes a good point when he states:

> A regrettable side effect of quackery, magnified in our era of instant communication, is that extensive efforts of responsible scientists are needed to test and expose irresponsible proposals and suggestions that promise "health" from overdosage with universal remedies. These efforts are diverted from more constructive activities, and society is the loser.[34]

A healthy person receiving an adequate diet has no need for routine vitamin supplementation. However, the use of multivitamin preparations produces little harm as long as the preparations are not used to excess. It is imperative to realize, however, that you cannot replace a missed meal, or inadequate protein, carbohydrate, or mineral intake, by the use of vitamins.

During periods of extra nutritional demand, such as pregnancy, lactation, or prolonged illness, vitamin supplementation may be in order. The American Medical Association suggests that one to one and a half times the RDA is appropriate during these times.[35]

Overdosage of vitamins, especially fat-soluble ones (particularly A and D), can cause severe toxicity. Thus the FDA restricts over-the-counter preparations of vitamin A and D to 10,000 IU and 400 IU respectively. The RDA for folic acid also should not be exceeded. Administered appropriately, vitamins are remarkably safe medications.

Much research is presently being conducted on the use of megadose vitamins as a form of therapy for many diseases, even those of a psychological nature.

Megadose vitamin use is usually tenfold or more above the RDA. In these amounts, vitamins are really serving as chemical therapy rather than as a vitamin.

Megavitamin Therapy

> Megavitamin therapy is sometimes termed ortho-molecular psychiatry. It is largely based on an ancient and cherished delusion of the laity: if a small dose of a medicament is good, a larger dose must be better. The procedure is in conflict with an elementary principle of pharmacology that states that increasing the dosage of a therapeutic compound leads to maximum effectiveness, and on further increase, to the production of toxic effects. This principle is routinely used by the FDA in setting tolerance levels for food additives.[36]

An American Psychiatric Association task force found megavitamin therapy no better than a **placebo**.[37] A recent report by the American Academy of Pediatrics concluded that "megavitamin therapy for learning disabilities and psychoses in children, including autism, is not justified on the basis of documented clinical results."[38]

The only use of megavitamin therapy that appears clinically justifiable is in such specific serious illnesses as rare vitamin-dependent genetic diseases and certain malabsorption syndromes.

REGULATING VITAMINS

A new law sharply restricts the FDA's authority to regulate vitamins and minerals. It forbids the agency to set maximum potencies on most vitamins and minerals and to limit the number of combinations of these products that may be sold. In passing the law, Congress has made it clear that the FDA should not attempt to provide economic protection for consumers by regulating vitamin and mineral supplements solely because they contain dosages the agency believes are greater than the body needs or can use, or because they contain added substances that the agency believes are nutritionally useless.

Under the new regulations, effective January 1978, the FDA's responsibilities are to:

1. Require minimum potency levels in nutritionally significant amounts.
2. Limit the composition of certain dietary supplements on the basis of safety. For example, high-potency preparations of fat-soluble vitamins A and D will remain prescription drugs, and the amount of folic acid allowable will continue to be limited.
3. Restrict the composition of combination products offered to infants, children, and pregnant or lactating women, setting maximum as well as minimum potency requirements.
4. Require the listing on the label of all ingredients, vitamins or otherwise, and where relevant, in terms of U.S. RDA and milligrams.
5. Restrict false or misleading claims.[39]

SUMMARY

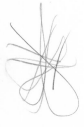

Wherein lies the answer to the vitamin maze? Researchers will someday discover how much is enough of a vitamin and how much is too much, whether some drugs have powers beyond that which is nutritional, and which diseases will respond to vitamin therapy. Until then, it is best to ignore elaborate claims and miraculous testimonials. Why don't we concentrate on eating well-balanced meals and getting the RDA? We are already aware of its benefits. If you are a picky eater or dieting, then a single multiple vitamin could do no harm, but never consider any vitamin a substitute for a well-balanced diet.

Remember, vitamins taken in excess, beyond the RDA, can be dangerous without proper direction. Consulting a reputable medical doctor is the wisest way to discover if one has a vitamin deficiency. Until more is known about vitamins and their healing powers, this should be the only way one would ever consider a significant increase of vitamin intake.

NOTES

1. Joseph DiPalma, "Vitamins: Facts and Fancies," *RN,* July 1972, pp. 57–66.
2. Leland Cooley and Lee Morrison Cooley, *Pre-Medicated Murder* (Radner, Pa.: Chilton Book Co., 1974), p. 118.
3. Jane Heenan, "Myths of Vitamins," *FDA Consumer,* May 1974, pp. 4–9.
4. Ibid.
5. Ibid.
6. Cooley, *Pre-Medicated Murder,* p. 118.
7. "Vitamins, Minerals, and FDA," *FDA Consumer,* September 1973, pp. 18–19.
8. DiPalma, "Vitamins: Facts and Fancies," pp. 57–66.
9. Food and Drug Board, National Research Council, *Recommended Dietary Allowances,* 8th ed. (Washington, D.C.: National Academy of Sciences, 1974).
10. DiPalma, "Vitamins: Facts and Fancies," pp. 57–66.
11. "Vitamins—What You Should Know," *American Druggist,* November 1974, pp. 34–40.
12. Edward G. Damon, "A Primer on Vitamins," *FDA Consumer,* May 1974, pp. 5–11.
13. Alan Fleischman and Laurence Finberg, "Vitamins: Too Much of a Good Thing," *Consultant,* August 1977, pp. 70–75.
14. "Who Needs Vitamin and Mineral Supplements," *Patient Care,* February 28, 1978, p. 108.
15. Dodi Schultz. "The Verdict on Vitamins," *Today's Health,* January 1974, pp. 54–60, 63.
16. Fleischman, "Vitamins: Too Much of a Good Thing," p. 70–75.
17. "Hazards of Overuse of Vitamin D," *Journal of the American Dietetic Association,* May 1975, p. 453.
18. Joseph R. DiPalma, "Vitamin Toxicity," *American Family Physician,* Vol. 18, No. 2, August 1978, pp. 106–109.
19. Institute of Food Technologists, "Vitamin E," *Food Technology,* January 1977, pp. 77–80.
20. National Research Council, "Supplementation of Human Diets with Vitamin E," *Nutrition Reviews Supplement,* July 1974, p. 38.
21. Jean Mayer, "Massive Dose Vitamins, the Newest Craze," *Family Health,* February 1972, pp. 25, 46, 48, 49.
22. "Vitamin Pills — You Don't Need, Can Kill You," *Consumer Digest,* July/August 1977, pp. 46–48.
23. "Vitamins—What You Should Know," pp. 34–40.
24. Ibid.
25. Reprinted with permission from Maria L. Fletcher, "Vitamin B-Complex and C," *Life and Health,* August 1977, pp. 18–21.
26. Ibid.
27. Ibid.
28. Mayer, "Massive Dose Vitamins, the Newest Craze," pp. 25, 46, 48, 49.
29. Terence W. Anderson, "New Horizons for Vitamin C," *Nutrition Today,* January/February 1977, p. 13.
30. Thomas H. Jukes, "Is Laetrile a Vitamin?" *Nutrition Today,* September/October 1977, p. 17.
31. Donald Kennedy, "Laetrile Warning," *Drug Bulletin,* November/December 1977, pp. 27–30.

32. Ibid.
33. Adolph Kamil, "How Natural Are Those 'Natural' Vitamins?" *Nutrition Reviews Supplement,* July 1974, p. 34.
34. Thomas H. Jukes, "Megavitamin Therapy," *JAMA,* August 11, 1975, Vol. 233, No. 6, pp. 550–551.
35. Phillip White, "Vitamin Preparations," *Postgraduate Medicine,* October 1976, p. 205.
36. Jukes, "Megavitamin Fad," *Drug Therapy,* pp. 550–551.
37. Ari Kiev, "The Megavitamin Fad," *Drug Therapy,* July 1976, p. 80.
38. Bennett Shaywitz et al., "Megavitamins for Minimal Brain Dysfunction," *JAMA,* October 1977, p. 1750.
39. Trisha Gorman, "Vitamins: Bringing Back That Glow of Health," *Drug Therapy,* February 1, 1977, p. 50.

4

The Truth About Minerals

When any food is burned, a powdery white residue called ash is left. This substance, representing the mineral content of the food, is only a fraction of its total weight. Comprising only 4 percent of our body weight, these minute amounts of mineral nutrients regulate many vital body processes, form molecules essential to good health, such as **hemoglobin,** and are incorporated into structural forms such as bones and teeth. Table 4-1 provides a list of the U.S. RDA of minerals known to be essential for body function. (The 1974 National Research Council RDA is outlined in Chapter 3, Table 3-1.)

Since the requirements for most minerals are very small, they are measured in milligrams (mg), one of which is equal to 1/1,000 of a gram. Trace minerals, elements needed by the body in even smaller amounts, are measured in micrograms (meg), one of which is equal to 1/1,000 of a milligram.

Our knowledge of human requirements for trace elements is incomplete, and the dietary recommendations for these nutrients are imprecise, for the difficulty of inducing deficiency of trace elements hampers attempts to isolate mineral action within humans. Yet researchers continue to identify uses of known elements and to discover other substances needed by the body for good health.

Table 4-1. U.S. RDA's for Minerals

	Unit	Infants (0-12 months)	Children under 4 years of age	Adults and children over 4 years of age	Pregnant or lactating women
Calcium	g	0.6	0.8	1	1.3
Iron	mg	15	10	18	18
Phosphorus	g	0.5	0.8	1	1.3
Iodine	meg	45	70	150	150
Magnesium	mg	70	200	400	450
Zinc	mg	5	8	15	15
Copper	mg	0.6	1	2	2.0

g = gram   mg = milligram   meg = microgram
1,000 meg (microgram) = 1 mg
1,000 mg (milligram) = 1 g

To understand the relative amounts needed,
it may be useful to know that 1 level teaspoon of white sugar weighs about 4 g.

Some minerals are needed in relatively large amounts in the diet: calcium, phosphorus, sodium, chlorine, potassium, magnesium, and sulfur. The "large" requirement may range from a hundred milligrams to one gram. Those minerals are generally classified as macrominerals.

The trace minerals, which are needed in smaller amounts, include iron, manganese, copper, iodine, zinc, cobalt, fluorine, and selenium. Some minerals, such as lead, mercury, and cadmium, are regarded as harmful.

Mineral elements have two general body functions—building and regulating. Their building functions affect the skeleton and all soft tissues. Their regulating functions involve a wide variety of systems, such as heartbeat, blood clotting, maintenance of the internal pressure of body fluids, nerve responses, and transport of oxygen from the lungs to the tissues.

MACROMINERALS

Calcium

Calcium is present in the body in greater amounts than any other mineral. Almost all of the two or three pounds of **calcium** present in the body is concentrated in the bones and teeth. Small amounts of calcium help to regulate certain body processes, such as the normal behavior of nerves, muscle tone, and blood clotting. Calcium is also an activator of a number of enzymes. Although growing children and pregnant and lactating women have the highest calcium needs, all people need calcium in their diets throughout life.

Milk and milk products are good sources of this mineral. Other good sources are green leafy vegetables (except spinach and chard), citrus fruits, and dried peas and beans. Meats, grains, and nuts, which are good sources of many other nutrients, do not provide significant amounts of calcium.

Phosphorus

Phosphorus is present with calcium, in almost equal amounts, in the bones and teeth, and is an important part of every tissue in the body. In combination with calcium, phosphorus contributes to the supportive structure of the body and is involved in a great variety of chemical reactions in the body. The ratio of calcium to phosphorus affects the **absorption** of each. Absorption is maximized when the two minerals are present in approximately equal amounts.

Phosphorus is present in nearly all foods, and deficiency apparently does not occur under normal conditions. Good sources are meat, poultry, fish, eggs, and whole-grain foods. Vegetables and fruits are generally low in this mineral.

Sodium and Chlorine

Sodium and chlorine are the two elements that combine to form sodium chloride (table salt), but each has separate functions in the body.

Sodium is found mainly in blood plasma and in the fluids outside the body cells, helping to maintain normal water balance inside and outside the cells. Sodium-rich foods come from animal sources such as meat, fish, poultry, eggs, and milk. Many processed foods, such as ham, bacon, bread, and crackers, have a high sodium content because salt or sodium compounds are added in processing.

Chlorine is part of hydrochloric acid, which is found in quite high concentrations in the gastric juice and is very important in digestion of food in the stomach.

The daily American diet provides a high intake of sodium, much of it added to food as salt. Salt (sodium chloride) consumption in the United States is estimated to range from about 6 to 18 grams a day. Even though the recommended allowance is 3 grams a day, the average requirement could normally be achieved without adding salt to any food.

Salt is added to processed food principally as a flavoring agent rather than as a preservative. In some instances it is the primary flavoring agent and may be used to mask other less appealing flavors. A reduction of salt intake is often prescribed by physicians to persons with kidney disease, cirrhosis of the liver, or congestive heart disease. A decrease in sodium intake can reduce the retention of water in the system (**edema**), which is typically associated with these health problems. Under conditions of heavy sweat losses or vomiting, salt intake may need to be increased, but the usual diet provides more than enough to cover losses from normal activities.

Salt has been found to cause **hypertension** (high blood pressure) in some individuals, but others do not seem genetically susceptible. There is some evidence that an imbalance with potassium intake may be a factor in hypertension. It has been estimated that 20 percent of the United States population, and up to 40 percent of older people, are susceptible to hypertension. The Select Committee on Nutrition has recommended reduction of salt intake as an important counter-measure:

> Millions of children and youths are moving toward hypertension. Excess dietary sodium is clearly an adverse factor in some, if not in most, people prone to hypertension. The evidence indicates that a systematic effort to reduce dietary sodium chloride intake and increase dietary potassium intake would result in the amelioration of much suffering among those who are prone and would increase both duration and quality of life for many millions of people.[1]

Researchers have also found possible connections between high salt intake and changes in levels of gastric acid secretion, stomach cancer, cerebrovascular disease, and migraine headaches. Even though no cause-and-effect relationships have been established, it would seem prudent to reduce one's salt intake.

Potassium

Potassium is found mainly in the fluid inside the individual body cells. With sodium, it helps to regulate the balance and volume of body fluids. A potassium deficiency is uncommon in healthy people but may result from prolonged diarrhea or from diuretic drugs (which cause higher urine volume). Deficiency has also been associated with extremely inadequate protein diets in children. Potassium is abundant in almost all foods, both plant and animal.

Magnesium

Magnesium is found in all body tissues, but primarily in the bones. It is an essential part of many **enzyme** systems responsible for energy conversions in the body. A deficiency of magnesium in healthy humans eating a variety of foods is uncommon, but it has been observed in some postsurgical patients, in alcoholics, and in individuals in certain other diseased conditions.

A magnesium deficiency may lead to neuromuscular dysfunction, hyperexcitability with tremor and convulsions, and sometimes behavioral disorders. Magnesium is found in a wide variety of foods, particularly plants.

Sulfur   Sulfur is also present in all body tissues and essential to life. It is related to protein nutrition because it is a component of several important amino acids. It is also a part of two vitamins, thiamine and biotin. The complete function of sulfur has not yet been established.

THE TRACE ELEMENTS

It seems unnatural that anything so very minute as a trace mineral could play an important part in the proper performance and maintenance of the human body. Yet time and experimental inquiry have proven beyond a doubt that these micro-elements are not only important but essential to many body functions. Most of them do not occur in the body in their free form, but are bound to organic compounds on which they depend for transport, storage, and function.

Scientists have known for more than one hundred years that iron and iodine are necessary for man. Between the years of 1928 and 1935, a period of rapid learning in the field of biochemistry, four more elements were found to be essential: copper, zinc, manganese, and cobalt. These findings can be credited to C. A. Elvehjem, E. B. Hart, and W. R. Todd from the University of Wisconsin. Then, in the next thirty years, three more elements also were found to be necessary: chromium, selenium, and molybdenum. In 1970, fluorine, silicon, tin, and vanadium were added to the list. What next? Time will tell.[2]

What do we know about trace minerals? Jean Mayer describes their function best:

> To understand the role of these trace elements—which we can now measure in fractions of a millionth of a gram—we must picture each cell in our bodies as a complex factory where thousands of chemical reactions go on at the same time to make us the living, breathing, growing, regenerating organisms that we are. In an ordinary factory, such chemical reactions could take place only with highly concentrated compounds at high temperatures. In the cells, they occur at body temperature, in watery fluids, with enzymes acting as catalysts. These enzymes, composed of complex protein molecules, have the amazing capacity of bringing specific molecules into the right position to react at the appropriate moment. Some of the enzymes contain vitamins as part of their own molecules, and many do not function except in the presence of the right trace mineral. Without such activators (and each enzyme requires a particular activator), no reaction takes place.[3]

Another fact that has come about through research is that the margin between what is beneficial and what is harmful is small. In most cases we are not sure where that line lies. For this reason most of our study of trace elements has been with animals.

Five of the elements found to be necessary to life were discovered through the painstaking efforts of Klaus Schwartz and his associates at the National Institutes of Health and now at the Veterans Administration Hospital in Long Beach, California. For over fifteen years, Schwartz's group has studied the effects and requirements of trace elements in rats and other small animals.

For his animals Schwartz constructed cages that are made entirely out of plastics in order to eliminate the contaminating effects of metal, glass, or rubber. Each isolator system housed thirty-two animals in individual cages. A highly efficient filter system sterilized the air of all trace elements that might be present. The diets were chemically pure amino acid instead of natural protein, and all other food was screened for metal contaminants. In this sterile environment the animals were raised from birth.[4]

With all these precautionary procedures, Dr. Schwartz was able to produce new trace element deficiencies in the animals and discover their various effects and cures. Because of the work of Schwartz and other equally devoted men and women, we can now discuss trace elements with a certain amount of understanding.

Iron is an essential part of the compounds necessary for transporting oxygen to the cells and putting the oxygen to work upon arrival. Because of its performance with the enzymes in the blood, iron is spread throughout the body, mostly in the blood, of course, with relatively large amounts in the liver, spleen, and bone marrow.   ***Iron***

Iron deficiency is a common scapegoat for many human ills. However, the only way a significant amount of iron can leave the body is through a loss of blood. Those who suffer periodic blood losses or those who are forming new blood have a greater need for dietary iron. Women most often fall into this category because of childbirth and monthly menstruation. Pregnant women often need an iron supplement to meet the increased demands of pregnancy. Older infants and children of preschool age are also particularly vulnerable to iron deficiency because they are suddenly weaned from the iron-fortified formulas of infancy to whole milk. Many parents are not as conscious of providing iron-fortified cereals and other iron-rich foods. Men seldom suffer from iron loss unless they bleed frequently because of an ailment such as a peptic ulcer. For adult males and for women past menopause, iron supplementation is generally unnecessary and potentially harmful.

Of all the minerals, iron is the most likely to be deficient in the diet because very few foods are really excellent sources. Eggs, liver, whole grains, dried fruits, and legumes (beans) are the best sources. Some foods, such as breads, rice, pastas, and breakfast cereals, are fortified with iron during processing. However, iron tends to alter food taste, and thus iron fortification in significant amounts is often commercially undesirable. One should select foods carefully to ensure an adequate amount of iron in one's diet.

Copper works hand in hand with iron. It is involved with the storage and release from storage of iron to form hemoglobin for red blood cells.   ***Copper***

The human body contains 100 mg of copper, an integral component of at least twelve enzymes.[5] The daily requirement for it is only 2 to 3 mg, though up to 25 mg/day may be consumed without hazardous effects. This level is unlikely to be reached, however, even using all possible avenues of exposure. Therefore, a buildup by way of consumption is very unlikely. Wilson's Disease, caused by excessive copper stores in the body, arises from faulty metabolism of the metal and not an increased intake.

Pure copper deficiency (hypocupremia) in humans was unknown until 1972, when Dr. Rashid Al-Rasald and John Spangler reported a case of a small, premature, but rapidly growing three-month-old infant with anemia and a central nervous system disorder. The baby, who showed laboratory and clinical signs of severe hypocupremia, responded to copper sulfate therapy.[6]

Copper occurs in most unprocessed foods. Organ meats, shellfish, nuts, and dried legumes are examples. Milk is a very poor source of copper. Although babies are generally born with a sufficient supply of this metal, they should not stay on milk alone for too long, even with vitamins. It is thought that if infants are fed only milk for the first seven to eight months of life, a copper deficiency may occur.[7]

Science has recently unveiled some interesting facts about copper. For instance, with age the copper level in the brain increases, while that in the liver, aorta, lungs, and spleen normally decreases with maturity.

Ofttimes, a copper deficiency is caused by disease rather than being the cause of disease. For example, multiple sclerosis frequently decreases the level of ceruloplasmin-bound copper in the body. Sheep and cattle with sway-back also show a marked deficiency in copper, but again copper is not the causative factor.

Future copper research may bring to light copper's connection with many diseases and its preventive and curative aspects.

Manganese

Manganese is needed for normal tendon and bone structure and is part of some enzymes, especially those involved in urea formation and pyruvate metabolism. Some blood proteins also contain manganese, which aids in the prevention of experimental atherosclerosis (produced in laboratory experiments with animals).[8]

Generous supplies of manganese are found in peas, beans, nuts, fruits, and whole grains, such as bran. In animals, manganese deficiency has led to fetal abnormalities; however, human deficiency is rare.

Manganese, as found in the emission of automotive fuels, may be the cause of neurologic symptoms similar to those of Parkinson's Disease. Chilean manganese workers frequently develop "Manganic Madness." It is characterized by "an abnormal gait, headaches, tremors, speech disturbances and an impulsive behavior; like Parkinsonism the disorder responds to L-Dopa."[9] It has been estimated that ten to twenty years' exposure is necessary before these symptoms occur.

Iodine

Until 1924, when iodized salt was introduced, many people suffered from **goiters** (enlargements of the thyroid glands). Today iodine is not mandatory, but under FDA regulation, noniodized salt must be labeled with the statement "This salt does not supply iodine, a necessary nutrient."

Iodine is required in extremely small amounts but is essential to the proper functioning of the thyroid gland, which controls the breathing rate of tissues. Without it, the tissues, and eventually the mind, slow down.

Seafoods provide the best supply of iodine, but for those without access to such, iodized salt will provide the necessary requirements for good health.

Zinc

Until recently, it was thought that zinc deficiency did not exist in the United States. However, recent studies show that people with a loss of a sense of taste, dwarfism, and delayed wound healing may be suffering from such a deficiency.[10]

Zinc is necessary for growth, **collagen** synthesis, wound healing, sexual maturation, protein digestion, **RNA** metabolism, and twenty enzymes. The blood, bones, kidneys, liver and voluntary muscles have the highest concentrations of zinc; analysis of hair indicates that the content increases during childhood and then progressively declines.[11]

Zinc is an important part of the enzymes that move carbon dioxide, via red blood cells, from the tissues to the lungs, where it can be exhaled.

Dr. Philip Walravens, of the University of Colorado, has found indications that zinc depletion is common in infants and young children. He cited a study in which 10 of 132 children, aged four to six years, showed definite deficiencies in the metal.[12] It is believed that in some isolated areas in Egypt, zinc deficiency is responsible for dwarfism in boys. After increased doses of zinc, the boys began to grow faster and mature sexually more rapidly.[13]

Maternal zinc deficiency in humans may be partially responsible for the number of spontaneous abortions and congenital malformations in countries with diets low in zinc.[14]

Zinc may be a means of medical therapy. Dr. George Brewer, of the University of Michigan Medical School, reports that it may be useful in treating sickle cell patients because an estimated one-fifth to one-third of patients with **sickle cell disease** have low zinc levels.[15]

Other studies show that high zinc supplements may depress platelet activity in animals and humans; hence, it might be useful in transplants and skin grafting in humans.[16]

Most recently zinc has been identified as an antibacterial factor in prostatic fluid, suggesting that the metal may act as a defense mechanism against chronic bacterial prostatitis and subsequent urinary tract infections. Further research is needed to determine the exact role of zinc in the immunity system.[17]

Zinc deficiency is also associated with impaired taste acuity and poor appetite, and has been implicated as contributing to the infant syndrome failure-to-thrive.

The FDA now recommends 15 mg/day of zinc. Zinc is usually associated with the protein foods, and good sources of this trace element are found in many common foods—fish, beef, chicken, whole grains, vegetables and oysters.

Cobalt

By itself, cobalt is not essential to the body, but it is a part of vitamin B_{12}, which is an essential nutrient. It is found therefore only in meat and meat products.

The bones and liver have the highest content of this element, which is present in metalloenzymes involved in the biosynthesis of DNA and amino acid metabolism. Cobalt is present in humans in very small amounts, only 10 mg. Excesses are excreted, so it is not highly toxic; however, large doses may cause diarrhea, vomiting, and nerve deafness.

Cobalt can be toxic when combined with excessive drinking and malnutrition. In Quebec in 1965-66, twenty men died because of so-called "inorganic cobalt toxicity." David Clegg tells the story:

> An inorganic cobalt compound was used in beer as a foam stablizer. The additive was authorized on the assumption that beer intake would not exceed

six bottles a day per man. However, in the Quebec outbreak, intake of beer frequently exceeded twenty bottles a day per man. Even at this level, the amount of cobalt permitted in the beer did not prove toxic to individuals on a nutritionally adequate diet.[18]

Chromium

Chromium works in some way with insulin. It is required for normal carbohydrate metabolism, growth, and lifespan. It is believed that a chromium deficiency is common in the United States. Processing and refining of such foods as flour and sugar remove much of the chromium from these products. Good sources of chromium are liver, beef, bread, mushrooms, and brewer's yeast. Green, leafy vegetables are the richest in chromium content, while dairy products, refined cereals, and sugars are the poorest.

Much has yet to be learned about chromium, but recent studies on this trace element and its work with glucose intolerance have been encouraging. Chromium in its simple form is poorly absorbed, but a natural complex element of it, called glucose tolerance factor (GTF) and found in brewer's yeast, seems to be very effective in small amounts.[19] Dr. Richard J. Doisy of State University in New York in Syracuse, has found that "brewer's yeast alleviates glucose intolerance in elderly people and lowers insulin requirements in some insulin-dependent diabetics."[20] Dr. Doisy, however, cannot prove his theory with brewer's yeast until he can discover a way to isolate the pure GTF. Dr. Doisy reports that "The only patients studied to date who have abnormal chromium absorption are insulin-dependent diabetics; we speculate that these patients are chromium deficient."[21]

Adequate chromium appears to prevent the serum cholesterol elevation that may occur with increasing age. In this connection it is interesting to note that chromium is one of the few minerals that have the highest concentration at birth and decrease continuously with increasing age.

Selenium

Dr. Klaus Schwartz and Dr. C. M. Foltz have discovered that selenium is essential to humans.[22] Though we know relatively little about this trace mineral, we do know that it is closely related to vitamin E, and without a daily intake of 0.1 meg, complications such as kidney damage, pancreatic **atrophy**, and liver **necrosis** may occur.

Selenium and other **antioxidants** like vitamin E have been implicated as cancer preventive agents. Cancer tends to be relatively low in areas of adequately seleniferous soil. The antioxidants may work either by protecting chromosomes from breakage or by decreasing damage to DNA, but this remains to be conclusively proven.

The human body contains up to 100 mg of selenium. But because it is excreted in the urine, the turnover of selenium is rapid. The amount available to us depends upon that available to the growing plants and animals we digest.

Too much selenium may prove harmful. Selenium is more lethal, in high doses, than is arsenic. In the Great Plains area, thousands of cattle died from eating plants containing excesses of selenium.[23]

There is no evidence at this time to suggest that the food supply in the United States contains either too little or too much selenium. There is reason, however, to suspect that indiscriminate selenium supplementation of the diet is potentially hazardous. A well-balanced diet is the best way to obtain selenium. Organ meats, muscle meats, and seafoods are the best sources of selenium. Grains and grain products also can contribute significant quantities of selenium, although the selenium content of these foods will depend heavily on where the grains were grown.

Fluorine runs a close second to iron as a subject of great controversy in the field of nutrition. Is it really beneficial to man? And, if so, how much and to what extent? *Fluorine*

Fluorine has been proven to be very useful when used in moderate amounts. It contributes to solid tooth formation and results in a decrease in dental cavities. In nearly all communities where fluorine is present in the water supply, dental cavities in children have been reduced by 50 percent or more.[24] Fluorine also aids in the retaining of calcium in the bones of older people. This element, like iodine, is found in small amounts in water, soil, plants, and animals.

Nickel, one of the newer elements, is found in the human body at a level of about 10 mg/person. It is found in small amounts in all food. Nickel is ingested and excreted at a similar rate, so no buildup occurs. *Nickel*

It has not yet been determined what significance it holds for the human body, if any, but nickel does seem to play a role in controlling prolactin and thus may affect lactation.

Good sources of nickel include grains, legumes, most vegetables, and cocoa.

One of the most poisonous elements, arsenic is also present in the human body. In fact, tests show that it exists at an amount of 20 mg/person, and daily intake is about 2 mg/person. However, it is not stored in the body, so no danger need be feared. *Arsenic*

Cadmium is considered the most "social" of metals because we come into contact with it through cosmetics, cigarettes, galvanized pipes, and foods grown with synthetic fertilizers. Individuals store about 30 mg; this amount increases with age. As of now we know of no metabolic function for this metal, and because of its firm retention in the body, it has been considered dangerous. *Cadmium*

Unlike cadmium, tin has a very low absorption rate, and it is remarkably nontoxic. Recent tests on animals indicate that tin may have some useful effects on humans. Rat studies show tin may be important for body growth and tooth development. In any case, the foods we eat amply cover any need for this element. *Tin*

Mercury is widespread in the human body. Although small amounts of metallic or inorganic mercury are safe, some organic compounds of this trace element put into the environment by industries have proven to be dangerous and insidious poisons. *Mercury*

In two separate incidents in Japan, rivers were contaminated heavily by factories with mercury. When fish and shellfish containing methylmercury were consumed by the population of fishing villages immediately downstream from the points of contamination, the result was widespread disease, many deaths, and many permanently disabled victims, including some who were congenitally poisoned. The symptoms, essentially irreversible, were paresthesia (abnormal sensations such as prickling that have no objective cause), progressive weakening of muscles, loss of coordination, constricted vision or blindness, deafness, and permanent mental retardation.

Lead

Unlike most of the trace elements, lead is well researched. We know that it is present in the human body in an amount of 100 mg/person. This is mostly deposited in the bones and is not considered harmful. However, lead is not essential and can be very harmful in excessive amounts. Toxic quantities comes from sources other than food, such as atmospheric dusts caused by cars which use leaded gasoline, paints, pica (nonfood objects eaten by children), and earthenware pottery. The amount of lead in food alone does not present any known hazard.

Vanadium

Vanadium is essential in the diet. It was found that rats on a diet that totally excluded vanadium suffered a retardation in growth of 30 percent. On the other hand, excessive doses of this element block the synthesis of cholesterol and reduce the amount of **phospholipid** and cholesterol in the blood.[25] Vanadium has also been shown to promote growth and teeth mineralization (excess minerals incorporated into the teeth). It may be found in bread, grains, and root vegetables.

Although the minerals have been treated separately for clarity, the various minerals are actually interdependent, and the extent of their relationships is still being investigated. For instance, we have known for fifty years that copper must be present for the proper metabolism of iron. Recently it was discovered that ceruloplasmin, a copper-containing protein of the blood, acts as the vital link between these two elements.[26] Copper absorption, on the other hand, can be greatly reduced by the presence of too much zinc or molybdenum. Thus many of the elements must work together for proper body functioning.

SUMMARY

While vitamins usually take center stage in any discussion of dietary supplements, minerals are also essential for good health and for growth. Just the right amount of minerals in our diets is necessary. Tamper with the supply, and we find ourselves with various types of deficiency diseases.

Macrominerals are those elements that are present in relatively large amounts in the body, and they are needed by the body in relatively large amounts as well. The macrominerals are calcium, phosphorous, sodium, chlorine, potassium, magnesium, and sulfur. A balanced and healthy diet will provide all the macrominerals necessary for proper body functioning. The macrominerals are important for well-developed bones and teeth, fluid balance and volume, digestive processes, energy conversion, and protein maintenance.

Researchers such as Klaus Schwartz have done much to add to our understanding of the presence and use of trace minerals in the body. However, there is still so much to learn. Meanwhile it is best to eat a well-balanced diet of a wide variety of foods, being certain to include unrefined foods such as vegetables, fruits, and whole grains, for no single food can act as a substitute for essential nutrients. Supplementation of the diet with any trace mineral should be discouraged unless under the directions of a physician. The margin between toxic and healthy levels is very small for many of the trace minerals.

Unlike the effects of bulk nutrients, the effects of excessive intake of trace elements are not immediately recognized. Even without producing obvious symptoms of toxicity, an increased intake of one element can adversely influence the availability of others, resulting in subtle imbalances.

NOTES

1. Select Committee on Nutrition and Human Needs, U.S. Senate, *Dietary Goals for the United States* (Washington: U.S. Government Printing Office, 1977), pp. 48–51.
2. Earl Frieden, "The Chemical Elements of Life," *Scientific American* Vol. 227, July 1972, pp. 52–60.
3. Jean Mayer, "Trace Minerals: Fact or Fad," *Family Health,* March 1971, pp. 54–55.
4. Morris Fishbein, M.D., "Trace Elements in Human Nutrition," Editorial, *Medical World News.*
5. "Essential Trace Elements," *MD Medical News Magazine,* Vol. 16, No. 11, November 1972, pp. 79–81.
6. Ibid.
7. Mayer, "Trace Minerals: Fact or Fad?" pp. 54–55.
8. "Essential Trace Elements," pp. 79–81.
9. Ibid.
10. Edward G. Damon, "A Primer on Dietary Minerals," *FDA Consumer,* September 1974, pp. 4–7.
11. "Essential Trace Elements," pp. 79–81.
12. "Trace Elements and Human Disease: Tracking an Insidious Flaw in Nutrition," *Modern Medicine,* September 16, 1974, p. 24.
13. "Essential Trace Elements," pp. 79–81.
14. Julie M. Jones, "Trace Elements in Human Nutrition: The Contribution of Cereals," *Cereal Foods World,* pp. 574–8.
15. "Trace Elements and Human Disease," p. 24.
16. Ibid.
17. "A Link Between Zinc and Immunity?" *Medical World News* February 7, 1977, pp. 57, 60.
18. David J. Clegg and Emil Sandi, "Trace Elements in Food," *The Canadian Nurse,* February 1973, pp. 38–42.
19. "Essential Elements," pp. 79–81.
20. "Trace Elements and Human Disease," p. 24.
21. Ibid.
22. "Essential Trace Elements," pp. 79–81.
23. Ibid.
24. Damon, "A Primer on Dietary Minerals," pp. 4–7.
25. Frieden, "The Chemical Elements of Life," pp. 52–60.
26. Ibid.

5

Digestion, Absorption, and Metabolism

Nutrients found in food provide energy sources, building materials, and regulatory substances that are essential to the life of every body cell. However, only a few substances contained in foods are suitable for body-cell use in their original form. **Digestion** is the process that prepares nutrients for absorption and use by the body tissues. Complex molecules are subdivided into simple, soluble nutrient materials which can pass through the digestive tract lining into the lymph and blood streams. Body metabolism then provides the energy to transform the nutrients into cell material.

The adult digestive tract is a hollow tube about 30 feet in length. It is in the lumen, or inner open space, that food is digested. (See Figure 5-1.) Of the six nutrient classes, water, vitamin and mineral elements, and a few simple sugars can be absorbed directly from food. Other food elements are modified in various ways as they pass through the gastrointestinal tract between the mouth and the small intestine until the nutrients are small enough to be absorbed across the tract walls.

Combining food with oxygen, the process that occurs when we burn food in our bodies, releases heat. This process is called metabolism. What would happen if all of our food was burned as soon as we ate it? It would release a blast of heat that would make us warm and comfortable for a while, and that would probably keep us alive for an hour or so. But we would need a constant source of food, and so we'd spend our lives eating. Such a system would be wasteful and inefficient.[1]

Instead, we have a system that will supply a steady source of energy. Our bodies store food in simple forms and capture the energy from food that has been burned, hoarding it in small reserves. When food is unavailable, our bodies extract those reserves of stored food and use them to keep us warm and to help us function.[2] Different kinds of food provide different kinds of energy, and the way our bodies process the food depends on the type of food.

Cooking enhances the flavor and digestibility of many foods, and the aroma of an appetizing, well-prepared meal will stimulate digestive secretions long before the food is eaten. But no matter how it looks, tastes, or smells, food is nothing more than a creative combination of three kinds of nutrients: carbohydrates, fats (triglycerides), and proteins, with a sprinkling of vitamins and minerals to add variety. Only a few foods consist of only one nutrient—egg white is pure protein, salad oil is pure fat, and sugar is pure carbohydrate. Most foods combine all three nutrients.

The breakdown of nutrients actually begins long before the food is ingested. Food processing and cooking softens cellulose and begins the breakdown of complex compounds, such as the starch and protein content of food.

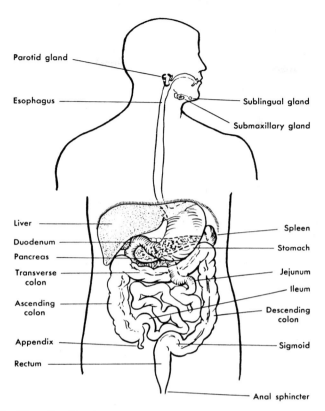

Parotid gland

Esophagus

Sublingual gland

Submaxillary gland

Liver

Duodenum

Pancreas

Transverse
colon

Ascending
colon

Appendix

Rectum

Spleen

Stomach

Jejunum

Ileum

Descending
colon

Sigmoid

Anal sphincter

Figure 5-1. The Digestive Tract

Fats and carbohydrates burn well. A calorie is the amount of heat needed to raise the temperature of a kilogram (2.2 pounds) of water one degree centigrade—one and a half calories would make a tablespoon of ice water boil. Fats yield nine calories per gram—over twice as many as carbohydrates.[3] Proteins provide four calories per gram. Part of the protein is nitrogen, which is excreted in the urine instead of being burned for energy by the body.

After food is digested, both mechanical and chemical processes break it down into absorbable forms.

DIGESTION

Enzymes are necessary in the chemical phase of digestion for the breakdown of: complex carbohydrates to simple sugars, fats **(lipids)** to **glycerol** and fatty acids, and proteins to amino acids. Enzymes are catalysts, or substances which can become involved in chemical reactions without undergoing changes themselves. They are secreted and mixed with food in the mouth, stomach, and small intestine as digestion progresses.

Large amounts of various juices are needed to digest food. However, in the absence of food, the enzymes in the juices may start to eat away at the digestive tract itself. To prevent enzyme activity in the absence of food, digestive secretions are coordinated with food ingestion by the nervous and **endocrine** systems.

In the Mouth   Food enters the digestive tract through the mouth, where it is ground by the teeth and mixed with saliva for moistening and lubrication. Saliva is secreted in response to nerve stimulation by food or other mechanical stimulators. (This explains why hikers often carry small stones in their mouths to stimulate saliva secretion when thirst is severe.) An acid, like vinegar, will chemically stimulate saliva secretion; even anticipation of food can stimulate the salivary glands.

An enzyme in saliva, called salivary amylase, begins to decompose the starches into simple sugars. Because the food stays in the mouth for such a short period of time, such enzyme action is the only "digestion" that takes place there.

Swallowing chewed food begins with a raise of the tongue that catapults the chewed food against the back of the throat. Muscles along the digestive tract walls take up the process next. The walls are made up of both circular muscular fibers, which squeeze and mix the food, and longitudinal fibers, which contract to push the food mass on through the system. These two muscle movements coordinate in a wavelike motion called **peristalsis.** The waves move food into the stomach. A muscle at the lower end of the esophagus keeps food from traveling back up the throat unless extra force is applied, as in vomiting.

Nervousness, anxiety, or fatigue can interfere with stomach movements and produce gastrointestinal disturbance. Strong emotions, such as fear or anger, can retard peristaltic movements or speed them up so that digestion is not properly completed.

In the Stomach   Food enters the upper portion of the stomach where the action of salivary amylase (ptyalin) continues until the stomach pH becomes too acidic. The stomach is an adjustable organ which can handle up to a liter of food comfortably. It dilutes, churns, partially digests and stores food until it is ready to feed into the intestine.

Most digestion takes place in the lower stomach, where gastric juices containing important enzymes are mixed with the food by the churning action of the stomach walls. Gastric proteases are enzymes that begin to split proteins into small amino acid chains called peptides. Lipases, or fat-digesting enzymes, are secreted but remain inactive at normal stomach acidity levels. The stomach lining cells also pour out hydrochloric acid, which stimulates the activity of the proteases. It also prevents carbohydrate digestion by inhibiting the action of the carbohydrate-splitting amylase swallowed along with the food. Hydrochloric acid is important for maintaining optimum stomach acidity and preventing bacteria from entering into the lower digestive tract.

Depending on diet and body composition, an ordinary meal remains in the stomach 3 to 4¼ hours. Gradually, the partially digested and highly liquefied food, now called chyme, is moved out of the stomach into the small intestine. Carbohydrate foods leave the stomach first, followed by proteins and then fats. This is why hunger sensations return more rapidly following meals high in carbohydrates but inadequate in protein and fats.

The stomach releases its contents intermittently at a rate that the small intestine can handle. If a meal is too concentrated, the stomach retains it until it is sufficiently diluted with gastric secretion. Meals with high content of glucose or fat are released slowly to prevent incomplete absorption. Indigestion (dyspepsia) and other common gastric complaints can often be traced to a stomach derangement: the musculature is not properly adjusting to the volume of food, or the stomach is discharging its contents too rapidly or too slowly into the **duodenum.**

Most digestion takes place in the small intestine, an organ measuring about twenty feet long. As the chyme passes into the duodenum (the first part of the small intestine), the intestinal juices, the pancreatic juices, and the bile from the liver combine to begin digestion. Complex carbohydrates are already partially digested by the process that began in the mouth with the salvia. The intestinal enzymes continue the process until all carbohydrates have been broken down into glucose, fructose, and galactose; the smallest possible sugars. See Figure 5-2 showing starch and disaccharide digestion.

In the Small Intestine

Protein digestion in the small intestine requires only one step: enzymes from the pancreas combine with enzymes in the small intestine to break proteins into their component amino acids; there is a mixture of twenty amino acids in most foods. Proteins broken down into the amino acids are then ready to be absorbed by the cells lining the walls of the small intestine. Figure 5-3 shows protein digestion.

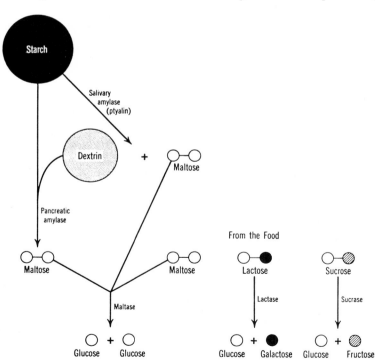

Figure 5-2. Starch and Disaccharide Digestion. From Eva D. Wilson et al., *Principles of Nutrition* (New York: Wiley, 1965).

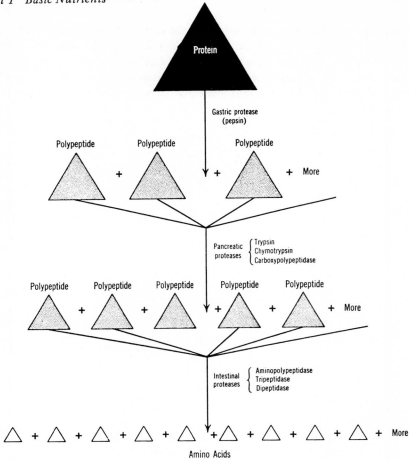

Figure 5-3.   Protein Digestion. From Wilson et al., *Principles of Nutrition.*

Fat digestion is the slowest of all digestive processes because of fat's complicated composition. It also slows down the flow of food from the stomach to the small intestine; the more fat eaten with a meal, the slower the stomach empties. As fat enters the small intestine it triggers the release of pancreatic enzymes that break down fat molecules into three fatty acids and glycerol. These fatty acids are not water-**soluble,** so they are unable to penetrate the layer of water on the surface of the jejunum (which is part of the small intestine) and reach the membrane of the absorptive cell. Bile, acting on the fat cells like a detergent combines with the fatty acids to form a soluble bubble that passes easily through the intestinal cell membrane. Once inside the cell, glycerol and fatty acids are reformed and combined with protein and cholesterol. The substances eventually enter the bloodstream via the fluid-filled vessels of the lymphatic system, and are carried throughout the body. Figure 5-4 sketches fat digestion.

Six hormones have been identified in the regulation of digestive-juice secretion in both the stomach and intestine. The hormones, produced in the gastrointestinal tract mucosae, are not directly secreted into the lumen of the digestive tract as the digestive enzymes are. Instead, they enter the bloodstream and are carried to their target organs. For example, hydrochloric acid from the stomach stimulates intestinal secretion of the hormone secretin, which enters the bloodstream and is carried to the pancreas. In response, the pancreas secretes its digestive juices into the intestine.

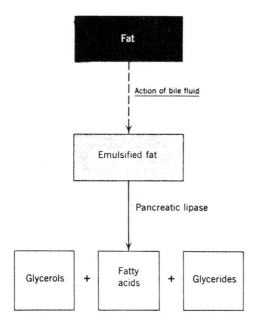

Figure 5-4.   Fat Digestion. From Wilson et al., *Principles of Nutrition.*

ABSORPTION OF NUTRIENTS

Although the gastric mucosae absorb small amounts of water, alcohol, simple salts, and glucose, most nutrient absorption takes place in the small intestine, particularly in the lower part of the duodenum and the first part of the jejunum. Nutrients are transferred from the lumen of the small intestine through the intestinal epithelium, where water-soluble nutrients enter the bloodstream and fat-soluble nutrients enter the lymph vessels for transportation to the body cells. Absorbable nutrients include amino acids, fatty acids, glycerol, simple sugars, minerals, and vitamins.

The surface of the small intestine is covered with finger-like projections called microvilli that secrete enzymes and absorb nutrients. Absorption is not automatic; the concentration of nutrients is higher inside intestinal cells than it is outside, and the cells must work in order to accomplish absorption. Each tiny villus—no more than 1/25 of an inch long—contains a blood vessel that carries away glucose and amino acids. These nutrients, once in the bloodstream, travel to every cell in the body. Vitamins are similarly absorbed into the bloodstream. The folding and pocketing of villi provides as much as 300 square yards of absorbable surface area. (See Figure 5-5.) Plenty of fluid is required for the process of absorption. About eight liters of fluid from the body daily pass back and forth across the intestinal membrane to keep the nutrients in solution. Diarrhea and other conditions causing dehydration may produce poor absorption.

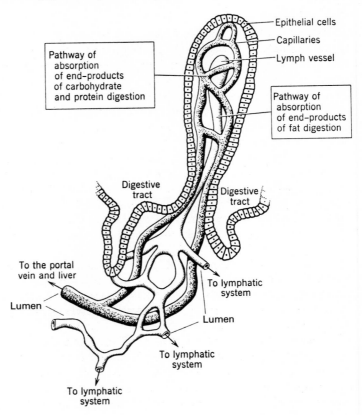

Figure 5-5. A Villus. From Wilson et al., *Principles of Nutrition.*

EXCRETION

The liquefied material that has resisted digestion passes into the large intestine or colon, where it is converted to more solid material and eventually excreted as the feces. No digestive enzymes are produced in this part of the tract, but there is some absorption of additional water and dissolved salts (minerals) into the bloodstream.

About 2/3 of the feces consists of water. The remaining mass consists of the nondigestible cellulose content of food residues from the digestive juices, cellular debris, and numerous bacteria. Usually the intestinal bacteria are harmless or even useful in producing substances such as vitamin K within the body. Few minerals or vitamins are excreted from the body, for they occur sparingly in foods and in a healthy individual digestion and absorption of energy nutrients is practically 100 percent efficient.

METABOLISM

By now the food is mostly digested—but it hasn't yet begun working for the body. The process that facilitates the working mechanism begins at this point. For about an hour and a half after glucose is absorbed from the small intestine, its level in the bloodstream increases steadily until it has risen from 30 to 40 percent. This in turn triggers cells in the pancreas to manufacture insulin and send it to the blood. Insulin remains in the bloodstream only until it reaches the liver, which it directs to store most of the glucose; muscles use the remaining glucose, either immediately or as storage. Glucose levels in the blood then begin to drop.

Although the muscles and the liver depend on insulin to digest carbohydrates and use the chemicals, the brain is able to absorb glucose independently—an important fact when the brain is forced to compete with other tissues for limited supplies of fuel. The amount of glucose in the brain never rises—no matter how much is in the bloodstream or how hard the brain works—but it can fall; anything greater than a 10-percent drop in the glucose level in the brain can be harmful or fatal.[4]

Amino acids also depend on insulin to find their way out of the blood and into the tissue; insulin gives them the push they need to penetrate cell walls.

The brain and certain nerves end up with about 70 percent of the carbohydrates consumed during the day; of the rest, 25 percent goes to muscle tissue, 2 percent to fat cells, and 3 percent to other tissues.

Getting fat into the cells is more complicated. The fat cells are still hooked up to the proteins they acquired in the small intestine (that enabled them to be absorbed into the small intestine). The globules of fat and protein circulate until they meet an enzyme whose sole function is to remove fat from circulation. Mimicking the earlier process of digestion, the enzyme breaks the fat back into the original three fatty acids and glycerol. These are returned to the liver.

DISPOSAL OF METABOLIC WASTES

The constant round of anabolic (building up) and catabolic (breaking down or disintegrating) metabolism produces chemical energy which can be converted to mechanical energy for work performed by the body muscles. All chemical energy produced in the body is eventually converted to heat energy, which maintains body temperature. Excess heat energy is given off by way of the skin, lungs, and excretions.

Carbon dioxide formed in the oxidative cycle is transported by the bloodstream to the lungs, where it is exhaled. Nitrogen from deaminated amino acids is synthesized into urea in the liver and is excreted by the kidney in urine, along with water formed in cellular metabolism. In an adult, up to 200 quarts of water may be removed daily from the blood by the kidneys. About 99 percent is reabsorbed into the blood by action of the antidiuretic hormone and only about 1 to 2 quarts eventually leaves the body in the urine.[5]

A minimum of 1½ to 2 cups of water is required daily to eliminate wastes; if it is unavailable for urine formation, metabolic wastes may accumulate and reach toxic levels. **Dehydration** may occur if too much of the water that normally would be reabsorbed by the blood is excreted. Water and some nutrients are also lost through the skin and lungs.

RESERVE ENERGY

If we eat too much—more energy than we need to consume to survive from meal to meal—we become fat, because the body stores all of the excess. If we eat too little, we dip into our fat and protein stores; the metabolism goes to work to keep the body alive for as long as possible. If we should be deprived of food for too long, we would deplete stored energy; the muscles, particularly the heart, would deteriorate, and other cells would lose their function, including brain cells. Long before they are harmed too much, though, cells curtail protein release—no one is sure how. The body begins to conserve its water, and less protein is lost through urea. Because of this process, we could live a week or two without food and water; if we did not have protein retention, we would die of dehydration within a few days. As less protein is burned, the body relies more and more on stored fat; a lean man who did not exercise could live off his body's stored fat for 60 to 70 days, and severely overweight people can fast for up to six months. The liver converts the fatty acids into ketone bodies, water-soluble substances that are used by the brain. In this way the brain receives vital substances without having to wait for the liver to manufacture glucose.

Approximately 40 to 50 percent of what we eat ends up as fat; this is simply because fat is the best way to store excess fuel, since it provides the greatest amount of heat when it is burned. The average 150-pound man has 20 to 30 pounds of fat on his body and some 13 pounds of stored protein—if he stored the energy contained in his fat as glycogen in muscle and liver cells, he would weigh over 300 pounds.[6]

How does the body retrieve the reserve energy? For up to eight hours after a meal, the liver converts stored glycogen into glucose and releases it into the blood; this glucose goes directly to the brain (since there is little insulin in the blood to direct the glucose to other body tissues). The liver's supply lasts only a few hours. If the body is deprived of food for longer periods, it draws on stored protein and eventually on stored fat.

Let's look at that process a little more closely. When the body needs to begin using the stored protein, muscle cells break down their protein into amino acids, which travel to the liver. Separating the nitrogen from the amino acids, the liver transforms these acids into glucose—used almost exclusively by the brain.

If food still doesn't arrive, the body turns to stored fat. Triglycerides that were converted by insulin return to simpler forms: the glycerol is converted to glucose in the liver, and the fatty acids circulate to all tissues in the body, where they become the body's major source of energy. Red and white blood cells also produce usable byproducts that are converted into glucose by the liver.

However, under normal circumstances we will have eaten another meal before the body is forced to rely on stored fat for fuel.

SUMMARY

The marvelous process of food ingestion, digestion, absorption, and metabolism is necessary for growth, maintenance, and repair of the body tissues as well as for the process of providing chemical energy to the body. Metabolism must be continual, or death will result. Table 5-1 summarizes the sequence of these actions, probably some of the most fascinating in the human body.

Table 5-1. Function of Chemical Secretions in Digestion

Organ of digestion	Secretion	Enzymes	Digestive function	Description of function
Mouth (salivary glands)	Saliva			Lubricating action of saliva aids in the swallowing of the food as it passes from the mouth to the stomach by way of the esophagus.
		Salivary amylase (ptyalin)	Carbohydrate digestion	Hydrolyzes starch to dextrin by splitting off molecules of maltose from the long carbohydrate chain.
Esophagus	None			Passageway to stomach. (Little digestion takes place here.)
Stomach (Gastric mucosa)	Gastric juice	Gastric proteases: Pepsin	Protein digestion	Mixed with food in lower part of stomach.
				(Present in inactive form—pepsinogen—to prevent digestion of stomach wall when stomach is empty.) Splits protein into smaller units of polypeptides which contain linked amino acids in groups of from three up to as many as several hundred.
		Rennin	Milk clotting	Believed to be present only in infant gastric secretion and only functional in early life period.
		Gastric lipase	Fat digestion	Inactive at normal acidity of gastric content. May digest highly homogenized foods such as milk and egg yolk.
	Hydrochloric acid (non-enzyme)		pH regulation	Creates optimum acidity in stomach for protein digestion.
			Protein digestion	Converts the inactive form of protein-splitting pepsinogen to the active enzyme pepsin.
			Carbohydrate digestion	Hydrolyzes some disaccharides.
			Mineral digestion	Increases solubility of calcium and iron, resulting in optimum absorption of these essential nutrients in the small intestine.
			Bacteriocide	Prevents entrance of bacteria into the lower digestive tract.
	Mucin		pH regulation	Protects stomach from hydrochloric acid by neutralizing strongly acid contents and forming protective covering on gastric epithelium.

Organ of digestion	Secretion	Enzymes	Digestive function	Description of function
Small Intestine	Pancreatic Fluid	Proteases: Trypsin Chymotrypsin Carboxypoly-peptidase	Protein digestion	Secreted into small intestine from pancreas. (Trypsin secreted in inactive form—trypsogen—to prevent digestion of intestine wall in the absence of food.) Further subdivide polypeptide chains into polypeptides of smaller units.
		Pancreatic amylase	Carbohydrate digestion	Converts remaining starch or dextrin to disaccharide maltose. Converts disaccharides (carbohydrate forms found in original food or end products of amylase action) to simple sugars for body absorption.
		Pancreatic lipase	Fat digestion	Hydrolyzes small fat globules into glycerol, fatty acid, and di- or monoglycerides.
	Bicarbonate (non-enzyme)		pH regulation	Neutralizes hydrochloric acid entering the intestine, creating a nonacidic environment ideal for catalyzing enzymes important in the remainder of the digestive process.
	Intestinal juices	Carbohydratase	Carbohydrate digestion	Split disaccharides to monosaccharides.
		Intestinal Disaccharides: Sucrase Maltase Lactase Lipases	Carbohydrate digestion / Fat digestion	Splits sucrose to glucose and fructose Splits maltose into two glucose units Splits lactose into glucose and galactose Removes fatty acids from fat molecules
		Aminopoly-peptidase Tripeptidase Dipeptidase	Protein digestion	Complete the digestion of proteins by liberating amino acids from peptides formed earlier in the stomach.
	Bile (liver secretion) Does not contain digestive enzymes		pH regulation Fat digestion	Neutralizes acidity of chyme. Bile salts emulsify fats into small globules of easily hydrolyzed pancreatic and intestinal lipases. Accelerates action of pancreatic lipase. Facilitates absorption of fat and fat-soluble vitamins.
Large intestine	None			Absorbs water and compacts non-digested material for excretion.

NOTES

1. Jerrold Olefsky, "What Happens to Your Lunch," *Human Nature,* April 1978, p. 38. Copyright © 1978 by Human Nature Inc. Used by permission of the publisher.
2. Ibid.
3. Ibid., p. 40.
4. Ibid., p. 43.
5. Thora J. Runyan, *Nutrition for Today* (New York: Harper and Row, 1976), p. 202.
6. Olefsky, "What Happens to Your Lunch," p. 46.

6

Getting Good Nutrition

Great-grandmother just wouldn't believe the things happening to food today. Frozen TV dinners, quickie hamburgers from the corner burger joint, "instant" cake, pudding and pie mixes, drive-in restaurants, fabricated foods—all this is a far cry from the three to five hours a day she spent preparing hearty breakfasts, lunches, and dinners for her brood.

Cooking and meal practices have changed drastically in recent years. Breakfast for many has become an almost nonexistent meal or, at best, a hurried, nonfamily affair. Lunch consists of a hamburger and shake from the local fast-food restaurant. Snack and convenience foods are increasing in popularity. Americans are less physically active and consume more calories from fat. Fat consumption has increased from 32 to 42 percent of our caloric intake; carbohydrates have decreased from 56 to 46 percent (protein has remained at a regular 12 percent).[1] Food companies spend over a billion dollars in national advertising each year, and their biggest campaigns are for the least nutritious foods. Children are a prime target for Saturday-morning television, where advertising is three times as dense as during adult programs. Candy, soft drinks, and sugar-covered cereals are popular items.

Despite the continual changes in food products, one factor remains constant—food is the only source of nutrition we have, regardless of how, when, and where it is prepared. The food industry introduces over 500 new food products each year. Nothing is wrong with this type of food supply—except for the flood of nutritional misinformation that accompanies it. We can't always dictate how food reaches us, but we can be nutritionally knowledgeable. We can learn to meet our nutritional needs in the reality of today's eating patterns.

A GOOD DIET

You'd have to spend years in intensive study to even begin to learn all we know about nutrition, but you don't need to know everything to be able to plan a well-balanced diet that will keep you healthy. Good nutrition sense can be developed through the study of a sound nutrition book, and your family doctor can help you understand possible deficiencies.

In planning a nutritious daily diet, you may wish to consult the Basic Four Food Groups chart (Table 6-1). Following this chart will usually assure that one receives the RDA for the various nutrients.

Table 6-1.

Guide to Good Eating...

A Recommended Daily Pattern

The recommended daily pattern provides the foundation for a nutritious, healthful diet.

The recommended servings from the Four Food Groups for adults supply about 1200 Calories. The chart below gives recommendations for the number and size of servings for several categories of people.

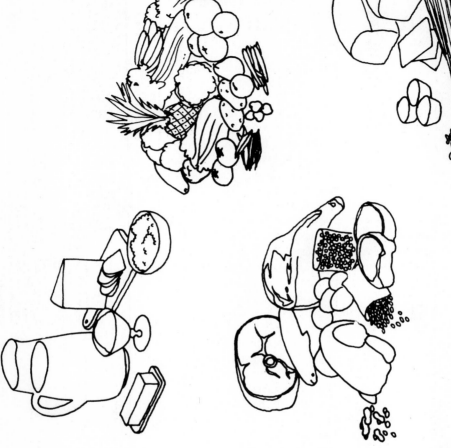

Food Group	Recommended Number of Servings				
	Child	Teenager	Adult	Pregnant Woman	Lactating Woman
Milk 1 cup milk, yogurt, OR **Calcium Equivalent:** 1½ slices (1½ oz) cheddar cheese* 1 cup pudding 1¾ cups ice cream 2 cups cottage cheese*	3	4	2	4	4
Meat 2 ounces cooked, lean meat, fish, poultry, OR **Protein Equivalent:** 2 eggs 2 slices (2 oz) cheddar cheese* ½ cup cottage cheese* 1 cup dried beans, peas 4 tbsp peanut butter	2	2	2	3	2
Fruit-Vegetable ½ cup cooked or juice 1 cup raw Portion commonly served such as a medium-size apple or banana	4	4	4	4	4
Grain, whole grain, fortified, enriched 1 slice bread 1 cup ready-to-eat cereal ½ cup cooked cereal, pasta, grits	4	4	4	4	4

*Count cheese as serving of milk OR meat, not both simultaneously.

"Others" complement but do not replace foods from the Four Food Groups. Amounts should be determined by individual caloric needs.

Courtesy of National Dairy Council.

Nutrients for Health

Nutrients are chemical substances obtained from foods during digestion. They are needed to build and maintain body cells, regulate body processes, and supply energy.

About 50 nutrients, including water, are needed daily for optimum health. If one obtains the proper amount of the 10 "leader" nutrients in the daily diet, the other 40 or so nutrients will likely be consumed in amounts sufficient to meet body needs.

One's diet should include a variety of foods because no *single* food supplies all the 50 nutrients, and because many nutrients work together.

When a nutrient is added or a nutritional claim is made, nutrition labeling regulations require listing the 10 leader nutrients on food packages. These nutrients appear in the chart below with food sources and some major physiological functions.

Nutrient	Important Sources of Nutrient	Some major physiological functions		
		Provide energy	Build and maintain body cells	Regulate body processes
Protein	Meat, Poultry, Fish / Dried Beans and Peas / Egg / Cheese / Milk	Supplies 4 Calories per gram.	Constitutes part of the structure of every cell, such as muscle, blood, and bone; supports growth and maintains healthy body cells.	Constitutes part of enzymes, some hormones and body fluids, and antibodies that increase resistance to infection.
Carbohydrate	Cereal / Potatoes / Dried Beans / Corn / Bread / Sugar	Supplies 4 Calories per gram. Major source of energy for central nervous system.	Supplies energy so protein can be used for growth and maintenance of body cells.	Unrefined products supply fiber—complex carbohydrates in fruits, vegetables, and whole grains—for regular elimination. Assists in fat utilization.
Fat	Shortening, Oil / Butter, Margarine / Salad Dressing / Sausages	Supplies 9 Calories per gram.	Constitutes part of the structure of every cell. Supplies essential fatty acids.	Provides and carries fat-soluble vitamins (A, D, E, and K).
Vitamin A (Retinol)	Liver / Carrots / Sweet Potatoes / Greens / Butter, Margarine		Assists formation and maintenance of skin and mucous membranes that line body cavities and tracts, such as nasal passages and intestinal tract, thus increasing resistance to infection.	Functions in visual processes and forms visual purple, thus promoting healthy eye tissues and eye adaptation in dim light.
Vitamin C (Ascorbic Acid)	Broccoli / Orange / Grapefruit / Papaya / Mango / Strawberries		Forms cementing substances, such as collagen, that hold body cells together, thus strengthening blood vessels, hastening healing of wounds and bones, and increasing resistance to infection.	Aids utilization of iron.
Thiamin (B$_1$)	Lean Pork / Nuts / Fortified Cereal Products	Aids in utilization of energy.		Functions as part of a coenzyme to promote the utilization of carbohydrate. Promotes normal appetite. Contributes to normal functioning of nervous system.
Riboflavin (B$_2$)	Liver / Milk / Yogurt / Cottage Cheese	Aids in utilization of energy.		Functions as part of a coenzyme in the production of energy within body cells. Promotes healthy skin, eyes, and clear vision.
Niacin	Liver / Meat, Poultry, Fish / Peanuts / Fortified Cereal Products	Aids in utilization of energy.		Functions as part of a coenzyme in fat synthesis, tissue respiration, and utilization of carbohydrate. Promotes healthy skin, nerves, and digestive tract. Aids digestion and fosters normal appetite.
Calcium	Milk, Yogurt / Cheese / Sardines and Salmon with Bones / Collard, Kale, Mustard, and Turnip Greens		Combines with other minerals within a protein framework to give structure and strength to bones and teeth.	Assists in blood clotting. Functions in normal muscle contraction and relaxation, and normal nerve transmission.
Iron	Enriched Farina / Prune Juice / Liver / Dried Beans and Peas / Red Meat	Aids in utilization of energy.	Combines with protein to form hemoglobin, the red substance in blood that carries oxygen to and carbon dioxide from the cells. Prevents nutritional anemia and its accompanying fatigue. Increases resistance to infection.	Functions as part of enzymes involved in tissue respiration.

There is no one diet that is ideal for everyone. However, observing a few basic principles when you select foods will ensure you a healthy diet.

1. Eat varied and balanced meals. For healthy functioning, your body needs many different nutrients—proteins, carbohydrates, fats, vitamins, and minerals. Not all foods contain all nutrients, so to receive adequate amounts of each, you should select a variety of foods from the four food groups: dairy products, meats and fish, cereals and grains, and fruits and vegetables.
2. Do not overeat. Depending on your size, rate of metabolism, and level of activity, your body requires a certain amount of calories per day to maintain your weight. Any extra calories you eat will be converted to fat and stored.
3. Eat less fat, salt, and sugar. Select fewer fatty meats and more fish and poultry. Also try to consume more polyunsaturated fats (vegetable oils) than saturated fats (meats, butter).

   Attempt to cut down on salt by taking the saltshaker off the table or by adding half the amount called for in recipes. If you usually cook with salt pork or fatback, cut the amount in half. Many commercially prepared foods contain a lot of salt.

   Nutritionists speak of sugar as "empty" calories—calories with no protein, fat, vitamins, or minerals. Additionally, sugar in sticky products may promote tooth decay. To reduce the amount of sugar you eat, cut down your consumption of cookies, cakes, candies, and sodas.
4. Eat more fruits, vegetables, and whole grains. Fruits and vegetables are good sources of vitamins and minerals. Whole grains supply not only carbohydrates, but also protein, vitamins, and minerals. They also have a high fiber content that may be beneficial in reducing your risk of intestinal disease.[2]

Additional guidelines for a healthy diet were provided by the report of the 1977 Select Committee on Nutrition and Human Needs of the U.S. Senate.[3] The committee stated: "In the view of doctors and nutritionists consulted by the Select Committee . . . changes in the diet amount to a wave of malnutrition—of both over- and underconsumption—that may be as profoundly damaging to the Nation's health as the widespread contagious diseases of the early part of the century." As a result of their investigation, the committee recommended the following dietary goals:

1. Increase carbohydrate consumption to account for 55 to 60 percent of the energy (caloric) intake.
2. Reduce overall fat consumption from approximately 40 to 30 percent of energy intake.
3. Reduce saturated fat consumption to account for about 10 percent of total energy intake; and balance that with polyunsaturated and monounsaturated fats, which should account for about 20 percent of energy intake each.
4. Reduce cholesterol consumption to about 300 mg a day.
5. Reduce sugar consumption by about 40 percent to account for about 15 percent of total energy intake.

6. Reduce salt consumption by about 50 to 85 percent to approximately 3 g a day.

Breakfast ends a night-long fast and is an important meal. Studies show that individuals who eat breakfast do considerably more work in the late morning hours than those who eat only a midmorning snack or omit breakfast completely.

A "good" breakfast depends on an individual's protein and calorie needs. Usually a meal which supplies about 25 percent of the daily nutrient requirement is recommended. Food served for breakfast should be evaluated in relationship to the other two daily meals in order to determine whether it is adequate in nutrition.

Instant breakfast drinks have become quite popular, due to their ease in preparation. These provide 25 to 33 percent of the daily nutrient needs except calories. When combined with eight fluid ounces of whole milk, a typical instant breakfast provides 300 calories and 17 to 18 g of protein. Vitamin and mineral contents vary.

If the other two daily meals contain a mixed variety of food to supply other major and trace nutrients, good instant breakfasts may be an effective, quick way to get nutrition. However, they are a poor way of developing good nutritional habits, particularly for children.[4]

Importance of Breakfast

In-between-meal snacks have always seemed to be unpopular with parents everywhere. However, regardless of the time of day food is eaten, it maintains its nutrient value and contributes to the daily total. Between-meal snacks can help provide a good nutrient balance, especially for children and teenagers. However, snacks are undesirable when they add only to caloric intake without providing comparable nutritional value. Some good snack suggestions (low in calories but high in nutrition) include:

Nutritional Snacks

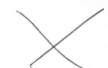

1. Sandwiches (peanut butter especially is high in polyunsaturated fats and protein).
2. Fresh Fruit—Apples, pears, apricots, peaches, cherry tomatoes, oranges.
3. Raw, Crisp Vegetables—Carrots, celery, cucumbers, radishes, lettuce.
4. Nuts—Dry-roasted peanuts, cashews, walnuts (high in protein and iron).
5. Popcorn—Made without butter, popcorn has only about 40 calories per cup. It can be popped in a small amount of vegetable oil.
6. Drinks—Orange juice, milk, ice water.
7. Soup.

Try to make sure snacks help meet the body's need for protein, vitamins, and minerals. Avoid foods high in carbohydrates, fats, and salt, such as pastries, sweet rolls, candy bars, soft drinks, potato chips.

Americans spend $50 million annually eating out, and much of this money is spent eating out at fast food restaurants. In fact, almost one-third of the typical American's cash is spent in fast foods. A recent Gallup Poll indicated that 33 percent of adults eat out every day, and 28 percent of these individuals eat at fast food restaurants. Further, 68 million Americans eat out two to three times a month.[5]

Fast Foods

Most of the appeal of the fast food restaurants is convenience; patronization of these establishments means no shopping, no food preparation, no clean-up, a minimum of decision-making connected with selection of food, and fast service. Others are drawn to fast food establishments because the food is generally consistent. For example, a hamburger bought at a McDonald's is basically the same everywhere—the consumer knows what to expect. Although eating at a fast food restaurant is not always as inexpensive as preparing food at home, it is generally cheaper than eating at any other type of restaurant. And finally, in many American families, both the mother and father work, which means that there is less time for cooking at home and more money to spend on eating out.[6]

There are some drawbacks to the fast food industry. Fast foods are high in carbohydrates and fats, which can be associated with high rates of heart disease, high blood pressure, and diabetes. Further, high consumption of carbohydrates and fats is now being linked to breast cancer, stomach cancer, and colon cancer. In addition, foods high in fat content can cause weight gain, because fat furnishes more calories per gram than either proteins or carbohydrates.

Further, health experts think that there may be additional dangers associated with the fats used in preparation of foods such as fish and french fries, for harmful substances can be produced when fat is heated and reused.

Fast foods are high in refined sugar. There is sugar in the sauces, ketchup, mustard, buns and rolls, ice cream, etc.[7] These refined sugars can be detrimental in that they may contribute to heart disease, diabetes, hyperactivity, cancer, obesity, and dental caries.

In addition, fast foods contain very little fiber—even in their bread products. Lack of fiber in the diet has been linked to gastrointestinal problems—especially colorectal cancers.

Finally, fast foods are low in essential vitamins and minerals and high in salt. Salt causes certain health problems and aggravates others.

Tables 6-2, 6-3, 6-4, and 6-5 show how specific foods served by fast food establishments stack up in the area of nutrition and nutrients.

Table 6-2. What's in a McDonald's Menu?

ITEM	Calories	Protein (gm)	Carbohydrates (gm)	Fat (gm)
Hamburger**	249	13	28	10
Cheeseburger	309	16	30	14
1/4 lb. Hamburger	414	27	33	19
1/4 lb. Cheeseburger	521	31	36	28
Big Mac**	557	26	41	32
Fillet of Fish	406	15	37	22
French Fries	215	3	28	10
Apple Pie	265	2	30	15
Chocolate Shake	317	11	52	7
Vanilla Shake	322	11	55	7
Strawberry Shake	315	10	50	8

Table 6-2. (Cont.)

ITEM	Protein	Vit. A	Vit C	Thiam.	Ribof.	Nia.	Cal.	Iron
				% of USRDA for Adults and Children over 4 years				
Hamburger	20	3	7	12	21	20	5	14
Cheeseburger	24	6	7	13	30	22	14	13
1/4 lb. Hamburger	41	5	5	15	37	36	7	21
1/4 lb. Cheeseburger	48	8	9	17	42	40	23	22
Big Mac	40	4	8	18	38	35	16	21
Fillet of Fish	23	*	3	15	21	16	9	9
French Fries	5	*	15	7	2	13	*	2
Apple Pie	3	*	3	*	2	2	*	3
Chocolate Shake	17	*	*	5	33	2	40	5
Vanilla Shake	17	*	*	5	31	2	35	*
Strawberry Shake	15	*	*	5	31	3	36	*

*Supplies less than 2% of the USRDA for these nutrients. ** Note that the bigger the burger, the bigger your intake of undesirable fats. Half of the big Mac's calories are derived from saturated fat.*

Table 6-3. Nutrients Deficient in McDonald's Meals (less than 1/3 RDA per meal)

RDA*	1/4 lb. Hamburger French Fries Chocolate Shake	Big Mac French Fries Chocolate Shake	Cheeseburger French Fries Chocolate Shake	Hamburger French Fries Chocolate Shake
	Percentage of Recommended Dietary Allowance in McDonald's Meals Males 14 to 18 years of age			
Vitamin A 5000 units	5.2	4.2	6.3	3.3
Vitamin B-6 2 mg	28.4	25.5	20.6	20.2
Vitamin D 400 units	20.2	17.2	15.2	13.2
Vitamin C 60 mg	20.0	22.6	21.3	21.0
Vitamin E 30 units	1.3	4.6	0.7	1.03
Folic Acid 0.4 mg	12.2	13.4	11.5	10.7
Thiamin 1.5 mg	27.6	30.3	25.6	24.3
Iron 18.0 mg	28.1	28.0	19.8	20.8
Magnesium 400 mg	21.9	22.6	18.9	18.5

Established by the U.S. Department of Health, Education and Welfare, Food & Drug Administration.
Source of Data: "Nutritional Analysis of Food Served at McDonald's Restaurants," WARF Institute, Inc.

Chart A	**McDonald's**	**Homemade**
Standard Hamburger on Roll	30 cents	20 cents
1/4 lb. Hamburger on Roll	70 cents	35 cents
Cheeseburger	37 cents	24 cents
1/4 lb. Cheeseburger on Roll	80 cents	39 cents
French Fries	25 cents	7 cents
Milk	20 cents	10 cents

(1978 prices)

Tables 6-2 through 6-5 from "The Fast Food Fantasy," *Consumers Digest*, May-June 1979, pp. 16–18.

Table 6–4. Protein and Calories at Fast Food Chains

RESTAURANTS (In alphabetical order)	MENU ITEMS (Main dish, side dish and beverage)	PROTEIN* (in grams)	CALORIES**
A&W	Super Papa Burger	19	448
	Small fries	3	249
	Root Beer Float	3	200
	TOTAL	25	897
BURGER CHEF	Super Chef	23	423
	Small fries	4	285
	Large Chocolate Shake	9	361
	TOTAL	36	1069
BURGER KING	Whopper	29	563
	Small fries	2	218
	Large Chocolate Shake	7	407
	TOTAL	38	1188
DAIRY QUEEN	Super Brazier	43	732
	Small fries	3	239
	Large Chocolate Shake	10	376
	TOTAL	56	1347
HARDEE'S	Deluxe Huskee	32	635
	Small fries	4	283
	Large Chocolate Shake	10	328
	TOTAL	46	1246
JACK-IN-THE-BOX	Jumbo Jack	28	558
	Small fries	2	226
	Large Chocolate Shake	13	540
	TOTAL	43	1324

(All data compiled by Jacobs-Winston Laboratories Inc., New York, N.Y.)

	*PROTEIN NEEDS		**CALORIC NEEDS	
	Female	Male	Female	Male
Adult Over 18	46	56	2000	2700
15 to 18 years	48	54	2100	3000
11 to 14 years	44	44	2400	2800
7 to 10 years	36	36	2400	2400

Table 6–5. A Pizza Lunch

Based on serving size, 1/2 10'' - pizza - 3 slices - two servings per 10'' pizza

	Beef	Pork	Cheese	Pepperoni	Supreme
Calories	490	470	440	460	480
Protein	31 gm	29 gm	26 gm	25 gm	29 gm
Carbohydrate	55 gm	55 gm	53 gm	54 gm	54 gm
Fat	16 gm	15 gm	13 gm	16 gm	16 gm
Percentage of U.S. Recommended Daily Allowances					
Protein	50	60	45	45	45
Vitamin A	15	15	10	10	10
Vitamin C (Ascorbic Acid)	Contains less than 2% of the USRDA of these nutrients				
Thaimine (Vitamin B$_1$)	30	25	20	30	25
Riboflavin (Vitamin B$_2$)	35	35	30	30	40
Niacin	30	40	20	30	40
Calcium	40	40	60	40	40
Iron	Contains less than 2% of the USRDA of these nutrients				

* As served by Pizza Hut.

GETTING HIGH-QUALITY FOOD

Although we can assume that fresh foods initially contain more nutrients than preserved foods, the nutrient value is probably about the same by the time fresh or prepared food reaches the table for consumption.

> Because of the large losses that occur in the home, the actual vitamin content of table-ready foods is frequently about the same regardless of the type of processing—or lack of processing the food has undergone. For example, a bowl of peas placed steaming on the table will contain 35–45% of its original "raw" vitamin C content regardless of whether it was prepared from fresh peas (45%), frozen peas (40%), or canned or freeze-dried peas (both 35%).[8]

Fresh produce which is shipped by train or truck several thousand miles to market loses nutrients during the days spent in transit. In any case, such produce is quite expensive if purchased out of season. Fresh vegetables from your own garden vary genetically in nutrient content and lose nutrients if they are stored for lengths of time. The most important factor is how food is handled during preparation rather than whether it is bought fresh, canned, or frozen.

People in ideal climates where fresh meat and produce are available year round might get along without using any preservative processes, but the general populace would face famine without stores of preserved foods. The availability of food is more important than the nutrient losses that take place during processing.

There are positive sides to food processing, too.

> Heat processing destroys the antidigestive factors in cereal grains, peas, and beans, thus making both the protein and carbohydrates in these products more utilizable by man. Heat processing also destroys the enzymes which bring about the destruction of vitamin B_1 in fish and fish products and the factors that would otherwise tie up the vitamins and iron in egg white.[9]

Food processing can also improve texture, flavor, and appearance of food. It also helps retain nutrients and encourages better diet.

Because of advanced technological processes, commercial food preparation tends to preserve nutrients slightly better than home processing does. Commercial processors also use special packaging to further conserve vitamin content. The difference is not great enough, however, to discourage sound home food preservation practices, especially when cost is considered.

Nature cultists claim that cooking food (and pasteurizing milk) destroys nutrients and makes the food impure. In reality, not all foods are more nutritious raw than cooked. Secondly, cooking is important to protect against bacteria and parasites as well as to add taste and tenderness to foods. The human gastrointestinal tract, unlike that of animals, does not retain microorganisms to break down the cellulose walls of many raw foods. Soft fruits and vegetables are easily digested, but harder, cellulose-rich vegetables (spinach, carrots, cauliflower, etc.) are more easily digested when cooked. Grains and meats also are cooked to soften the fiber, develop flavor, and promote digestibility.

*Raw versus
Cooked Foods*

Avoiding Nutrient Loss

Food is bound to lose nutrients during preparation. Here are some suggestions which will help you keep nutrient loss to a minimum.

Washing.   Wash all raw food thoroughly. Washing does not cause nutrient loss. The main danger in eating raw foods, especially organic foods, is from bacterial or parasitic contamination.

Trimming.   Keep trimming to a minimum. Trimming somewhat diminishes nutritive values of both fresh and processed food. There is more vitamin C in the peel (which is often discarded) and just under the skin of apples, tomatoes, and citrus fruit than on the inside. The tip end of asparagus has more vitamin C than the butt, and the outer green leaves of cabbage, lettuce, and similar vegetables contain carotene while the inner leaves have little. You lose small amounts of niacin from carrots and riboflavin from potatoes when you peel them.

Slicing and Dicing.   Whole fruits and vegetables are usually more nutritious than bits and pieces of such foods, since some vitamins may escape when food is exposed to air. Slice food immediately before serving, and store it afterwards in airtight containers.

Cooking.   Most nutrient loss occurs during the final cooking preparation in the home. Water-soluble vitamins (vitamin B_1, riboflavin, and niacin) are particularly vulnerable to leaching. Losses of the fat-soluble vitamins and vitamin C generally occur during heating and storage in the presence of air. However, vitamins are neither created nor destroyed—most of them merely pass out of the food into the cooking water and are still in the pan or can until you drain the liquid into the sink. Cook vegetables with small amounts of water and little exposure to air. Use leftover liquids for gravies, sauces, vegetable cocktail, or soup. Different cooking methods cause various degrees of nutrient loss. Baking potatoes whole, for instance, retains a good proportion of vitamin C. But the vitamin C in potatoes does not survive mashing or frying of thin slivers as in french fries or potato chips. The baking of bread or cooking of rice does not affect nutrient content. If the way you prepare food seems to eliminate taste, you may be destroying some valuable chemicals.

Use fresh products as quickly as possible. Rotate canned storage items regularly. Store frozen foods at a temperature as close to $0°$ F. as possible. Thawing of frozen vegetables can cause nutrient loss—put frozen vegetables into a heated pot directly from the freezer and eat defrosted items immediately after thawing.

The Best Way to Buy Meat

Meats (especially organ meats) are excellent sources of iron, protein, and B vitamins. All the meats you buy should be government inspected, and you should keep them refrigerated. Jean Snyder offers the following tips for consumers who want not only to buy the best available meat for their families, but also to help make sure that their governmental agencies are doing all they can to protect consumers:

1.   Buy only federally inspected and graded meat. You can tell it by the purple "roll stamp" that appears on all large pieces. Usually the grocer

will aid you by adding his own label reading "USDA Prime," "USDA Choice," or some other indication that the meat comes from federally approved plants. You are better off with USDA-inspected meat in spite of the system's failings.

2. Never buy meat that is distinctly "two-toned." The darker portion is likely to be old or spoiled.
3. Never buy meat in packages that are torn or broken.
4. If you want the best possible ground beef, grind it yourself or have it ground to order by your butcher.
5. If you see anything wrong with the meat, let your butcher know about it. If you don't see the cut you want with a federal stamp, ask for it. Let your butcher know that it makes a difference to you.[10]

GOOD NUTRITION NO CUREALL

Although a good diet permits us to avoid deficiency diseases like rickets or scurvy and to forestall some of the great killers of our time, such as heart disease, even the best nutrition will not keep us young forever, help us shed weight without effort, or eliminate all fatigue, headaches, and minor miseries of life. Nor can diet prevent such diseases as arthritis, multiple sclerosis, or muscular dystrophy.

Surprisingly, an estimated 10,000,000 Americans believe that certain foods work wonder cures. Some of the favored foods, such as whole grains, wheat germ, and blackstrap molasses, provide high-quality nutrition. They do not, however, have special health-giving powers. For example, blackstrap molasses cannot cure illness and has no special uses as a food. It is a concentrated sugar food with a high content of iron and calcium (much more than honey). But, in normal usage in small amounts, it does not make an important contribution to the diet.

DIETS FOR SPECIAL NEEDS

There are certain times during the life cycle when there are special nutritional needs. Usually these times occur when there are special demands on the body, and generally these needs take the form of a requirement for more calories or a special type of food. Once the demand has been eliminated, one can resume previous eating habits. Pregnant and breastfeeding women often require special foods and an increase in calorie intake. The elderly have a special need for high-quality foods rather than a high quantity of food.

Pregnancy

Sound nutrition is especially important before and during pregnancy. Studies show that birth defects can be initiated by deficiencies of protein, vitamin C, thiamine (vitamin B), pantothenic acid, folic acid, vitamin B_{12}, and various minerals.[11] A large proportion of the estimated miscarriages, cases of mental retardation, and physical deformities occurring in the United States could be prevented if optimal nutrition were ensured in expectant mothers.

Women should be on a good diet at all times, for the first few weeks of fetal development occur even before a woman knows she is pregnant and the mother's nutritional status during this time is crucial. The infant's baby teeth, for example, are formed in the first few weeks of the embryo's life, and permanent teeth begin formation five months before the child is born. The mother, if malnourished, must sacrifice her own skeleton to build up her child's teeth. X-ray studies of the jaws of newborn infants show that tooth development is much better if the mother has been on a nutritionally sound diet, rich in calcium (milk and cheese), phosphorus (dairy and animal products, fruits, vegetables) and fluoride (in water supply or by dentist's prescription) during pregnancy.

A woman's metabolism changes during pregnancy. She may need an average of an extra 200 calories a day to satisfy requirements for vitamin A, thiamine, ribo-flavin, niacin, and iron. Proper maternal nutrition may mean a lifetime of health for the expected baby.

Weight Gain. Infant mortality and **morbidity** are much greater in low-birth-weight infants; and the more weight the mother gains during pregnancy, the bigger the infant tends to be at birth.

The realization of these facts has led several nutrition groups to recommend that a woman gain 20 to 25 pounds during a normal pregnancy.[12] Pregnancy is not time for a crash diet, even if the mother is overweight. Overweight women also need to gain 20 to 25 pounds during pregnancy.

During the first trimester there is little or no need for additional calories in the diet. Normal gain during the first thirteen weeks is from 2 to 4 pounds. During the second and third trimester, however, there is an average gain of .9 pound each week, and the recommended dietary allowances for this period suggest a 400-calorie-per-day increase to meet this need. The second trimester gain is chiefly the "temporary" gain of maternal tissues; the infant does most of its gaining during the third trimester.[13]

General Nutritional Guidelines. The following suggestions provide a general overview for good nutrition during pregnancy:

1. Increase the intake of milk, cheese, fruit, fruit juices, yellow and green vegetables, whole-wheat bread, whole-grain cereals, fish, and lean meat.
2. Decrease the intake of sugar, candy, pastries, cakes, and large amounts of unnecessary fats.
3. Drink plenty of fluids, especially milk and water (preferably fluoridated).
4. Eat plenty of high-fiber foods—vegetables, fruits, cereals.
5. Salt intake need not be restricted unless by a physician's advice. However, avoid excess amounts of salt or highly salted foods like anchovies, potato chips, and salted nuts.
6. Do not take vitamin or mineral supplements unless prescribed by a physician. Excess amounts of vitamins can cause unpredictable side effects. Most physicians will prescribe a vitamin supplement with iron.
7. Exercise regularly.
8. Do not smoke, use alcohol, or take drugs unless prescribed by a physician who knows you are pregnant.

Cravings and Nutrition. The world-famous cravings of pregnant women need not be nutritionally harmful. No one knows exactly why women experience such strange hunger pains for various substances from strawberries and pickles to clay. While it's true that a woman's metabolism changes during pregnancy, most doctors agree that cravings for specific foods are largely psychological in nature.

Cravings are not harmful unless their indulgence causes other problems. Eating too much ice cream, which is high in calories, for example, may lead to improper weight gain. Pickles, peanuts, and pretzels contain large quantities of salt which may contribute to toxemia (problems in metabolism during pregnancy which cause circulating toxins; underlying cause is unknown). Of course, if a woman eats laundry soap or clay, she runs the risk of anemia or blockage and possible rupture of intestines.[14]

After delivery, the nutritional needs of the infant are still very important. Where possible, breastfeeding with human milk seems to be superior to other methods of feeding for a number of reasons. Breast milk contains more whey proteins (which provide essential amino acids) than cow's milk, is free from bacteria, and is easier to digest because of the close biochemical relationship of human milk proteins to serum proteins.

Breastfeeding and Nutrition

Milk formulas are adequate, but cow's milk may cause allergies (eczema, ulcerative colitis) in the newborn. Also, cow's milk contains 40 percent less iron and vitamins A and D than human milk. This means that anemia or vitamin A and D deficiencies may develop sooner in infants receiving cow's milk than in breastfed babies. Vitamin C is adequate in human milk but is insufficient in cow's milk. Also, heating of cow's milk reduces the vitamin C content by about 50 percent. Thus after the second postnatal week, formula infants should receive additional vitamin C.

Breastfeeding is also favored because of the protective substances in human milk:

> Clinicians see the breast as a second placenta, performing a function—the transfer of immune "killer cells" to the fetus—that the placenta may have found too dangerous to complete in utero. A mother's protective antibodies can cross the placenta to the fetus, usually in five times the concentrations existing elsewhere in her body. These protective antibodies persist in the infant for four or five months after birth, on the alert for infection.
> There's about a two-week delay between the time an invader enters the infant and the time his own killer cells go into action. If the baby is being breastfed, the mother's lymphocytes can come to his rescue.[15]

Breastfed infants are less susceptible to respiratory and gastrointestinal infections than formula babies. Premature babies have a lower mortality rate and are less susceptible to infection with breastfeeding.[16]

For breastfeeding to be successful, the mother must be in good health, maintain an adequate diet during both pregnancy and lactation, and not take drugs potentially dangerous to the baby. The mother should not have a history of breast cancer. Most important, she must want to nurse the baby.

So breastfeeding, with vitamin supplementation, should be encouraged because of its many nutritional and immunologic advantages. Modern knowledge of the psychophysiology of breastfeeding points to the overwhelming advantage of human milk. But if for some reason parents opt for the bottle, they should be cautioned against overfeeding the baby or propping bottles. Bottle propping may result in overfeeding, because a child may take in more milk than he or she would if held by the mother. It may also lead to dental problems, because the child may fall asleep with the bottle in his or her mouth, leaving a coating of lactose (milk sugar) on the teeth. Also, parents should not introduce solid foods until the infant is at least three months old. The combination of formula and/or milk solid foods may lead to obesity.[17]

Old Age   Although old age can not be avoided through nutritional means, some diseases associated with aging may be caused by nutritional deficiencies. Nutritional requirements do not decrease with advancing age, although the quantity of food needed may do so. However, nutrition often declines among the elderly, for a variety of reasons.

Some of the causes of nutritional problems are as follows:

1. Limited income.
2. Loneliness, apathy, depression, or bereavement lessens the appetite.
3. Reduced activity.
4. Elderly persons living in urban areas are particularly prone to social isolation, which leads to mental and physical deterioration.
5. Food fads and fallacies or chronic alcoholism paves the way for poor nutrition.
6. Chronic invalidism.
7. Poor dental health.
8. Mental disturbances.[18]

Diseases that accompany old age are called degenerative because they occur as a result of breakdown in body tissues. As people age, they become less active and their desire to eat also decreases, but their need for vital nutrients does not decline. As nutrition declines, tissue inevitably breaks down.

Protein requirements of the aging are as great as those of younger groups. Although osteoporosis (which may result from a calcium deficiency or old age) cannot be reversed by high dosages of calcium, the calcium need in old age does not decrease. Iron is also still required in normal amounts — iron deficiency anemia is all too common among the aged.[19]

Vitamin deficiency is also prevalent among this age group. It is believed that a partial deficiency in the B vitamins is often responsible for the mental confusion experienced by old people.[20]

There are certain things that can be done to improve the nutritional well-being of older people. For example, they should be encouraged to follow balanced diets that have a slightly reduced number of calories and are relatively low in salts and saturated fats, high in fiber, and rich in iron, vitamin B_{12}, and calcium. Exercise is ever important, as it cuts down the risks of obesity and elevated blood pressure.

Even though animal studies cannot always be applied to humans, it is interesting to know that the longevity of rats can be extended with dietary manipulation. Life expectancy of laboratory animals has been lengthened by chronic, severe underfeeding. In fact, the *higher* the intake of food regardless of composition, the *shorter* the lifespan.[21] Perhaps future research will allow us to identify the mechanisms involved and in some way apply them to humans.

SUMMARY

Good nutritional practices are not difficult to maintain if one follows certain practices, such as eating balanced meals; not overeating; eating small amounts of fat, salt, and sugar; and eating a lot of fruits, vegetables, and grains.

Breakfast is one of the most important, yet most neglected, meals of the day. It has been shown that people who eat breakfast perform more work later on in the morning than those who do not eat breakfast. Instant breakfasts have become popular of late, and although they may supply adequate nutritional needs (provided the other meals of the day are balanced), they do not teach good nutritional habits.

Snacking has become a way of life in America. It has boosted the market of "junk foods" substantially. However, there are nutritionally sound foods that can be eaten for snacks, such as fruit, vegetables, nuts, and sandwiches.

Adequate and balanced nutrition is especially important during pregnancy and lactation. Sound nutrition during pregnancy and lactation protects both the mother and her developing baby. It is also particularly important that the elderly be properly nourished. And yet it is during old age that an individual is most likely to be poorly nourished, for income is limited, loneliness prevents proper nutrition, there is a reduction in activity, physical and mental infirmity hamper food preparation, and apathy and depression impair the appetite.

NOTES

1. Alan T. Spiher, "Food Shoppers' Beliefs: Myths and Realities," *FDA Consumer,* October 1974, pp. 13-15.
2. "What Is a Good Diet," *Patient Care,* February 28, 1978, p. 127. Copyright © 1978, Patient Care Publications, Inc., Darien, Ct. All rights reserved.
3. Select Committee on Nutrition and Human Needs, U.S. Senate, *Dietary Goals for the United States* (Washington, D.C.: U.S. Government Printing Office, 1977).
4. "Instant Breakfasts—Nutritious Junk Food," *Consumer Reports,* June 1977, pp. 324-327.
5. "Fast Food Chains," *Consumer Reports*, September 1979, p. 508; "The Fast Food Fantasy," *Consumers Digest,* May/June 1979, p. 14.
6. "Fast Food Chains," pp. 508-513.
7. "The Fast Food Fantasy," pp. 14-19.
8. "The Effects of Food Processing on Nutritional Values. A Scientific Status Summary by the Institute of Food Technologists' Expert Panel on Food Safety and Nutrition and the Committee on Public Information." *Nutrition Reviews,* Vol. 33, No. 4, April 1975, pp. 123-126.

9. Ibid.

10. Jean Snyder, "About the Meat You Are Buying," *Today's Health,* December 1971, pp. 38–39, 67-69.

11. Jean Mayer, "When You're Eating for Two," *Family Health,* October 1976, pp. 31, 46.

12. Myron Winick, "The Pregnant Patient: How Much Weight Should She Gain?" *Modern Medicine,* October 15, 1977, pp. 108-111.

13. Elizabeth Holey, "Promoting Adequate Weight Gain in Pregnant Women," *The American Journal of Maternal Child Nursing,* March/April 1977, pp. 152-157.

14. Susan Lyons Middaugh, "The Food, (and Other) Cravings of Pregnant Women," *Science Digest,* January 1975, pp. 29-31.

15. "New Evidence Favors Breast-Feeding," *Medical World News,* June 16, 1975, pp. 26-28.

16. Derrick Jelliffe and Patrice Jelliffe, "Breast Feeding Is Best for Infants Everywhere," *Nutrition Today,* May/June 1978, pp. 12-16.

17. Myron Winick, "When the Patient Asks About Breast Versus Bottle Feeding," pp. 83, 87, 90.

18. Dodda B. Rao, "Problems of Nutrition in the Aged," *Journal of the American Geriatrics Society,* Vol. XXI, No. 8, August 1973, pp. 362-367.

19. Jean Mayer, "Aging and Nutrition," *Geriatrics,* May 1974, pp. 57-59.

20. Ibid.

21. Select Committee, *Dietary Goals for the United States.*

UNIT 2

CONTEMPORARY ISSUES IN NUTRITION

7

The Sensible Side of Cereals, Breads, and Flour

Although we know that one cannot live by bread alone, bread is still the staff of life, and as such it has attracted much attention through the ages. During certain periods of history, white bread held great prestige; its consumption was largely by those of the upper class. To continually serve white bread meant wealth and position. Later, as modern milling techniques made white flour easier to produce, white bread became available to people from all walks of life, and the masses reacted by adopting white bread as the staple food and resolutely refusing to eat other kinds. Today white bread has become the scapegoat for many of our ills.

WHAT IS THE DIFFERENCE BETWEEN WHEAT AND WHITE FLOUR?

Perhaps the best way to answer this question is to describe the principal parts of the wheat grain, and then explain what happens to the berry during the processing that produces white flour as we know it.

Whole-grain bread, cereal, or flour contains the three principal parts of the wheat grain. As shown in Figure 7-1, they are (1) the **endosperm**, which constitutes 82 percent of the bulk of the kernel; (2) the **bran**, which is the outer covering; and (3) the small embryo or **wheat germ**, constituting 3 percent of the weight. The bran consists of the aleurone layer, which immediately surrounds the endosperm and makes up 7 percent of the weight of the kernel, and the outer protective coatings, which constitute 8 percent of the weight. The aleurone layer is actually separate from the bran, but it is so thin and firmly attached to the bran that it is lost when the bran is removed.

During the milling process, the outer covering (bran) and the wheat germ are usually removed, leaving only the white starchy portion of the kernel, the endosperm. Although this portion does constitute the bulk of the kernel and contains rich supplies of protein, the largest concentration of vitamins and minerals has been swept away, leaving a relatively inferior portion for use. Table 7-1 shows that nutrients are distributed unevenly throughout the kernel and that about 25 percent of protein and most vitamins are stripped away in the milling process. Large amounts of minerals and a large portion of the amino acid lysine, already in a small amount, are also lost.

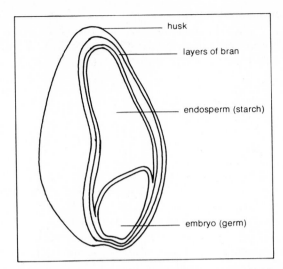

Figure 7-1. A Kernel of Wheat. From *Health Perspectives,* 2nd edition, by Hafen, Thygerson, and Rhodes, Brigham Young University Press, 1979, p. 128.

Table 7-1. Nutrients Available (as Percentages of Amounts in the Whole Grain) in the Endosperm, Bran, and Germ of Wheat

Nutrients	Endosperm (Percent)	Bran (Percent)	Germ (Percent)
Protein	70–75	19	8
Pantothenic acid	43	50	7
Riboflavin	32	42	26
Niacin	12	86	2
Pyridoxine	6	73	21
Thiamine	3	33	64

From *Health Perspectives,* 2nd edition, by Hafen, Thygerson, and Rhodes, Brigham Young University Press, 1979, p. 128.

The bran and germ layers, with their rich supplies of vitamins and minerals, only constitute about 20 percent of the entire weight of the kernel. These portions are generally made into feed for cattle, following their removal from the whole grains. The bran contains most of the fiber; even though it is not a nutrient per se, it is needed for a healthy diet.

The government became concerned about the nutritional loss during processing, and in 1943 the first mandatory food enrichment act was passed. This was the start of a long list of amendments and acts passed to improve the general nutritional content of bread.

WHAT IS ADDED TO ENRICHED BREAD AND FLOUR?

In 1974, an act by the Food and Drug Administration mandated that enriched bread produced in the United States must contain 40 mg of iron per pound and all other enriched bread must contain 25 mg of iron per pound.[1] The only other nutrients restored in enriched bread and flour are thiamine, riboflavin, and niacin. The levels of enrichment are controlled carefully by the FDA. The following figures give the approximate percentage loss of certain nutrients in the refining of wheat:[2]

*Thiamine	86
*Riboflavin	70
*Niacin	86
*Iron	84
Vitamin B_6	60
Folic acid (B vitamin)	70
Pantothenic acid (B vitamin)	54
Biotin (B vitamin)	90
Calcium	50
Phosphorus	78
Copper	75
Magnesium	72
Manganese	71

The starred nutrients are restored in enriched flour.

IS ENRICHED WHITE BREAD LESS NUTRITIOUS THAN WHEAT BREAD?

This is a difficult question which has been the subject of much debate. We do not have proof that the eating of white bread is injurious as many food faddists would have us believe. Nor does white flour poison the body or cause alcoholism, as some people claim. We do know that there are advantages and disadvantages to both white bread and wheat bread.

Because of a loss of nutrients during the milling process, many believe that white bread and flour are obviously inferior. But Sidney Margolius states, "At 1972, enrichment levels (before the new increase in iron became effective) about four slices of enriched bread (close to four ounces) provided a young woman with all of her daily calcium needs; about fifteen percent of protein needs; twenty-five percent of thiamin; nineteen percent of niacin, and thirteen percent of riboflavin and iron."[3]

Table 7-2 shows the nutritional value of various breads.

"But," argue the whole-grain advocates, "what about the other vitamins and minerals not restored in enriched bread?" This is a good question. Most vitamins and minerals are not as plentiful in restored white flour as in whole-wheat flour. Although iron is restored in enriched flour, the trace elements, such as copper, manganese, and zinc, are largely removed. Many nutritionists feel, however, that this is not important, as those additional nutrients can be amply supplied by the rest of the diet, if it is well-balanced.

Jean Mayer cites one report that shows no superiority of wheat bread over white:

> After World War II, two highly competent British nutritionists examined groups of German orphans who got over seventy percent of their daily calories from bread. The researchers could find no difference in health, growth, and development between youngsters who ate whole-grain bread and those whose bread was white enriched. The rest of the diet was high in milk, meat, and vegetables.[4]

Table 7-2. Nutritional Value of Various Breads

Food	Measure	Grams	Percent Water	Calories	Net Total (Lipids) Grams	Saturated (Total Grams)	Fatty Acids Unsaturated Oleic	Linoleic
Cracked Wheat Bread	Loaf, 1 lb. 20 slices	454	35	1,190	10	2	5	2
French or Vienna Bread, Enriched	Loaf, 1 lb.	454	31	1,315	14	3	8	2
White Bread, Enriched, 2% Nonfat Dry Milk	Loaf, 1 lb. 20 slices	454	36	1,225	15	3	9	2
White Bread, Unenriched, (1–2% Nonfat Dry Milk)	Loaf, 1 lb. 20 slices	454	36	1,225	15	3	9	2
Whole-wheat, Graham, Entire-wheat Bread	Loaf, 1 lb. 20 slices	454	36	1,103	14	3	7	4

Food	Measure	Protein (Grams)	Carbo-hydrates (Grams)	Calcium (Milli-grams)	Iron (Milli-grams)	Vitamin A (Inter-national Units)	Thiamin (Grams)	Riboflavin (Grams)	Niacin (Grams)	Vitamin C (Grams)
Cracked Wheat Bread	Loaf, 1 lb. 10 slices	39	236	399	3.0	Trace	.53	.42	3.8	Trace
French, or Vienna Bread, Enriched	Loaf, 1 lb.	41	251	195	10.0	Trace	1.26	.98	11.3	Trace
White Bread, Enriched (1–2% Nonfat Dry Milk)	Loaf, 1 lb. 20 slices	39	229	318	10.9	Trace	1.13	.77	10.4	Trace
White Bread, Unenriched, (1–2% Nonfat Dry Milk)	Loaf, 1 lb. 20 slices	39	229	318	3.2	Trace	.40	.36	5.6	Trace
While-wheat, Graham, Entire-wheat Bread	Loaf, 1 lb. 20 slices	45	216	449	10.4	Trace	1.17	1.03	12.9	Trace

U.S. Department of Agriculture.

Professor Robert S. Harris of the Massachusetts Institute of Technology studied the nutrient content of 44 typical national breads. American white enriched bread came in second, topped only by nonenriched semi-white wheat bread from Finland.[5] Indeed, despite what many may want to believe, enriched white bread is a satisfactory source of many nutrients.

Another recent study by Consumers Union showed that despite processing, many white enriched breads contain enough of the essential and accompanying nutrients not only to support life of test animals, but also to encourage their health and growth.[6] One would expect that the whole-wheat breads, with their superior quantity of many nutrients, would support life and encourage health and growth at a better rate than white breads. However, this was not the case; in fact, the test animals showed better growth on some of the more processed breads than on the whole-grain breads. Consumers Union speculated on the test results as follows:

> We know that whole-grain flours contain phytic acid, a substance that can prevent the body from using many of the flours' minerals. (Phytic acid is milled out of white flour.) The presence of phytic acid, then, might account for the poor nutritional performance of some of the lower-ranked whole-grain breads.
>
> But what of the whole-grains that performed better nutritionally? Our guess is that the phytic acid in those breads may have been rendered less effective because of the way the breads are made. But that's only a speculation. In fact, speculate is all we can do about the results of our bread testing since we could find no pattern of ingredients to characterize the various Ratings groups and no valid explanation for why one brand of bread proved to be so much better for the rats than another.[7]

On the whole, however, evidence continues to grow in favor of whole grains, the cereals with the highest extraction rate. The extraction rate is the percentage of the kernel removed in processing—a flour with 90-percent extraction rate has lost 10 percent of the total kernel and 10 percent of the wheat's original weight. Whole-grain flour has a 100-percent extraction rate. White flours and white bread flours have approximately a 70-percent extraction rate. Commercial pastry flours may be as high as 40 percent. At low extraction rates, vitamins and minerals are lost rapidly. A 70-percent extraction rate leaves only about 1/5 to 1/3 the B vitamins, and the mineral content also drops rapidly. This is why highly refined flours need to be enriched.

It has been recommended by some nutritionists that we return to whole-grain flours with an extraction rate of 80 to 85 percent, even though the flour may be a grayish white rather than the white-white of more refined flours.[8]

ARE THERE ANY DANGERS CAUSED BY THE ADDITIVES IN COMMERCIAL ENRICHED BREAD?

All additives put into processed food in the United States must be approved by the FDA. Those added to bread are no exception.

Bleaching agents are added not merely to color the flour, but to give the flour its stability and desirable baking quality. These agents also permit the **gluten** to retain the leavening gas more effectively.

Additives keep breads and cereals from spoiling rapidly. Some molds are known to be toxic. Bread made without preservatives will usually get moldy in three or four days at room temperature.

Indeed, the additives in bread are helpful and certainly safe if used at FDA approved levels.

IS THERE ANY ADVANTAGE TO STONE-GROUND BREAD?

One of the latest crazes is that of **stone-ground** breads. Advocates of this fad state two advantages. First, stone grinding is slower and therefore cooler. This prevents heat from destroying any of the nutrients in the grain. Second, stone grinding distributes and crushes the grain more evenly, causing no loss of the wheat germ.

However, Stanley C. Roy, vice president of Elam's, a mill producing stone-ground flour, states, "Provided that all of the wheat grain is ground into flour, I doubt that there is any difference in the nutritional value of stone-ground whole-wheat flour vs. whole-wheat flour that is ground some other way. Where methods other than stone grinding are used, I believe there is a stronger possibility that part of the grain is taken away, however."[9]

WHAT ABOUT CEREALS?

Many Americans have made the mistake of thinking breakfast cereal is a meal in and of itself. Parents hand the child a bowl of cereal in the morning and feel they have done their duty. No food in and of itself is nutritionally balanced. As breakfast is one of three meals eaten in a day, it should contain one-third of an individual's nutritional needs. So if cereal is your choice of breakfast foods, make a complete meal of it. Add some orange juice or fruit and an egg or some meat, for better nutrition.

When served with milk, cereal can be a good supply of calcium; however, as consumer reporter Sidney Margolius stated, "If milk is the main nutritional value in eating dry cereals, then obviously there are easier ways to drink it than with a spoon."[10]

Cereal is an excellent source of carbohydrates, but it is best to avoid those cereals with the sugar coating if for no other reason than to cut down on tooth decay. In addition, although we think of cereals as being mainly starch, they also add protein. Even though cereal protein does not contain enough of the amino acids lysine and tryptophane, with the addition of milk these amino acids are provided in sufficient quantity.

The loss of nutrients from processing cereals is similar to that from processing flours and breads. There are only minor variations in what happens to wheat when it is milled versus what happens to rye, oats, rice, barley, and corn. It is difficult to get a sufficient quantity of iron, trace minerals, and the B vitamins, such as thiamine, if cereals are too refined or unenriched. Thus enriched cereal product standards have been established for thiamine, riboflavin, niacin, iron, and, in some cases, calcium and vitamin A.

The best way to judge the quality of a breakfast cereal is to carefully read the list of ingredients on the label, realizing that ingredients must be listed in order of predominance. See Table 7-3 comparing various cereals.

A properly enriched cereal can be an effective part of a well-balanced diet. A recent study illustrates the role of ready-to-eat breakfast cereals on the nutritional content of various breakfasts chosen by children.

A sampling of the breakfast choices of 250 four- to twelve-year-old children indicated that:

- When breakfasts including ready-to-eat cereals were compared with non-cereal breakfasts (those including eggs, bacon, and juice, for example), the

Table 7-3. The Great Cereal Debate

Cereal (1 cup)	Calories	Protein	Calcium	Iron	Vit. A	B_1	B_2	Niacin	C
Bran, Fortified	144–179	7.6+	50.00	5.8	2,820	.70	.55+	7.0+	21+
40% Bran Flakes, Fortified	106	3.6	19.00	12.4	1,650	.41	.49	4.1	12
Raisin Bran Fortified	144	4.2	28.00	17.7	2,350	.58	.71	5.8	18
Corn Flakes	97	2.0	1.0+	0.6	1,180	.29	.35	2.9	9
Corn, Puffed Plain	80	1.2	3.00	0.8	0	.35	.42	3.5	11
Fortified	114	1.7	9.00	3.5	1,410	.35	.42	3.5	11
Farina, Regular, Instant, Quick Cooked	103	3.2	0.20	0.0	0	.10	.07	1.0	0
Oats, Maple Flavor Cooked	166	6.2	24.00	1.4	0	.14	–	–	0
Oats, Rolled Cooked	132	4.8	0.22	1.4	0	.19	.05	0.2	0
Oats, Puffed Fortified	139	2.3	63.00	0.9+	1,180	.29	.35	2.9	9
Rice Krispies Plain	60	0.9	3.00	0.3	0	.07	.02	0.7	0
Fortified	175	1.9	16.00	0.8	2,120	.41	.63	5.2	16
Wheat Flakes	106	3.1	12.00	3.5+	1,410	.35	.42	3.5	11
Wheat, Puffed Plain	54	2.3	4.00	0.6	0	.08	.03	1.2	0
Sugar Coated, Fortified	132	2.1	7.00	1.2	1,650	.41	.49	4.1	0
Wheat, Shredded Plain	177	5.0	22.00	1.8	0	.11	.06	2.2	0
Fortified	146	3.6	16.00	14.1	1,880	.46	.56	4.6	14

Nutritive Value of American Foods in Common Units, Agriculture Handbook #456, USDA. Compiled by Richard Salazar.

caloric, protein, and mineral contents were similar, but the vitamin and iron contents were *much higher* in the cereal breakfasts. Thus, the cereal greatly improved the nutritional content of the actual breakfasts chosen by children in this study.

- The fat content in the noncereal breakfasts was *two times as much* as in the cereal breakfasts, and the cholesterol content was nearly *five times as much.* The fiber and sucrose contents of the cereal breakfasts were somewhat higher than in the noncereal ones, but these differences were of much less magnitude than those of fat and cholesterol.
- The frequency of eating and of skipping breakfast was also analyzed. Those children who ate no ready-to-eat cereals skipped breakfast 20

percent of the time—*three times as often* as those who did eat these cereals.[11]

Thus, if carefully monitored for nutritional content, the ready-to-eat cereals can play an important role in the breakfasts of many Americans.

WHAT SHOULD I LOOK FOR WHEN SHOPPING FOR BREAD?

When buying bread read the ingredients list carefully. Some "natural" or "wheat" breads are really just white bread with caramel food coloring.

If you're dieting, don't automatically eliminate bread. Contrary to what most people think, the average slice of bread contains only about sixty calories. Not only that, but breads (particularly high fiber) tend to help dieters attain **satiety**. A weight-reducing diet can only be considered suitable if, in addition to allowing effective weight reduction with a diet of physiologically balanced nutrient composition, sufficient satiation can be achieved. The number of calories in a slice of bread is offset by the amount of crude fiber and nutrients, and the time it takes to digest it.

Buying the store brands of breads and cereals is usually cheaper than the national labels. The only way you can be sure is to compare based on weight, not size. A larger loaf that weighs less is not going to provide more nutrition.

Remember that the more instant a product is, the more it has been refined. Breads and cereals cooked at home are usually much less expensive than the ready-to-serve kind. Consumers Union suggests the following for more nutritious home-baked bread:

1. Instead of using whole-grain flour, use unbleached, enriched flour. Essential minerals, such as magnesium, zinc, calcium, and iron, can be bound up by phytic acid, which may be found in relatively high levels in whole-grain flour. This makes these minerals less available for human metabolism. In contrast, enriched white flour contains little, if any, phytic acid. The quantity of some vitamins and minerals is reduced in enriched white flour, but with the enriching process these are replaced, some of them at higher levels than before.
2. Yeast should be used generously. It is an excellent source of B-complex vitamins, phosphorus, iron, magnesium, and many trace elements that are needed for good health. Double the amount of yeast you use in a recipe. You may like the yeastier taste, too.
3. Find recipes that use plenty of milk and eggs. The more you use, the more nutritious the bread will probably be. Different forms of eggs and milk are all rich in nutrients.[12]

SUMMARY

The discussion of advantages and disadvantages of whole-wheat and white flour and bread could go on for volumes. It basically is a matter of personal preference. For those eating a nutritionally balanced diet, there is virtually no advantage of wheat over white. Many prefer the texture of the whole grain, since it does contain the bran, which adds fiber and roughage and may help prevent some gastrointestinal disorders. Yet others who have gastrointestinal disorders believe thay cannot handle the roughage; therefore, they avoid it.

If you prefer white bread, then enjoy it. Just make sure it is enriched and that you eat a well-balanced diet all the time to supplement it.

As for cereals, it is best to use those that are less refined with little or no sugar coating.

NOTES

1. Jean Mayer, "The Best Bread in the World," *Family Health,* October 1972, pp. 25–26.
2. Reprinted from "Concerning Cereals," by Lydia Sonnenberg, M.A., *Life and Health,* May 1976, p. 32, © 1976 by the Review and Herald Publishing Association. Used by permission.
3. Sidney Margolius, *Health Foods—Facts and Fakes* (New York: Walker and Company, 1973), pp. 111–113.
4. Mayer, "The Best Bread in the World," pp. 25–26.
5. Ibid.
6. Consumers Union, "Bread: You Can't Judge a Loaf by Its Color," *Consumer Reports,* May 1976, pp. 256–260.
7. Ibid.
8. Jean Mayer, "The Whole Wheat Story," *Family Health/Today's Health,* May 1976, pp. 45, 68, 69.
9. Margolius, *Health Foods—Facts and Fakes,* p. 114.
10. "Which Cereals Are Most Nutritious?" *Consumer Reports,* February 1975, pp. 76–82.
11. Gravini, Robert B., "Cereals in Today's Breakfasts—A Realistic View," *Health Values: Achieving High Level Wellness,* Vol. 2, No. 2, March/April 1978, pp. 101–108.
12. Consumers Union, "The Bread Brouhaha," *Consumers Report,* October 1976, pp. 576–577.

8

Sugar in the Raw

Another nutritional controversy centers around one of the least understood foods of all time—sugar. From one group you hear, "Sugar is a must for energy." Yet from another group, "Sugar is poison." Where is the average consumer to turn for the correct answers? Actually, neither is completely correct, but both contain some sweet truths.

Western civilization has not always had sugar. We knew very little about this sweet substance until the fifteenth century, when the Portuguese introduced sugar cane into Africa. Not until they brought it from Brazil in the sixteenth century did it become a normal commodity among Europeans.[1]

Time was when sugar was a great luxury, rather than a staple. In 1830, England, which has to import most of its sugar, consumed 5 pounds per person per year. Today the average Englishperson devours 125 pounds per year. In the United States the rate of consumption has gone from nothing, when the Pilgrims first landed at Plymouth Rock, to a high of 128 pounds per person per year.[2]

Various kinds of sugar accounted for only about 32 percent of total carbohydrate consumption in the period 1909 to 1913. However, by 1978, sugar (sucrose, fructose, lactose) had replaced starch, or complex carbohydrates, as the predominant carbohydrate energy source. Moreover, while the amount of sugar we eat has been increasing, the average per-capita consumption of flours and grains has dropped by more than half over the course of this century. Therefore we're getting more and more of our carbohydrates from sugar—the carbohydrate supplying the fewest nutrients.

The largest components of the sugar category are refined sugar and syrups, and then molasses and honey, accounting for about 14 percent and 4 percent of total calories, respectively. The remainder occurs naturally in fruit and milk products.

The greatest factor in increased sugar use has come from the addition of refined sugar to processed foods.

Page and Friend report:

Use in processed food products and beverages has increased more than threefold from nearly 20 to 70 pounds, while household purchase has dropped one-half from a little more than 50 to about 25 pounds. Currently, food products and beverages account for more than two-thirds of the refined sugar consumed—70 pounds out of a little over 100 pounds. Moreover, beverages now comprise the largest single industry use of refined sugar in the United States diet, or nearly 23 pounds. Furthermore, the amount used in beverages has increased nearly sevenfold since early in the century when 3½ pounds per person per year was used in these products. Use of refined sugar in beverages is now second only to household use.[3]

Soft drink consumption in the United States has doubled since 1960, rising from 13.6 gallons a year to 27.6 in 1977. This translates into 221 sixteen-ounce cans and 21.5 pounds of sugar a year.

The increase has evidently been made at the expense of more nutritious beverages. Since 1962, soft drinks have become the second most highly consumed beverage, displacing milk. Currently, soft drinks compete with coffee for first place.[4]

A look at product ingredients on supermarket shelves reveals the difficulty of finding almost any type of prepared food product without sugar in it. It is used not only in sweet baked goods and desserts, but also in sauces, many baby foods, almost all fruit drinks, salad dressings, canned and dehydrated soups, pot pies, frozen TV dinners, bacon and other cured meats, some canned and frozen vegetables, most canned and frozen fruits, fruit yogurt, and breakfast cereals.

The presence of sugar in processed foods may provide more than sweetness. Sugar, in some foods, can help retain and absorb moisture, depress the freezing point, act as a preservative, and enhance the appearance. However, the Senate Select Committee on Nutrition reported that "increased use of sugar is traceable in large part to the desire of food manufacturers to create unique food products with a competitive edge."[5]

DOES THE BODY REQUIRE SUGAR?

Contrary to popular belief, the body does not require table sugar (sucrose). It does require carbohydrates, which can be found in either sugar or starches. The interesting thing about carbohydrates is that they are not all the same. Those found in sugar are made of smaller molecules, which can go to work faster but appear to be more harmful to the body than the longer-chain molecules of starch origin. Although both supply energy, only starches provide other essential nutrients.

IS SUGAR NEEDED AS A SOURCE OF ENERGY?

What happens to all this sugar in the body? Consumers Union answers that question in their report "Too Much Sugar."[6] Basically, it is digested and used like any other carbohydrate. Nearly all carbohydrates are ultimately converted into glucose, the primary fuel of the body. Glucose, or "blood sugar," is delivered by the bloodstream to the liver, where it is converted and stored as glycogen until needed by the body. With the help of the hormone insulin, blood glucose then enters nearly all cells of the body and is used as an energy source. The glucose that is not needed by the cells is metabolized in the liver into fatty substances called triglycerides, which are transported in the bloodstream to the fat depots of the body. The body can later draw upon those stores of fat if it needs energy during fasting or dieting.

Why, then, in view of the body's basic need for energy, is there anything wrong with eating sugar? The problem is that sugar, unlike most other sources of carbohydrate, contains no nutrients only calories. It is a classic component of "junk food"—generally, a processed food that is relatively high in calories, lacks any significant amounts of protein, vitamins, or minerals, and contains comparatively large quantities of fats or sugar. Essentially, there is absolutely no dietary requirement for sugar (sucrose) that cannot be satisfied by other more nutritious foods, such as fruits and vegetables. In fact, if no dietary carbohydrate is available, protein can be converted into glucose.

There is not even a need for sugar for so-called quick energy, to fuel a morning of tennis, skiing, or the like. Unless you fast for more than a day or two, your body has sizable reserves of liver glycogen to call upon. If you eat sugar before exercising, the sugar will quickly be metabolized and move into storage with your other fuel reserves.

If you get 20 percent of your calorie requirement from sugar, you have to rely on the other 80 percent of your diet to supply the nutrients you need—no dietary feat for most people, but a neat trick for anyone trying to lose weight.

In a recent report, the Senate Select Committee on Nutrition called for a 45 percent reduction in sugar consumption. I see little sense in picking an arbitrary percentage, but many people would do well to pay attention to the amount of sugar they are consuming. A lot of sugar certainly does you no good nutritionally, and it may contribute to a variety of health problems.

CAN EATING SWEETS CAUSE SUBSTANTIAL WEIGHT GAINS?

Yes. It is interesting to note that while the consumption of meat and bread declined in the 1970s, the intake of sugar remained the same. Thus we find more obesity among Americans and fewer people who are adequately fed.[7] Ten to 20 percent of children in the U.S. are overweight and from 35 to 50 percent of all middle-aged Americans.

Alexander Woolcott once said, "Everything that's fun is either illegal, immoral, or fattening." This is certainly true of sugar. Dr. Bela Szepesi has been doing some testing on rats and finds that those fed on sugars gain more weight than those fed on starches. Another researcher, Dr. Carolyn D. Bernaner, explains the difference between starches and sugars this way:

> One would expect starch, commonly believed to be fattening, to produce as much fat as sugar. But the human metabolic system could be compared to a network of highways, with a main road where food molecules normally travel toward transformation into energy, and side roads for use when the main highway is crowded—as when people overeat. Starch molecules and fat molecules are made up of the same individual units, but starch is a long chain and sugar only two links. The starch molecules break down slowly, so they stay on the main road. On the other hand, the sugar molecules spill over easily onto the side roads where much more of the molecules can be changed into fat.[8]

It's the total amount of excessive calories rather than sugar itself that causes weight gain. Carbohydrates, including sugar, contain 4 calories per gram, or 113 per ounce. Sugar-sweetened foods tend to be those that are already highly concentrated with calories—cake, pies, etc. Remember, a person trying to lose weight will reach satiation more quickly with a pound of apples than with a two-ounce candy bar, even though they contain about the same number of calories.

WHAT PART DOES SUGAR PLAY IN DENTAL DECAY?

Authorities all agree that sugar can promote tooth decay and gum disease. Although tooth decay is not by any means deadly, it can be painful and is expensive. The Army indicates that for every 100 inductees, 600 fillings are required, 112 extractions, 40 bridges, 21 crowns, 18 partial dentures, and 1 full denture.[9] That's a lot of dental work. Americans today spend about 2 billion dollars a year treating tooth decay. Dr. Abraham E. Nizel, of the Tufts University School of Dental Medicine, states that if everyone had the dental work done that needs to be taken care of, we would be paying the dentists in this country 8 billion dollars a year.[10]

One government survey indicates that:

> In nations of the Far East, where sugar intake per person per year ranged (at the time) from twelve to thirty-two pounds, the national averages for decayed, missing or filled teeth in adults twenty to twenty-four years old ran from 0.9 to 5. By contrast, in South American nations, where sugar intake was high (forty-four to eighty-eight pounds per person annually) the averages for decayed, missing or filled teeth in the same age group ran from 8.4 to 12.6. As for the United States today, it has been estimated that ninety-eight percent of American children have some tooth decay; by age fifty-five about half of the population of this country have no teeth.[11]

Progressively, tooth decay has become more common as we use grain rather than flesh and fruit as our main sources of food, as we make refined flours and sucrose abundantly available, and, most recently, as we vastly increase use of the packaged ready-to-eat sweetened snacks and candies that flood the modern market. Ordinary sucrose or sugar plays a dominant part in the high frequency of decay. Sucrose is particularly cariogenic, because it is not only easily fermented to acid but also readily changed to sticky polysaccharides by oral bacteria, thereby promoting their adherence to the teeth.[12] In fact, the important matter is not the amount of sugar eaten, but the kind. Sweets such as sticky candies tend to adhere to teeth more than others. Table 8-1 illustrates the sugar content of various types of foods and beverages.

The decay process begins with colonies of bacteria (called dental **plaque**) that stick to your teeth. When you eat, the bacteria break down your food and change the sugar to acid. The sticky bacterial plaque then holds the acid to the tooth surface, allowing it to attack the enamel on your teeth, resulting in tooth decay.[13]

Another causative factor in dental caries is frequency of intake. Dr. Abraham Nizel explains,

> Each time the dental plaque on the tooth surface is exposed to sweets, twenty to thirty minutes of acid is produced. So, if five lozenges or cough drops are eaten, one after another, within a space of fifteen minutes, they might produce thirty-five minutes of acid. On the other hand, if they are eaten twenty minutes apart, they will produce one hundred minutes of acid.[14]

Table 8-1. Hidden Sugar

Food	Approximate Sucrose Content By Weight, expressed in percentage
Candy and Gum	
Average candy bar	20–60
Hard candy	20–85
Non-chocolate candy	25–90
Gum	45–85
Cookies and Cakes	
Chocolate cake	30–60
Cake (angel food)	20–30
Chocolate and fudge cookies	25–50
Non-chocolate or fudge cookies	16–48
Doughnuts	15–30
Ice Cream Products*	
Popsicles	10–15
Sherbets	15–20
Ice cream	7–15
Ice cream sandwichs	15–25
Soft Drinks	
Soda pops	2– 9
Punches	2–10
Cough Drops and Lozenges**	23–68
Breads, Crackers and Wafers	
Breads	0– 4
Crackers and wafers	0–25
Fruits and fruit juices*	0– 8
Dried fruit	.6– 6
Vegetables and vegetable juices	0– 5
Snack Foods	
Potato chips and corn chips	0– 3
Pie	12–30
Cupcakes, etc.	15–40
Puddings	7–20
Dry Breakfast Cereals	1–70
Most range from	10–50

Remember, if you're concerned about calories—foods contain calories from protein, carbohydrates, and fats.

*This represents sucrose content only and does not include natural sugars, such as fructose and lactose.

**There are several brands that contain as little as 2 to 5%. However, most are as indicated in the chart.

The dental plaque that is formed from a sugar-concentrated diet can also lead to periodontal problems (gum disease). Plaque contains bacterial irritants which cause the gums to bleed. In addition, if the plaque is not removed daily, it can harden by mixing with the salts in the saliva. The hardened plaque (calculus) collects on the teeth below the gumline and irritates the inside skin. This creates a pocket where more infection can occur. If left unchecked, the infection can destroy the supporting bone and the tooth can be lost.[15]

Sugar eaten as a part of a meal tends to cause less damage to teeth than the same amount of sugar consumed during a between-meals snack. To reduce the risk of decay, dentists recommend rinsing your mouth or brushing your teeth soon after consuming anything sweet and avoiding sweets between meals. If you must snack, select foods containing artificial sweeteners. Particular items to avoid include cough drops, breath mints, and candies, which remain in the mouth for a long time, feeding the bacteria and prolonging the acid attack.

IS IT TRUE THAT SUGAR IS THE CAUSE OF MANY FATAL ILLNESSES?

No definite answer to this question can be found at present.

Heart Disease

Dr. John Uydkin, nutritionist at the University of London, makes the highly controversial claim that sugar is involved in coronary artery disease, and that the evidence against sugar is even more conclusive than it is against cholesterol. He believes that those who suffer heart attacks consume more sugar than those who don't.[16]

Another strong advocate of this view is Dr. Aaron M. Cohen of the Hadassah University Hospital in Jerusalem. His studies take place in what is known by researchers as the "living laboratory," a community in Jerusalem which consists of two neatly divided populations. One group comprises people who have recently emigrated to the city from the wild nomadic country of Yemen. They are presently in a process of transition from their life as herders to the life and atmosphere of modern Israel. The other group is made up of Yemenites who have been in the city for a generation. Both consume the same diets of fat-laden meat and milk products, yet the earlier settlers have high blood levels of fat and cholesterol and a high incidence of heart disease. The newcomers do not. What makes the difference? Dr. Cohen feels that it is the fact that the earlier group has become accustomed to the practice of eating sweets, while the new arrivals have not.[17]

You may say, "Well, a lot of factors involved in urbanizing besides dietary changes can cause tension and bring about heart trouble." This is true. In addition, a high-sugar diet has not been shown to cause heart disease in research animals, whereas a high-fat and/or high-cholesterol diet has. Thus the controversy over this matter has not yet been resolved.

Cancer

Jean Mayer, a well-known nutritionist, does not feel that present evidence provides any suggestion that sugar is a cause of cancer. Concerning cancer of the colon, he explains:

There has been speculation that it [sugar] might have some link to bowel cancer, but current research suggests that diets low in fiber and high in meat, milk, eggs, and refined flour and sugar promote cancer of the colon and rectum. Eating high-roughage foods such as salads and bran cereals—and decreasing intake of refined cereals and sugar—may be the answer. But this is a far cry from saying "sugar causes cancer."[18]

The present evidence seems to implicate total dietary fat more than just a diet high in refined carbohydrates and sugar.

Diabetes   The sugar-diabetes relationship is a subject of much controversy and little real knowledge. In his study of the Yemenite cultures Dr. Aaron Cohen observed that those newly arrived in Jerusalem showed no cases of diabetes, yet after 25 years in a civilized environment, incidence of diabetes had risen to the normal 3.5 percent.[19]

Along these same lines, Dr. Berndanier testified before the United States Senate, Ninety-third Congress, that his investigations have led him to conclude that certain individuals are sensitive to high sugar intakes. These are the individuals who may acquire diabetes at some time in their lives. Since other individuals do not respond to high sugar intake, this would point toward a genetic tendency in diabetes.[20] In other experiments, laboratory rats prone to diabetes developed the disease on a high-sugar diet—but not a sugar-free diet.

In any case, there is evidence that links obesity and adult-onset diabetes. It appears that the insulin resistance of cells increases when excess weight is lost. So keeping weight down and sugar intake low is the best way to treat or prevent at least some cases of maturity-onset diabetes.

ARE ALL SUGARS THE SAME?

If you read labels carefully in a health-food store, you would no doubt conclude that white refined sugar is rated on a par with DDT and arsenic. But that does not mean you will not find sugar in "health-food" products. So-called health breads, for instance, are often chock full of honey, molasses, brown sugar, or "raw" sugar. It's just white refined sugar that is considered to be the villain.

Is there any truth to the notion that one sugar is somehow better for you than another? Some sugars are not quite as bad for your teeth as sucrose. Otherwise, there is virtually no difference among them worth worrying about. To understand why, it is necessary to look at the way the most common commercial types of sugar are produced.

There are more than one hundred substances identified as sugars. These include fructose (fruit sugar), dextrose (one of the sugars made from corn starch and chemically identical to glucose), lactose (the sugar in milk), and maltose (malt sugar, formed from starch by the action of yeast). But the word sugar is commonly used to refer to sucrose, which comes from sugar cane or sugar beets. In a typical manufacturing operation, the sugar cane is shredded into small pieces, crushed, and the juice separated. Processing causes the sugar in the juice to crystallize, forming sugar crystals and syrup. These are separated by a mechanical device into the end products, raw sugar and molasses. Then comes a washing and filtering, and the raw sugar is turned into refined white sugar.

Raw sugar is banned in the United States, for good reasons: it contains such contaminants as insect parts, soil, molds, bacteria, link, and waxes. When it's partially refined to make it sanitary, it can be sold as turbinado sugar. Brown sugar consists of sugar crystals coated with some molasses syrup. Most refiners make it by spraying syrup onto refined white sugar.[21]

DOES BROWN SUGAR CARRY
ANY ADVANTAGE OVER WHITE?

No, not really. Brown sugar retains some of the molasses from which purified sugar crystals are separated and therefore does contain small amounts of the minerals found in molasses. If brown sugar were the sole source of sugar in a diet it would provide iron, yet at quantities relatively small compared to caloric intake. A half cup of brown sugar contains 370 calories, which would only amount to 2.6 milligrams of iron. Brown and turbinado sugar may look more healthful because of their dark color and distinctive odor; however, the few additional nutrients they contain are so minuscule in quantity that for all practical purposes they are worthless. The nutrients simply are not present in the usable parts of the sugar cane or sugar beet plant. See Table 8-2 comparing the nutritional value of honey, molasses, sugars, and syrup.

IS IT HEALTHIER TO USE HONEY INSTEAD OF SUGAR?

Honey is formed by an enzyme from nectar gathered by bees. Depending on where the nectar comes from, honey can differ in composition and flavor. But all honey is a blend of a number of different sugars, largely fructose and glucose. Like brown sugar, honey has a few nutrients—mainly potassium, calcium, and phosphorus. But, again, they are scant. You would have to eat 91 tablespoons of honey each day to get your recommended daily requirement of potassium, 200 for calcium, and 267 for phosphorus. The only nutrient of any significant value found in honey is iron. And still one would need to eat over five tablespoons of honey (310 calories) to obtain 0.9 mg of iron—the amount found in one medium egg yolk.[22] There's no evidence that honey is easier to digest than other sugars. When you eat table sugar, your body breaks the sucrose down into fructose and glucose, the two leading ingredients of honey.

What about substituting honey for sucrose in cooking or in your coffee to get more sweetening power per calorie? It is true that some batches of honey can be as much as 40 percent sweeter than sugar (although other batches can actually be less sweet). A cup of honey has only 23 percent more calories than a cup of sugar. So with a little luck, you do get more sweetening power per calorie. Substituting honey will change the character of the food you're preparing, however, so you might have to alter the cooking time or some other aspect of the recipe.

Table 8-2. Honey, Molasses, Sugars, and Syrup Compared

Food Items	Calories	Protein (mg)	Calcium (mg)	Phos. (mg)	Iron (mg)	A (mg)	B_1 (mg)	B_2 (mg)	Niacin (mg)	C (mg)
Brown Sugar										
1 cup	820	0.0	187	42	7.5	0	0.02	0.07	0.4	0
1 Tbs	51	0.0	12	2.8	0.5	0	Trace	Trace	Trace	0
White Sugar										
1 cup	770	0.0	0	0	0.2	0	0.0	0.0	0.0	0
1 Tbs	46	0.0	0	0	Trace	0	0.0	0.0	0.0	0
Honey										
1 cup	1031	1.0	17	20	1.6	0	0.02	0.14	1.0	3
1 Tbs	64	0.1	1	1	0.1	0	Trace	0.01	0.1	Trace
Syrup (Table Blends)										
1 cup	951	0.0	151	52	13.4	0	0.0	0.0	0.0	0
1 Tbs	59	0.0	9	3	0.8	0	0.0	0.0	0.0	0
Molasses (Black Strap)										
1 cup	699	—	2244	276	52.8	—	0.36	0.62	6.6	—
1 Tbs	43	—	137	17	3.2	—	0.02	0.04	0.4	—

CONCLUSION: Black strap molasses is the most nutritious form of sugars, and the difference between sugar and honey is so slight it does not merit concern — and sugar is considerably less expensive.

Nutritive Value of American Foods in Common Units. Agriculture Handbook #456, USDA. Compiled by Richard Salazar.

The idea that honey is natural and, therefore, nutritionally wiser than sugar is a great hoax. In fact, the late Dr. Adelle Davis admits:

> Despite the fact that honey is a natural sweet, it contains only traces of nutrients and appears to cause tooth decay as quickly as does refined sugar. Persons who are convinced that honey is "good for them" often eat large amounts, gain unwanted pounds, and spoil their appetite for more nutritious foods.[23]

HOW SAFE ARE SUGAR SUBSTITUTES?

If you are worried about calories, sugar substitutes look great, with little or no calories per serving. Then, we face the question of their safety.

Cyclamates

Most of the scare over sugar substitutes arose when cyclamates were banned by the FDA in 1969, after researchers discovered cancer in animals fed large doses. Since that time a big dispute has gone on over how the cyclamates were used in those tests. Cyclamates might be back on the market soon if the National Cancer Institute would agree with the scientists who say it is not a cause of cancer.

However, in 1976, the FDA announced that because of "unresolved safety questions," it will not lift the ban. This followed a report by a six-member committee assembled by the National Cancer Institute that said that a definitive assessment of cyclamate's cancer-causing potential for humans is not now possible because of "state-of-the-art problems we have had and will continue to have with compounds that at worst may be weakly carcinogenic in animals."[24] The feeling was that, even with negative data in animal tests, the possibility of cancer in a treated group could not be excluded. Although the evidence did not establish that cyclamate causes cancer, there was concern over "statistically significant increases in tumors in cyclamate-treated animals from several studies."[25]

Saccharin

In 1977, the Food and Drug Administration announced a proposal to prohibit the use of saccharin in foods or beverages and as a tabletop nonnutritive sweetner. The ban was proposed as a result of studies conducted by the Health Protection Branch of the Canadian government, which showed that high dosages of saccharin fed to rats were associated with increased incidence of malignant bladder tumors. The proposed ban has created much confusion among consumers and professionals.[26]

At the present, products containing saccharin must carry a warning label advising people the artificial sweetener may cause cancer. Buyers in restaurants will find the notice printed on little sacks of sugar substitute; those drinking diet pop—which accounts for 74 percent of all saccharin in food—will find the statement on the side or top of cans. And all stores selling foods containing saccharin must post the following notice:

> SACCHARIN NOTICE. This store sells food including diet beverages and dietetic foods that contain saccharin. You will find saccharin listed in the ingredient statement on most foods which contain it. All foods which contain

saccharin will soon bear the following warning: Use of this product may be hazardous to your health. This product contains saccharin which has been determined to cause cancer in laboratory animals.

Even though there is as yet no proof of a cause-effect relationship between saccharin and cancer in humans, a study conducted by the Canadian counterpart of the U.S. National Cancer Institute has provided statistical evidence of an association between saccharin use and cancer in humans. Scientists compared artificial sweetner use in 480 men who had bladder cancer and in a carefully matched control group without bladder cancer. They found that the men who consumed saccharin had a significantly higher incidence of bladder cancer than the men who did not. The higher the consumption of saccharin, the greater were the chances for getting bladder cancer.[27] Similar studies in the United States, however, have not produced the same results.[28]

A panel of scientists who studied saccharin for the Congressional Office of Technology Assessment said saccharin was a relatively weak carcinogen (substance that induces cancer).[29] "Weak," however, refers to the number of cancers caused, not to the seriousness of the cancer. Cancer caused by a weak carcinogen is no less deadly.

The Office of Technology Assessment panel also pointed out that the potential risk of this weak carcinogen could be large if many people are exposed to it. Unquestionably, many people are exposed to saccharin. Some 6 million pounds of the artificial sweetener are used in the United States annually, three-quarters of it in diet soft drinks and most of the rest in dietetic foods and table sweeteners used in place of sugar. The Office of Technology Assessment study estimated that if 200 million people drank one can of diet soda per day, anywhere between 600 and 15,000 additional cancers a year would result.

There are some professionals who feel a great injustice would be done by banning saccharin because of its value for diabetics and those using it for weight control. However, there are those who point out that there is no evidence that saccharin is beneficial for weight control and that diabetes can be managed without saccharin.

Saccharin advocates feel that when a risk is associated with a popular product like saccharin, the best course of action is to require a warning label and let consumers decide for themselves whether they want to use the product. But when the risk involved is cancer, that is not an easy course to follow. Public opinion polls show that Americans fear cancer more than any other calamity—even war—and with good reason. Each day 1,000 Americans die from cancer. Each day 1,600 new cases of cancer are detected. And scientists now agree that the majority of cancers, perhaps as many as 80 or 90 percent, are caused by substances in our environment—substances in the food we eat, the air we breathe, the water we drink, and the products we make and use.[30]

It is in this context that the final decision about saccharin will be made.

Whatever the outcome, the saccharin controversy does have its beneficial side. It has drawn public attention to the whole process of regulating environmental hazards—from methods scientists use for testing potential carcinogens to the consumer protection laws and how they work. Saccharin has influenced people to look at some of the products they use in a new light, causing them to focus on not only the benefits but the risks as well.

This growing awareness is valuable because scientists will continue to raise hard questions, not only about new and exotic products but about old friends such as saccharin. And when scientific questions are raised, people must decide where to draw the line between the individual desire for free choice and the collective need for protection.

If cyclamates and saccharin worry you, there are other artificial sweeteners now on the market and in the process of being released. If you are faced with the decision between artificial sweetener and pounds, or artificial sweetener and diabetes, maybe the answer is to use saccharin. But please be moderate.

SHOULD SUGAR BE ELIMINATED
ALTOGETHER FROM MOST DIETS?

In the first place, sugar is an integral part of all living substances. It is produced in plants through photosynthesis. Animals eating the plants also contain sugar in their makeup. Therefore, we cannot escape it. However, only lactose (milk sugar), fructose (sugar found in fruits), and glucose (blood sugar) are essential to life. Sucrose (table sugar) can be eliminated from the diet almost completely, and, at least in the case of many diabetics, probably should be.

However, the American consumption of carbohydrates looks something like this: 50 percent from starch; 40 percent from sucrose from the sugar cane or sugar beet; 5 percent from lactose, and 5 percent from other sugars, mostly glucose, fructose, and sucrose from fruits and vegetables.

The impact on health of increasing sugar use is not well understood. The most immediate problem is the danger in displacing complex carbohydrates, which are high in micronutrients, with sugar, which is essentially an energy source offering little other nutritional value. This not only increases the potential for depriving the body of essential micronutrients, but, noted Dr. Jean Mayer, may actually increase the body's needs for certain vitamins:

> [Sugar calories] increase requirements for certain vitamins, like thiamine, which are needed [for the body] to metabolize carbohydrates. They may increase the need for the trace mineral chromium as well.
> Thus, a greater burden is placed on the other components of the diet to contribute all the necessary nutrients—other foods need to show extra-ordinary "nutrient density" to compensate for the emptiness of the sugar calories.[31]

Complete elimination of sugar is not necessary in normal cases, but one should seriously consider cutting down on daily intake.

Here are some tips that might be useful.

1. Make a continuous effort to cut down on those fattening and sugar-laden treats we all enjoy so much, like cakes, pies, candies, and soda pops.

2. Inspect the labels of packaged goods and buy those with the least amount of sugar. For instance, get fruits canned in their own juices as opposed to those in heavy syrup.
3. Cut down on the amount of sugar you add to such things as tea, coffee, and breakfast cereals. Better yet, don't use any sugar at all.
4. Cut down on between-meals snacks. If you feel a need for them, eat things like fruit, raw vegetables, popcorn, or nuts.
5. Beware of preprepared foods—over 75 percent of our sugar consumption comes from this area.
6. Most important, remember moderation.

One important thing to remember is that fanaticism in any direction is foolish. Don't be scared into fads by the numerous reports floating around. Eat nutritionally balanced meals from the four basic foor groups, don't overindulge, and then enjoy what you eat!

Remember, sucrose is a "natural" substance; it comes from a plant. In the same way, nature has put sugar in other fruits and vegetables. Just because a bottle of apple juice says "unsweetened" or "no sugar added," this doesn't mean that sugar wasn't there in the first place. The natural sugars in orange, apple, and many other fruit juices make them slightly higher in total sugar than a bottle of Coca Cola. But there are two important differences: The fruit juices give you other nutrients besides calories, and one of the principal sugars (fructose) is somewhat easier on tooth surfaces than sucrose.[32]

Meanwhile, even if you want to substitute nutritious foods for that one-third of a pound, or six hundred calories, of sugar the average American eats daily, you may still find yourself thwarted by the lack of information on product labels. Manufacturers can use several different sugars to avoid putting the word sugar at the head of their ingredients list. Until a government agency acts to require a clear revelation of sugar percentage in processed foods, all you can do is to check the label to see which sugars have been added. As a key, look for any word ending in "ose," such as maltose or dextrose. Corn syrup or corn sugar is a commonly used sucrose substitute. Ultimately, they all mean the same thing: You're buying sugar.

SUMMARY

Americans have drastically increased their sugar intake over the centuries. The big increase in the consumption of sugar has come in the areas of soft drinks and the so-called junk foods.

There are certain problems that may be linked to high sugar consumption. One that is of increasing concern to health and medical personnel is the problem of overweight. It is the excessive number of calories in sugar rather than the sugar itself that causes weight gain.

Sugar is also a major factor in the promotion of tooth decay and other oral diseases. Sugar and plaque bacteria combine in the mouth to form acids, which erode tooth enamel.

The relationship of sugar to coronary artery disease is a controversial issue, indeed, some experts feel that this relationship is even stronger than that between cholesterol and coronary artery disease. Others feel that factors such as stress are more directly responsible for heart disease.

Also unresolved is the question of whether diabetes and cancer can be related to excess sugar consumption.

Many people feel that it is more healthful to use honey rather than the many forms of sugar on the market today. However, there is no basis for this assumption.

Sugar substitutes have been under fire for the past several years—ever since cyclamates were taken off the market. If you use an artifical sweetener, it is best to use a chemical sweetener other than saccharin or a cyclamate. But any artificial sweetener should be used with moderation.

Basically, if you're concerned about nutrition or your teeth, try to satisfy your craving for sweets with fresh fruits and fruit juices.

NOTES

1. Jean Mayer, "Scale Down Your Sugar," *Family Health,* April 1974, pp. 74–75.
2. Ibid.
3. Select Committee on Nutrition and Human Needs, U.S. Senate, *Dietary Goals for the United States* (Washington, D.C.: U.S. Government Printing Office, 1977), pp. 43, 45.
4. Ibid.
5. Ibid.
6. "Too Much Sugar," *Consumer Reports,* March 1978, pp. 136–142. Copyright 1978 by Consumers Union of United States, Inc., Mount Vernon, N.Y. 10550. Reprinted by permission from *Consumer Reports,* March 1978. Reprints of "Too Much Sugar" are available from Consumers Union, Reprint Division, Orangeburg, N.Y. 10962.
7. Edward Elelson, "Sugar Is Not So Sweet," *Family Health,* March 1971, pp. 27–32.
8. Ibid.
9. Select Committee, *Dietary Goals for the United States,* pp. 43, 45.
10. Michael Jacobson, "Our Diets Have Changed, But Not for the Best," *Smithsonian,* April 1974, pp. 96–102.
11. Select Committee, *Dietary Goals for the United States,* pp. 43, 45.
12. James P. Carlos (ed.), *Prevention and Oral Health,* Fogarty International Center and National Institute of Dental Research, DHEW Publication No. 74-707, pp. 35–36.
13. Excerpted from "Diet and Health," a booklet by the American Dental Association, 1975, pp. 3–4. Copyright by the American Dental Association. Reprinted by permission.
14. Lou Joseph, "Foods and Drinks That Will Cause You the Fewest Cavities," *Today's Health,* October 1973, pp. 41–43.
15. American Dental Association, "Diet and Health," pp. 3–4.
16. Elelson, "Sugar Is Not So Sweet," pp. 27–32.
17. Ibid.
18. Mayer, "Scale Down Your Sugar," pp. 74–75.

19. Select Committee on Nutrition and Human Needs, U.S. Senate, *Nutrition and Disease* (Washington, D.C.: U.S. Government Printing Office, 1973), p. 201.
20. Ibid.
21. "Too Much Sugar," p. 142.
22. American Medical Association, "Let's Talk About Food," (Action, Mass.: Publishing Sciences Group, Inc., 1974).
23. Sidney Margolius, *Health Foods—Facts and Fakes* (New York: Walker and Company, 1973).
24. "Cancer Unit Submits Report on Cyclamate," *FDA Consumer,* October 1976. p. 24.
25. Ibid.
26. News release, U.S. Department of Health, Education, and Welfare, Food and Drug Administration, March 9, 1977.
27. R. W. Morgan and M. G. Jain, "Bladder Cancer: Smoking, Beverages, and Artificial Sweeteners," *Canadian Medical Association Journal,* Vol III, 1974, pp. 1067-1070.
28. "Saccharin—Where Do We Go From Here?" *FDA Consumer,* April 1978, pp. 16-21.
29. Ibid.
30. Ibid.
31. Select Committee, *Dietary Goals for the United States,* pp. 43, 45.
32. "Too Much Sugar," pp. 136-142.

9

The Fiberless Folly

Not too many years ago, fiber (or roughage, as Grandma would have called it) was not considered when carbohydrates in the diet were analyzed, as most of it remains in its original state throughout the system and is not absorbed into the intestinal tract. Yet researchers are discovering a possible loophole in this theory big enough to kill hundreds of Americans yearly and cause many thousands of others to suffer.

EXACTLY WHAT IS DIETARY FIBER?

Dr. Denis P. Burkitt describes fiber as follows:

> Dietary fiber is that part of the structure of all plant food which is not broken down by intestinal enzymes and so reaches the large bowel undigested. Because fiber is not digested, it has no nutritional value and has been thought of as more of a contaminant than as a food. In fact, until quite recently, it was thought that removing fiber added to the quality of food.[1]

Thus dietary fiber includes those parts of a plant that are resistant to digestion by secretions of the gastrointestinal tract. Dietary fiber can include **celluloses,** hemicelluloses, mucilages, waxes, pectins, gums, and lignin. These substances are not found in all plants and may vary considerably, especially when comparing fresh material with dehydrated or toasted material. The substances also vary greatly in their capacity to hold water and trace minerals.

Refined foods, sugar, flour, and fats have been criticized for years because of all the dangerous debris they contain, yet the real hazard is what they lack. Most of these food stuffs are completely digested and absorbed, leaving no appreciable food residue.[2] Cereal foods in particular suffer from the removal of fiber, which is essential for certain physiological functions. One of the major functions of dietary fiber is to retain water in the large intestine. Consequently, persons who are on fiber-rich diets usually pass larger and softer stools, whereas those on fiber-depleted diets pass smaller and firmer ones. The smaller stools cause the colon to over-contract, since it is made to handle large amounts of bulk. This overcontraction causes a spasm in the colon, which in turn causes a generalized disturbance in the entire tract. Eventually on a fiber-free diet, the bowel muscle will hypertrophy because of the pressure required to move the feces.

See Table 9-1 for a list of common higher-fiber foods.

Table 9-1. High-Fiber Foods

High-fiber foods

Biscuits and cakes	Whole-meal flour or rye, oatmeal or rolled oats, dried fruit and nuts can all be included in one's cooking.
Bran	Weight for weight, bran has the highest fiber content of all the readily available foodstuffs. Unprocessed bran (8 to 10 teaspoons/day) is the cheapest available. Bran can be mixed with flour for homemade bread, cakes, biscuits, or muffins, and mixed in sauces, puddings, or stewed fruit.
Bread	Whole-wheat, raisin, cracked wheat, and whole-rye breads, and any made from whole-wheat or whole-rye flour of 100% extraction. Extra-high fiber bread can be made by adding additional bran.
Breakfast cereals	All-Bran, Puffed Wheat, 40% Bran Flakes, Bran Chex, Raisin Bran, Shredded Wheat, porridge oats.
Flour	Whole meal, such as whole wheat or whole rye. Use only flour containing 100% of the whole grain.
Fruits and nuts	All kinds in generous amounts. Raw and dried fruits, skins included, are preferable.
Rice	Use brown or polished rice if available; otherwise, bran can be added to white rice.
Vegetables	All kinds in generous amounts, including plenty of raw vegetables . Potatoes should be baked or boiled in their skins.

From *Current Prescribing,* July 1978, p. 59.

WHAT ARE SOME OF THE DISEASES BELIEVED TO BE A RESULT OF THE LOW-FIBER DIET?

Infectious diseases, once the greatest cause of mortality, have become much less prominent through the miracle of modern medicine. On the other hand, non-infectious diseases now dominate the mortality profile.

Much of this can be blamed on the affluent western life style. In Africa and other rural areas, many of the infirmities that cause such havoc in the West are virtually unknown. It is only when these people adopt the urban way of life and dietary habits that these diseases begin to take their toll.[3] Part of the problem associated with urbanization is the lack of cereal fiber in the diet. Let's consider some of the afflictions that may be associated with this type of diet.

Coronary Artery Disease

In 1910, William Osler considered coronary heart disease a rarity. In 1925, it was considered "newsworthy" by Sir John McNee, when he described two cases of this "rare condition" he had seen in the United States. Today it is one of the leading causes of death.[4]

Many specialists feel that the removal of fiber from the diet raises the serum cholesterol level, a noted forerunner of coronary heart disease. One study has shown that adding fiber to the diet will reduce serum cholesterol in both animals and man.[5]

Dietary fiber has the potential to bind bile acids, fats, including cholesterol, and certain minerals, such as zinc, iron, and calcium. The more rapid transit time induced by high-fiber intake may have some effect on removing cholesterol from the system. However, a recent study showed that serum triglyceride levels increase during high fiber intake in patients with hyperlipemia.[6] Also, the binding properties of dietary fiber may lead to loss of some nutrients such as zinc and iron.

Appendicitis

Appendicitis, although discovered by Parkinson in 1812, did not become common until after 1880.[7]

When the stool is not kept transitory, it collects in the colon. The appendix, which is an appendage to the colon, also collects the immobile waste products; because of existing acids, the appendix may become inflamed. This probably is caused by pressure in the appendix, which increases when the appendix gets blocked with little masses of fecal material as a result of constipation due to low dietary fiber. The raised pressures within the appendix can also cut off the blood supply of the lining, which then becomes devitalized. Bacteria can then invade and cause appendicitis.[8]

Diverticular Disease of the Colon

Diverticular disease has become a real clinical problem only in the last fifty years.

The small, hard stool of a low-fiber diet is not easily propelled through the intestine, and therefore requires high peristaltic pressure. Half a lifetime of generating these pressures causes **trabeculation** of the sigmoid (the lower part of the colon) and herniation of its mucosae. The raised pressures within the colon force little "out-pouches" or "knuckles" of the lining out through weak spots in the overlying muscle.[9] (See Figure 9-1.) The pouches can trap feces, which can cause inflammation resulting in nausea, vomiting, chills, fever, and lower abdominal pain.

Diverticulosis was once thought to be asymptomatic. Today, however, it is known that symptoms ranging from mild dyspepsia (indigestion) to severe colic can be associated with diverticulosis. These symptoms are caused by the abnormal contractions of the colon and probably the rest of the intestine. The thickened sigmoid can cause recurrent attacks of pain, so severe that sigmoid colectomy is performed in the mistaken belief that inflammatory diverticulitis is present. Subsequent examination of the specimen fails to reveal evidence of infection. This condition has been called "painful diverticular disease."

Soft Bulky Feces

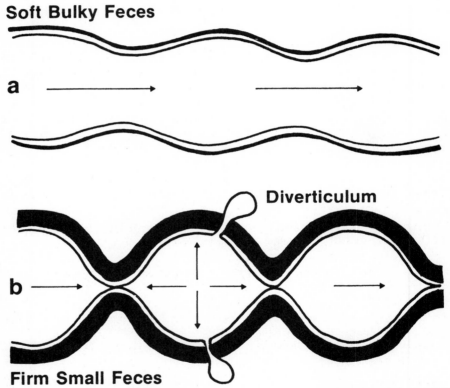

Firm Small Feces

Figure 9-1. Reproduced with permission from *Cereal Foods World* 22(1): 8, 1977.

Varicose Veins   There is no history of the beginning of varicose veins, but as it is similar in its distribution to that of deep vein thrombosis, it too may date from the turn of the century.

Dr. Burkitt describes lack of fiber as it relates to varicose veins:

Constipation causes both increased pressure within the lumen of the large intestine as it contracts to propel its abnormally viscid contents, and also increased pressure within the abdomen during straining to evacuate small, hard stools. The raised intra-abdominal pressures might well be an important factor in the causes of varicose veins, and hiatus hernia. Raised intra-abdominal pressures can be transmitted to the veins of lower limbs when the valves have become incompetent.[10]

When the leg veins are no longer protected by valves, the inside pressures increase, with resulting dilation and varicose veins.

Hiatus hernia is a condition where the top end of the stomach protrudes through a hole in the diaphragm and into the thoracic cavity. It has been recognized as a common condition only during the last thirty years.

Hiatus Hernia

It is felt that intra-abdominal pressures produce hemorrhoidal veins, and that this same intra-abdominal pressure also contributes to the production of hiatus hernia.

Little is known as to the beginning of hemorrhoids as a medical problem. However, it is interesting to note that hemorrhoids generally proceed varicose veins in occurrence, possibly because hemorrhoidal veins have no valves and are not protected from intra-abdominal pressures during defecation.

Hemorrhoids

Abdominal straining forces blood from the large veins in the abdomen into smaller veins that surround the anal canal. It is thought that the stretching and dilating over long periods of time create the hemorrhoid problem.[11]

With low-fiber diets, there are more **anaerobic** bacteria (those that thrive in an environment without oxygen) in the stool. These degrade bile salts, and the results are toxic. Since a low-fiber diet also increases transit time, the intestinal mucosae are exposed to those toxic agents for longer periods of time.[12] Dr. Burkitt feels that these toxic products are carcinogenic when combined with slow transit time.

Tumors and Cancer of the Colon

On the other hand, there is no firm evidence that bile-acid metabolites can cause cancer in humans, although they do resemble some potent carcinogens in structure and may be cocarcinogenic in animals.[13]

Art work shows that obesity is a new scourge of western society. It did not become common until about two hundred years ago.

Obesity

Fiber in the diet will cause a feeling of satiety before you have eaten many more calories than you need, because bulk foods connect other wastes in the intestine, absorb moisture, and generally take longer to eat. When foods are refined, we require more food to achieve a feeling of fullness; this adds more calories. Thus although there has not been enough research as yet to determine whether a high-fiber diet actually contributes to weight reduction, there is no question that such a diet tends to satisfy hunger more quickly.

One recent study did show that a high-fiber diet will help to reduce plasma glucose levels in diabetics. The investigators think that fiber acts by releasing the absorbed glucose to the bloodstream more slowly, as it takes a longer time for bulky foods, compared to refined foods, to be digested. Thus there is no bolus of available glucose in the blood at one time.[14] This effect may help healthy persons with weight control; the subject needs more research.

WHAT CAN FIBER DO IN THE DIET?

Only two points concerning a high-fiber diet can definitely be proven. First, fiber relieves constipation and its unpleasant effects. Second, a high-fiber diet can manage diverticular disease—unprocessed bran can relieve symptoms and discomfort and restore bowel habits to normal.

Jean Mayer has stated:

> Recent studies done in Britain and the United States, however, have shown that when patients suffering from diverticulitis are fed an appropriate amount of bran, several things happen. One of their symptoms—mild diarrhea—is reversed. (Apparently, the fiber absorbs some of the free liquid.) Also, since the softer stool moves more freely, the patient no longer has to strain. Gradually, the "irritated bowel syndrome," which results from exaggerated muscle contractions, disappears. Finally, bowel movements become regular, and the need for a laxative drops.[15]

Recent research shows that the recommended medical management of diverticulosis includes (1) adequate bulk in the diet to prevent marked pressures and (2) antispasmodic drugs.[16]

However, studies of various other problems connected with a low-fiber diet seem to indicate that fiber can do much more. Dr. Burkitt, Dr. Painter, and their colleagues observed that in African rural areas where the diet is quite coarse, the people do not experience the discomforts of constipation, cancer of the colon, irritable bowel, diverticulosis, or even appendicitis.[17]

ARE THERE PROBLEMS WITH A HIGH-FIBER DIET?

Whatever the scientific merits of the high-fiber theory, consumers have already been eating a little more fiber than they may realize. For more than a decade, cellulose processed mainly from wood pulp or cotton has been added in minute quantities to dozens of foods. It has been used in ice cream to prevent crystals from forming, in low-calorie salad dressings to keep the ingredients from separating, and as a stabilizer in whipped cream toppings and powdered and liquid egg substitutes. Cellulose is added to reconstituted foods, such as frozen fish sticks, to hold the tiny bits of food together.

Cellulose also is used to give thickness to diet drinks and to prevent flavorings such as chocolate from settling out of solution. Such additives have gone unnoticed because purified cellulose does not change the color, flavor, or aroma of the product.

Lately, larger amounts of cellulose have been added to bread, and claims have been made that such loaves have 50 to 400 times more fiber and 25 to 33 percent fewer calories than competing brands. Some manufacturers also are experimenting with adding wood pulp to cookies, macaroni, rolls, cakes, and even meats.

Some people, swayed by the publicity for a high-fiber diet, may think they can solve their health or weight problems by eating food to which this wood pulp fiber has been added. Wood pulp fiber is not the same as the dietary fiber in brans, grains, fruits, and vegetables, and no one knows what the long-range effects of eating it will be. Moreover, wood pulp has no nutritive value. Eating foods to which wood pulp fiber has been added while sharply curtailing foods that provide essential nutrients could have very serious effects on the health.

Under the food and drug laws, manufacturers of products containing added cellulose cannot claim that eating such food will prevent disease or in any way improve health. For those who wish to increase their fiber intake, the Food and Drug Administration recommends eating more whole-grain breads and cereals and fresh fruits and vegetables. Even dietary fiber that occurs naturally in food should be taken in moderation. Fiber advocates themselves warn against too sudden a change in the diet; it takes time for the digestive system to adapt.

Scientists have not yet determined how much fiber anyone should eat. There are no Recommended Daily Allowances (U.S. RDA) for fiber. The source of the fiber is also important. Bran, for example, has a laxative effect, but some fruits and vegetables do not. Bran should never be eaten dry because it can clog the digestive system.

Eating a high-fiber diet can have some distressing side effects, such as a feeling of being stuffed or bloated. Stomach rumblings, usually frowned on in polite society, are caused by changes in the material passing through the intestines.

Large amounts of fiber can impair the body's ability to absorb certain important minerals such as iron, copper, and calcium. Eaten over a long period of time, large amounts of indigestible material such as fiber can lead to a condition called volvulus of the sigmoid colon, which requires surgery.

Experts in nutrition point out that fiber is just one part of a properly balanced diet. Adding fiber to a poor diet probably will cause more problems than it will solve. Much more research is needed before anyone can say with certainty what the full role of fiber is in the human diet.[18]

SUMMARY

There has been an explosion of interest in and research on dietary fiber. Its role as a preventive agent for some problems of the digestive and circulatory system is supported by epidemiology (the science of investigation and the cause of disease — particularly epidemic diseases), direct experimentation, and some ethnic and socioeconomic dietary patterns. However, although an increase of fiber in the typical American diet may be indicated, the idea that some chronic diseases can be cured by a high-fiber diet is simplistic. We do not yet know how much fiber is best in all situations, and claims made for the value of increased dietary fiber in preventing diseases such as varicose veins, heart disease, cancer, appendicitis, and hemorrhoids need to be substantiated by further research.

Meanwhile, following are a few good pointers just in case:

- Start the day with a bowl of bran or whole-grain cereal. Wheat, rye, barley, corn, and oats are all good, but rolled oats and wheat are best. It is wise to buy the long-cooking kind instead of the instant type. "Instant" generally means highly refined.

- Begin eating more fresh fruits and leafy or fibrous vegetables. Shorten cooking time when preparing them, as heat has a tendency to break down fiber.
- Finally when eating bread, use the whole-grain wheat. These few tips may do more to keep the doctor away than the proverbial apple.

NOTES

1. Denis P. Burkitt, "Western Civilization, Diet, and Disease," *Drug Therapy,* January 1974, pp. 51–62.
2. "Diverticulosis," *The Health Letter,* Vol. 5, No. 6, March 28, 1975.
3. Denis P. Burkitt, A. R. P. Walker, and N. S. Painter, "Dietary Fiber and Disease," *Journal of the American Medical Association,* Vol. 229, No. 8, August 19, 1974, pp. 1068–1074.
4. Ibid.
5. "On the High-Fiber Diet," *Executive Health,* Vol. 10, No. 7, p. 3.
6. P. J. Palumbo, et al., "High-Fiber Diet in Hyperlipemia," *Journal of the American Medical Association,* July 21, 1978, Vol. 246, No. 3, pp. 223–227.
7. Burkitt et al., "Dietary Fiber and Disease," pp. 1068–1074.
8. Denis P. Burkitt, "Food Fiber," *Cereal Foods World,* January 1977, pp. 6–9.
9. Burkitt, "Food Fiber," pp. 6–9.
10. Burkitt et al., "Dietary Fiber and Disease," p. 1071.
11. Burkitt, "Food Fiber," pp. 6–9.
12. "Roughage in the Diet," *Medical World News,* September 6, 1974, pp. 35–42.
13. Robert A. Levine, "High-Fiber Diets—The Theories and the Facts," *Current Prescribing,* July 1978, p. 54.
14. Jean Mayer, "Fiber: The Neglected Nutrient," *Family Health,* March 1973, pp. 41–42.
15. Ibid.
16. Thomas D. McCaffery, "Managing the Patient with Diverticulosis: Can Fiber Help?" *Modern Medicine,* August-September 1978, pp. 95–97.
17. "Roughage in the Diet," *Medical World News,* pp. 35–42.
18. Barbara Harland and Annabel Hecht, "Grandma Called It Roughage," *FDA Consumer,* July/August 1977, pp. 18–19.

10

The Burdensome Beverages

Liquids are important in the diet for body fluid replacement and valuable calorie and nutrient additions. Coffee, tea, alcohol, and cola have become some of the most popular beverages consumed throughout the world. Unfortunately although these beverages make significant caloric contributions to the diet, they do not make comparable nutrient additions. In fact, these beverages are practically devoid of food value, and may create dependence in the user. If you consume colas, coffee, tea, alcoholic beverages, or even cocoa, here are some important nutritional facts you should understand about these popular but burdensome beverages.

THE CAFFEINATED BREWS

For ages, people have brewed beverages from plants for pleasure consumption. The most popular of these brews today is, of course, coffee. The average American consumes three cups of coffee daily, or about 16 lb of coffee each year. Any coffee drinker can tell you about the nice pick-me-up feeling, the increased work output, the quieted nerves, and the relief from headache pain which accompany coffee consumption. Although coffee has no food value to provide energy sources to the body, studies show that coffee consumption (without sugar or cream) is accompanied by brain wave arousal, increased respiration, rising blood pressure, and increased reflex activity. But if only food can provide more energy for body functions, how does coffee accomplish all this?

Coffee and tea, cola and cocoa, contain the drug caffeine, a nervous system stimulant belonging to a class of alkaloids known as xanthines, which belong to the same **analeptic** (invigorating) drug group as speed pills, pep pills, and amphetamines. The xanthines also include theophylline, which is in tea, and theobromine, which is in cocoa and chocolate. The theophylline in tea is known to dilate coronary blood vessels, thus antagonizing blood vessel constriction, a well-known effect of caffeine. Theobromine is less potent than caffeine as a central nervous system stimulant, but it is more active as a cardiac stimulant and diuretic. Chocolate beverages often contain ten to twenty times more theobromine than caffeine.

The Active Ingredients

Caffeine is a natural plant substance found in small amounts in coffee beans, tea leaves, cocoa beans, and cola nuts. It can, however, be synthesized from dimethylurea and malonic acid. In a pure hydrated form, caffeine is a white, powdery solid much like cornstarch. It is odorless, very bitter to the taste, and slightly soluble. It is legal to buy and sell because it is not a physically addicting drug.

Caffeine manipulates the release of energy into the blood from body stores by blocking normal energy cut-off systems which stop certain body activities at a given point. In one body system, for example, a chemical called cyclic AMP (adenosine monophosphate) facilitates the release of sugar into the blood. During normal body function, another chemical, phosphodiesterase (PDE), terminates the flow of cyclic AMP when the ideal amount of sugar is reached. When caffeine is added to the system, it inhibits PDE activity so that the cyclic AMP continues releasing unnecessary sugar. This excess energy is available for immediate use, thus explaining the pick-me-up feeling coffee gives. Since as little as two cups of coffee significantly raises blood sugar, caffeine can aggravate diabetes or cause hyperglycemia.

Unfortunately, the body pays for the sudden energy loss several hours later with undue fatigue and decreased efficiency and alertness. A hangover effect is also produced one to three hours after the stimulant is taken — mental efficiency drops below normal values after having been improved. The feeling of well-being and increased performance is obtained at the expense of decreased efficiency later.

Coffee.   A cup of coffee contains anywhere from 100 to 500 mg of caffeine. (A single medicinal dose of the drug varies from 100 to 200 mg.) Caffeine content of coffee varies with the method of preparation. Drip and vacuum coffees contain the least amount of caffeine among the ground coffees. Percolated coffee (approximately 150 mg/cup) retains slightly more caffeine than does drip coffee, and boiled coffee contains more than either drip or percolated. Instant contains the lowest amount of caffeine, about 80 to 90 mg per cup. The strength of the original coffee beans also affects caffeine content. At present, no method has been devised to remove all the caffeine from coffee. However, decaffeinated coffee contains about .05 percent caffeine (15 to 25 mg per cup or about 3 percent of the original amount) as compared to 1.5 to 1.9 percent caffeine in regular coffee. Dr. Lawrence E. Lamb, a noted cardiologist, is of the opinion that coffee is so damaging to the central nervous system that eventually it will be recognized as one of the major health hazards of our society.[1]

Tea.   Tea leaves and coffee beans both contain about 1.5 percent caffeine, with tea leaves usually yielding a slightly larger proportion. However, in its final form most tea contains about half as much caffeine as coffee. Some teas contain up to 110 mg, but the usual amount is 50 to 75 mg per cup. In any case, Americans drink on the average only ½ cup of tea a day.

Cola Soft Drinks.   Caffeine is a natural constituent of the cola bean and is a legally required ingredient of the cola drinks. The FDA Standard of Identity for Soda Water requires that the presence of caffeine in cola beverages not exceed .02 percent by weight. Caffeine content in soft drinks varies from 2.4 mg to 6.0 mg per ounce. Two ten-ounce bottles of an average cola drink contain about the same amount of caffeine as one cup of coffee. The effect of the caffeine in cola drinks is the same as that of the caffeine in coffee.

Cola drinks are devoid of nutrients but rich in calories. They also supply sugar for decay-producing bacteria in the mouth.

Cocoa and Chocolate.   Many people don't realize that a single cup of cocoa contains 50 mg of caffeine (about half the amount in a cup of coffee), as well as theobromine. For a child, cocoa can be equivalent to coffee, since children's bodies are more sensative to drugs. Cocoa is also found in chocolate bars. The average 1½-oz. chocolate bar contains around 25 mg. Four such bars would equal a single cup of coffee in caffeine value. White chocolate contains the same amount of caffeine as milk chocolate, though it may contain a slightly smaller amount of theobromine than milk chocolate.

Coordination and Metabolism. Although caffeine speeds up mental stimulation, it impairs motor coordination and reduces accuracy. Recently acquired manual skills or those requiring fine muscular coordination may be particularly affected.

Effects of Caffeine

Caffeine and the other xanthines increase the resting metabolic rate 10 to 15 percent and accelerate food-burning for energy, which requires greater oxygen supplies. Caffeine may be helpful in weight reduction. When calories are severely restricted, the body decreases metabolism as a protective measure, which lessens weight loss. Caffeine stimulates metabolism to counteract the body mechanism, reduces appetite, and helps maintain energy.

A single cup of coffee containing as little as 50 to 100 mg of caffeine can produce numerous body reactions. Caffeine is a nervous system stimulant which temporarily relieves fatigue, and improves thinking and idea association. It can increase sensitivity to light, touch, and other stimuli to the point where the sensations become unpleasant or even painful. This prolonging and magnification of nerve messages may explain the tremors, agitation, and occasional convulsions experienced with large amounts of the drug.

The Heart. Recent studies have not shown a causal relationship between caffeine and heart disease. However, even if caffeine is not the direct cause of heart attacks, it may be related in several ways.[2] Caffeine stimulates heart muscle fibers, and excess amounts can increase heart rate, an important indication of heart function, even in young, healthy persons. People with resting heart rates below 70/minute have much less chance of suffering a heart attack than those with rates over 80/minute. Both coffee and cigarettes increase heart rate in sensitive people. Because of stress, anxiety, excitement, poor physical condition, and ingestion of harmful drugs, some sedentary office workers have resting heart rates of over 100.

Caffeine consumption lessens a person's maximum physical capacity by forcing the heart to work harder. Because metabolism speeds up, circulation must deliver more oxygen to cells, which means the heart must pump more blood. This is expecially detrimental for persons who already have heart disease. Caffeine and related drugs also worsen heart irregularities (**arrhythmia**) described as the heart's "skipping a beat" or "turning over" and sudden attacks of fast heartbeat. To relieve the pain due to heart disease, physicians attempt to lower body metabolism to decrease the body's need for oxygen and to lower thyroid function. Physical rest and avoidance of caffeine and other similar drugs which increase body metabolism are prescribed.

Caffeine causes a drop in a special enzyme which removes fat from the blood. An increase in free fatty acids and sugar in the blood is associated with greater risk of high blood pressure. In other parts of the circulatory system, caffeine causes a constriction of the blood vessels in the brain, with a decrease in cerebral flow.

Caffeine may not be the only consideration in the link between coffee and heart disease, however. The *Journal of the American Medical Association* warns:

> If you're convalescing from a heart attack, don't drink hot beverages. They can cause a slowing of the rate and premature contractions of the heart.
>
> Sixty patients who had suffered acute heart attacks were monitored at St. Vincent's Medical Center of Richmond, Staten Island, New York, after swallowing glasses of hot and cold water. Sixteen of the 60 heart attack patients who drank the hot water showed marked changes in heart action. One patient had problems after both hot and cold drinks. None of the group of 40 controls who also were given the beverages showed any change.
>
> The control group was drawn from persons who had survived for at least six months after a heart attack, in addition to some entirely healthy subjects.
>
> Administration of a drug, atropine sulfate, prior to drinking the hot water warded off the danger of poor heart action.[3]

Digestion. Caffeine stimulates the formation of acid-pepsin digestive juice in the stomach. Excessive acid digestive juice may lead to peptic ulcers, particularly of the duodenum. If coffee is drunk alone without food, as it often is in the United States, the caffeine stimulates high levels of acid secretion without the buffering action of food. Patients with peptic ulcer or a predisposition to ulcer disease may be more sensitive to coffee. Ulcer patients especially should avoid coffee.

Flavor oils in coffee are also irritating to the digestive tract and can cause diarrhea in susceptible persons. Even decaffeinated products have irritating coffee oils and should be avoided by patients with digestive disturbances. The tannin in tea has the opposite effect and can cause constipation. This is why tea is administered during acute diarrhea.

Others who should avoid coffee are those on bland diets and those with abdominal pain as seen in spastic or irritable colon, diverticulosis, or diarrhea. Some individuals with overactive bowels who experience spasm of the colon, diarrhea, and abdominal pains precipitated by emotional tension are given tranquilizers and agents to decrease the overactive contractions of the colon. Coffee should not be drunk while one is on this medicine because it causes the opposite effect of these medicines and thus negates both the tranquilizing and antispasmodic actions.

In one study of 11,000 former college students who were daily coffee drinkers (one to two cups), it was found that the users, compared to abstainers, were at one to four times the risk of developing peptic ulcers later in life. The risk was the same for cigarette smokers compared to nonsmokers. Habitual coffee consumption was a better predictor of subsequent peptic ulcer than the cigarette habit. However, the combination of coffee drinking and cigarette smoking yields a risk 1.6 times that of abstinence.[4]

There are some who feel the above-described effects may be the result of other substances in coffee besides or in combination with caffeine.

There are a few studies that have also linked coffee and other caffeine containing beverages with bladder cancer. However, this is strictly a statistical relationship at this time, with no evident cause and effect relationship.

Chromosome Damage. Caffeine can cause chromosomal damage (breakage and fragmentation) in humans as well as in lower animals. However, at the present time caffeine would probably be considered a weak mutagen. Caffeine can pass freely from the blood to the ovaries and testes and from the blood of a woman who is seven to eight weeks pregnant to the fetus. However, it is not known whether this has an effect on birth defects.

The Center for Science in The Public Interest did find that some animals fed equivalents of the caffeine present in eleven cups of coffee gave birth to offspring with cleft palates, missing digits, and malformed skulls.[5]

Although the levels of caffeine consumption that caused defects in animal studies are levels to which a small minority of pregnant women are likely to be exposed, the Center has suggested to the U.S. Department of Health, Education, and Welfare that women, especially those in the first three months of pregnancy, be advised to minimize their consumption of coffee, tea, cola beverages, and non-prescription drugs containing caffeine, even though the studies do not prove that caffeine causes birth defects, miscarriages, or infertility in humans. It has also been found that heavy caffeine use by pregnant women may cause their babies to be less active at birth and have poorer-than-average muscle tone.[6]

Therapeutic Uses of Caffeine. Although caffeine's main use is in caffeinated beverages, it also is ingested as a main or secondary ingredient in many non-prescription **therapeutic** drugs. For example, No-Doze contains about 110 mg of caffeine while Excedrin contains 60 mg. Caffeine and its related drug compounds possess some important pharmacological properties.

Uses and Misuses

Both caffeine and theophylline lower venous blood pressure and increase cardiac output. Only theophylline is used to treat congestive heart failure, however, because of the stimulating effects caffeine has on the central nervous system. The xanthines may also be used to relieve paroxysmal **dyspnea** (sudden periodic attacks of labored, painful breathing) associated with left heart failure. They are also used to lessen the frequency and severity of attacks of **angina pectoris** and in the management of **coronary** thrombosis.

In large doses, caffeine is used to rouse patients from coma. Because it stimulates heart rate, blood flow, and the central nervous system, it is used to treat aspirin, barbiturate, morphine, and alcohol poisoning. It acts as a mild respiratory stimulant, especially in morphine-induced depression. Also, it is used to rouse patients from abnormal functioning of the pancreas.

Caffeine and the other xanthines are widely used to treat headaches. In this case, caffeine is combined with an **analgesic** such as a salicylate to treat ordinary headaches or with ergot alkaloid to treat migraines. During a migraine, dilated arteries in the head stretch the small nerve fibers in the artery walls; caffeine induces vaso-constriction to relieve such pain. The average dose for treatment of migraine headache is 150 to 500 mgs taken orally.

The xanthines relax smooth muscles of the bronchi, and theophylline especially is used to treat bronchial asthma. They are also used to control biliary (pertaining to the bile ducts, gallbladder, hepatic ducts, or liver) spasm which has been produced by injection of morphine, dihydromorphinone hydrochloride, or codeine. The xanthines increase specific muscle contraction; caffeine especially increases the capacity to do work. A new use being researched is the treatment of **hyperkinetic** children with caffeine.

Individual Differences.   Individual response to caffeine, as with any drug, varies widely. For some individuals, a single cup of coffee can cause a whole night of sleeplessness. Others can drink three or even five cups and sleep soundly. The effects of drugs are also more profound and concentrated in children. A 70-pound ten-year-old who drinks four colas and eats three chocolate bars during the day consumes more caffeine per kilogram of weight than does a 170-pound man who drinks seven cups of coffee per day.

Early morning wakenings and difficulty getting to sleep are problems that particularly plague the elderly who use caffeine products.

Dependence Syndrome.   Caffeinated beverages, especially coffee, induce dependence upon the stimulating effects of the drug contents. When deprived of their usual morning coffee, users suffer mental craving, irritability, nervousness, and severe headaches. These symptoms will disappear with several days abstinence as the body readjusts to function without caffeine. Withdrawal symptoms can be relieved instantly with a single cup of coffee. Heavy drinkers who drink to lessen lethargy and the discomfort of headaches, irritability, and nervousness may find it easier to taper their coffee consumption rather than quit it all at once when they decide to stop using caffeinated beverages.

At a recent American Psychiatric Association meeting, Dr. John Greden, director of psychiatric research at Walter Reed Army Medical Center, said, "Too much coffee can produce 'caffeinism.' And 'caffeinism' can masquerade very well as a psychiatric disorder. According to Dr. Greden, large doses of caffeine can mimic chronic anxiety, a disorder normally treated with psychotherapy and tranquilizers. Symptoms include headaches, irritability, restlessness, insomnia, hallucinations, muscle twitching, vomiting, and diarrhea.[7] The result is that doctors try to treat the disorder with still more drugs when they should be getting rid of one.

The aforementioned symptoms can be produced in some people with as little as 250 mg. of caffeine, a dosage frequently exceeded by many people on a daily basis. Dr. Greden said: "For example, three cups of coffee, two headache tablets and a cola drink consumed in one morning, approximate 500 mg. of caffeine intake. Among heavy coffee or tea drinkers, ingested dosages frequently exceed this by gross amounts." He concluded by saying: "All medications including caffeine have potential for abuse and many individuals clearly ingest symptom-producing doses daily through use of tea, coffee and medication."[8]

Caffeine Poisoning.   Caffeine poisoning can result in death, but fatality is rare. Usually caffeine poisoning reaches only the stage of neurasthenia (depressed state characterized by a sense of weakness or exhaustion), which incapacitates a person to work. The toxic dose for humans, about ten grams, is so large that caffeine overdose is rare. A person would have to drink about 70 to 100 cups of coffee to reach that amount. Central nervous system depressants, such as short-acting barbiturates, are given to counteract caffeine poisoning.

Unpleasant reactions to caffeine can take place with even a one-gram dose (insomnia, restlessness, and excitement that may progress to mild delirium). Caffeine combined with other substances can also trigger adverse reactions. It is wise when taking any new medicine to quit taking old drugs. This includes the caffeine found in tea, colas, coffee, and cocoa.

Caffeine Cure for Drunkenness. Many Americans believe the popular notion that coffee is useful to sober up drunks. In actuality, there is no substance that can speed up the metabolism of alcohol in the body or combat its effects. All caffeine does is wake up the drunk and perhaps relieve headache caused by overdilation of the arteries in the brain and head region.

ALCOHOLIC BEVERAGES AND NUTRITION

About 70 percent of the adult American population drink alcoholic beverages. Twelve percent are heavy drinkers who drink almost daily. Alcohol itself is a drug and can be classified as a sedative, tranquilizer, hypnotic, or anesthetic depending on the quantity consumed. Unfortunately, like the caffeinated beverages, alcohol does not contain a fair share of nutrients to justify the number of calories it contains. In fact, except for minute amounts of B vitamins and traces of minerals in wines and beer, alcoholic beverages contain no nutrients. Most of the nutrients originally present in the grains, grapes, or other fruits are lost during processing. Table 10-1 lists the nutritional content of alcoholic beverages.

Table 10-1. Nutritional Content of Alcoholic Beverages

Food nutrient*	Type of beverage and quantity†					
	Beer 12 oz.	Rum 1.5 oz.	Whiskey 1.5 oz.	Martini 2 oz.	Manhattan‡ 2 oz.	Wine§ 4 oz.
Calories	175.0	150.0	110.0	160.0	160.0	160.0
Calories from alcohol	125.0	150.0	110.0	110.0	110.0	145.0
Protein (grams)	2.0	0.0	0.0	0.0	0.0	0.0
Fat (grams)	0.0	0.0	0.0	0.0	0.0	0.0
Carbohydrate (grams)	12.0	0.0	0.0	0.0	0.0	4.2
Thiamine (milligrams)	0.1	0.0	0.0	0.0	0.0	0.0
Nicotinic Acid (milligrams)	0.75	0.0	0.0	0.0	0.0	0.0
Riboflavin (milligrams)	10.0	0.0	0.0	0.0	0.0	0.0
Ascorbic Acid (milligrams)	0.0	0.0	0.0	0.0	0.0	0.0
Folic Acid (milligrams)	0.0	0.0	0.0	0.0	0.0	0.0

*Approximate amounts only.

†Quantities — as most often consumed.

‡Only accounts for caloric content of mixer.

§Dry wine — 20 percent alcoholic content.

Alcohol does contain plenty of calories—about two hundred calories per fluid ounce. Alcohol contains about seven calories per gram as compared with four calories per gram for either carbohydrates or proteins, or nine from fat. Moreover, in beer, some additional calories, about four per ounce, remain from the surviving cereal content of the original grain that was fermented.

Alcoholic beverages containing appreciable amounts of carbohydrate in addition to the alcohol are the highest in calories. These include sweet liquors, dessert wines, drinks mixed with ginger ale or sweetened soda, and special beverages with additional cream, sugar, chocolate, and coconut.

Alcohol is a major factor in obesity; its consumption sabotages efforts to control fat through diet and exercise. For social drinkers who have a tendency to gain weight, one or two daily cocktails make the difference between success and failure in a weight control program.

Malnutrition

If alcohol becomes one of the major sources of calories in the diet, as often happens with heavy drinkers, serious nutritional complications can result. Over 15 million Americans consume enough alcohol to account for at least 75 percent of their daily caloric intake.

Even the circumstances surrounding alcoholic consumption encourage poor food selection, irregular meals, and the purchase of expensive but nutritionally poor food snacks. **Gastritis** caused by heavy alcohol consumption also diminishes the appetite for normal foods. An average alcoholic consumes a diet consisting of about 9/10 of the needed calories, 2/3 of the needed protein, 1/2 the B-vitamin requirement, and 1/4 of the needed amount of magnesium, phosphorus, and zinc.[9]

Heavy alcohol consumption causes injury to the absorbing surface of the small intestine. Even though the body may need nutrients, the intestine is able to absorb only 1/2 the B vitamins, thiamine, and folic acid, and about 2/3 of the amino acids present. Alcohol also increases the urinary loss of some amino acids and minerals, including magnesium, zinc, potassium, and phosphorus. Frequent intestinal upsets resulting in diarrhea and vomiting account for further mineral loss. Folic acid, pyridoxine, several of the B vitamins, and other nutrients are depleted in meeting the increased need to burn off the alcohol. A combination of alcohol and a deficiency of essential nutrients, special proteins, and certain vitamins may predispose heavy drinkers to **cirrhosis** of the liver.[10]

Alcohol also interferes with the normal utilization and metabolism of food, and this can lead to numerous nutritional disorders. In the liver, alcohol metabolism will have priority over metabolism of foodstuffs. Thus, there is a type of competition in which alcohol will win, so that some of the food eaten cannot be properly utilized by the body.

Factors in Alcohol Absorption

Under ordinary conditions, the alcohol in any beverage is absorbed relatively quickly through the stomach walls and the small intestine and then distributed throughout the body. The absorption can be markedly influenced by a number of physical and psychological factors.[11]

Alcohol Concentration. The greater the alcohol concentration of the beverage—up to a maximum of about 40 percent (80 proof)—the more rapidly the alcohol is absorbed and the higher are the resulting peak blood-alcohol concentrations. With identical amounts of alcohol swallowed, the highest blood-alcohol levels are produced by undiluted distilled spirits, and the lowest by beers.

Other Chemicals in the Beverage. The greater the amount of nonalcoholic chemicals in the beverage, the more slowly the alcohol is absorbed. For this reason, the alcohol in distilled spirits—especially vodka and gin—is absorbed most rapidly, and that in table wines and beers most slowly.

Presence of Food in the Stomach. Eating with drinking has a noticeable effect on the absorption of alcohol, especially when alcohol is consumed in the form of distilled spirits or wine. When alcoholic beverages are taken with a substantial meal, peak blood-alcohol concentrations may be reduced by as much as 50 percent.

Speed of Drinking. The more rapidly the beverage is ingested, the higher the peak blood-alcohol concentrations will be. Thus, these levels are lower when the beverage is sipped or taken in divided amounts than when it is gulped or taken in a single dose.

Emptying Time of the Stomach. In a number of clinical conditions, such as that marked by the "dumping syndrome," the stomach empties more rapidly than is normal, and alcohol seems to be absorbed more quickly. Emptying may be either slowed or speeded by fear, anger, stress, nausea, and the condition of the stomach tissues.

Body Weight. The greater the body weight of an individual, the lower the blood-alcohol concentration resulting from ingestion of a standard amount of alcohol will be. The blood-alcohol level produced in a 180-pound man consuming four ounces of distilled spirits, for example, will generally be substantially lower than that occurring when the same amount is taken by a 130-pound man in the same length of time.[12]

The most notable and dramatic effects of alcohol are attributable to its action on the brain and are related solely to its concentration in the blood.

Inhibitions. Alcohol tends to reduce people's inhibitions or shyness and loosen self-control, although they may feel this effect as stimulation. Some of the feelings that may be released include anger, hostility, sensations of inferiority or superiority, overconfidence, love, generosity, tenderness, and jealousy. All of these feelings may result in unusual (for the drinker) behavior, such as crying, fighting, yelling, hugging, laughing, nagging, and taking risks. However, people with no major hang-ups may experience no important changes in behavior when they drink.

Thinking. While small amounts of alcohol with food will not normally affect most people's ability to think clearly, increasing amounts tend to make it harder for people to make judgments, concentrate, and understand. In particular, alcohol may prevent inexperienced drinkers from realizing that their ability to think clearly and act normally has diminished.

Psychological Effects

Performance.   Generally speaking, the more alcohol a person drinks, the more difficulty he or she will have doing physical tasks. However, moderate amounts of alcohol (one or two drinks) do not seem to hurt many people's ability to act sensibly. For some people and some tasks, small amounts of alcohol may help them to do things better, perhaps because it relaxes them by removing tension or nervousness which sometimes inhibits behavior. For example, a couple of drinks can make sexual activity easier for some people—but larger amounts of alcohol make sex difficult and often impossible.

Physiological   As previously mentioned, the speed of alcohol absorption generally affects the rate
Effects   at which one becomes intoxicated. Conversely, the speed of alcohol metabolism affects the rate at which one becomes sober again.

Once absorbed into the bloodstream and distributed throughout the body, alcohol undergoes metabolic or oxidative changes. It is first converted into acetaldehyde, a highly irritating, toxic chemical. However, this substance rarely accumulates, since it is quickly oxidized to acetate, which is transformed into a variety of other compounds and eventually oxidized completely to carbon dioxide and water. Although between 2 and 5 percent of the alcohol is excreted chemically unchanged (mostly in the form of urine, breath, and sweat), most of the ingested alcohol is oxidized by the liver at the rate of about one-third of an ounce of pure alcohol per hour. Individual differences do exist because the rate of metabolic processes may vary a little. Alcohol affects various parts of the body in a number of ways.

Stomach.   A small amount of alcohol tends to increase the flow of juices and starts mild activity that is often felt as hunger. If a person has ulcers, the added flow of juices can be harmful. Heartburn may be a sharp irritation of the lining, caused by these juices, and resulting from the absence of enough food to neutralize them. Heavy drinkers may have a chronic inflammation of the stomach lining.

Liver.   After one indulges in prolonged heavy drinking, the liver can become swollen and tender (acute hepatitis). In severe cases, cirrhosis may occur. Incidence of cirrhosis is increasing, and about 10 percent of alcoholic persons develop the disease. Cirrhosis is characterized by diffuse scarring of the liver. Duration and amount of alcohol consumption correlate with this disabling and potentially fatal complication.

Kidneys and Other Glands.   Alcohol increases urinary activity. This activity is caused by the effect of alcohol on the pituitary gland. Alcohol inhibits the secretion of an antidiuretic hormone produced by the pituitary gland; therefore, the kidney forms more urine. This gland normally acts as a brake on the production of urine. Alcohol suppresses the secretion of another pituitary hormone that is normally involved in the production of labor in pregnant women; thus, it can delay childbirth.

Water Balance.   Laboratory experiments have shown that after an individual has been drinking, his or her water balance shifts. Water moves from inside the cells to the space around them and causes a feeling of thirst. It is not known whether this shift has any other effect on the body. Alcohol causes dehydration because of a suppression of the antidiuretic hormone. Prolonged drinking leads to cellular retention and severe depression of cellular functions.

Heart and Circulation. Alcohol produces an effect known as "blood sludging." Alcohol causes red blood cells to stick together in clumps, which may entirely plug capillaries. When sludging is extensive, cells in entire areas of an organ will starve for oxygen. This has been identified particularly in the eye. It is possible that this mechanism causes other damage to the body. Alcohol causes an increase in heartbeat and blood flow, and the blood vessels near the surface of the skin become dilated, producing a feeling of warmth. However, this actually causes the body to lose a slight amount of heat. A higher rate of heart disease among former drinkers than among nondrinkers suggests a need for further research.

Alcohol-precipitated heart conditions usually occur in cases of heavy drinking or a preexisting heart condition. Some recent information in popular literature suggests that one to two drinks of alcohol per day may decrease the risk of having a heart attack. However, data supporting that claim have not been duplicated in extensive experimentation. Further research is now being conducted.

Disease Syndromes. Heavy drinkers have long been known to have lowered resistance to pneumonia and other infectious diseases. Since lowered resistance may occur in well-nourished heavy drinkers, it appears to result from a direct interference with immunity mechanisms. Recent research suggests that there is a relationship between heavy drinking and cancer of the mouth, pharynx, and esophagus.

Unless permanent organ damage has occurred, most heavy drinkers can recover their health quickly by discontinuing alcohol consumption and returning to an adequate diet. The nutritional complications of alcohol ingestion comprise only a small portion of the medical and social problems caused by alcohol. The National Council on Alcoholism (NCA) states that the effects of alcohol are responsible for more deaths in the United States than any other problem except heart disease and cancer.

SUMMARY

Caffeine is a constituent of beverages such as coffee, cola drinks, chocolate drinks, and tea. Caffeine is a nervous system stimulant, a cardiac stimulant, and a diuretic.

Caffeine affects many body functions. For example, it speeds up mental stimulation, but it impairs motor coordination so that accuracy is reduced.

The theory that there is a relationship between heart disease and caffeine has not been substantiated. However, even if caffeine is not a direct cause of heart disease, there is probably at least some minor relationships between the two. Caffeine can elevate the heart rate because of its stimulant action, and has been known to produce heart palpitations.

Caffeine can affect digestion by causing the digestive organs—especially the stomach—to produce more enzymes and acids than necessary. This can result in various gastrointestinal upsets.

Caffeine can cause chromosome damage in humans and in animals. Animals that ingested excess caffeine have produced offspring with such birth defects as cleft palates, missing fingers and toes, and malformed skulls.

Excessive use of caffeine can produce various symptoms such as insomnia, restlessness, and tremulousness. Caffeine has, on the other hand, been used therapeutically to alleviate migraine headaches.

Alcohol abuse has become one of our major health problems in the United States, with 12 percent of the population being heavy drinkers. Even though alcohol contains many calories, it has very little nutrient value; thus heavy drinkers may develop nutritional deficiencies.

Alcohol absorption is affected by several factors, such as the concentration of the alcohol in the beverage, other chemicals present in the beverage, whether or not there is food in the stomach, how fast the alcohol is ingested, how quickly the stomach empties, and the drinker's body weight.

Psychologically, alcohol affects the inhibitions (so that a person feels less inhibited and will do things that he or she normally would not do), thinking (so that it is harder to make judgments, concentrate, and comprehend), and performance (so that it is harder to perform physical tasks).

Physically, alcohol affects the liver (which is the major organ for metabolizing alcohol), the stomach (which produces increased gastric juices), the kidneys (which become more active), water balance (so that some degree of dehydration occurs), and the heart, and lowers resistance to disease.

NOTES

1. Leon H. Abrams Jr., "Caffeine—A Paradigm of Subliminal Cultural Drug Habituation," *Journal of Applied Nutrition,* September 1976, pp. 33-40.
2. O. Paul et al, "A Longitudinal Study of Coronary Heart Disease," *Circulation,* Vol. 28, 1963, pp. 20-31.
3. "Extrinsically Induced Arrhythmia in Acute Myocardial Infarctions," *Journal of the American Medical Association,* May 20, 1974, p. 1021.
4. "The Medical Effects of Coffee," *Medical World News,* January 26, 1976, pp. 63-73.
5. "Coffee May Perk Up Pregnant Mom, but Not Her Baby," *Medical World News,* April 17, 1978, pp. 8, 13.
6. Ibid.
7. Greden, "Caffeinism Can Mimic Chronic Anxiety," *American Journal of Psychiatry,* Vol. 131, 1974, p. 1089.
8. Ibid.
9. Communications, Inc., *The Health Letter,* Vol. 1, No. 4, 1973.
10. Ibid.
11. National Institute on Alcohol Abuse and Alcoholism, *Facts About Alcohol and Alcoholism,* DHEW Publication No. (ADM) 74-31, 1974, pp. 1-44.
12. *People Do Drink and Drive* (Washington, D.C.: American Driver and Traffic Safety Education Association, 1973), pp. 1-25.

11

Vegetarianism—Health or Hazard?

Anyone who subscribed to the vegetarian lifestyle fifty years ago would have been considered an eccentric, a fanatic or perhaps even a crackpot. But within recent years vegetarianism has become a way of life for over 10 million Americans, a number that is increasing daily.[1] With so many people adhering to such a philosophy, one is naturally inclined to ask, "Can this be merely a fad? Or is there some sound reasoning behind such a forbearing diet?"

WHO'S WHO IN THE VEGETARIAN HALL OF FAME?

Actually, vegetarianism has had its disciples throughout history. A story is told of a woman who was invited to dine at the home of Leo Tolstoy. Upon arriving, she was shocked to find a live chicken tied to her chair. When she inquired about the matter, Tolstoy told her, "My conscience forbids me to kill it. As you are the only guest taking meat, I would be greatly obliged if you would undertake the killing first."[2] Gandhi stated, "I hold flesh to be unsuited to our species."[3] The great athletes of ancient Greece also followed vegetarian diets. Other names to be added to this list are Voltaire, Milton, Newton, Shelley, Schweitzer, and George Bernard Shaw, to mention a few.

WHY DO PEOPLE BECOME VEGETARIANS?

Never have so many people sought to make vegetarianism a way of life at one time for so many varying reasons. These include: ethics, philosophy, aesthetics, economics, and nutrition.

Ethics

Numerous arguments in favor of vegetarianism could be listed under ethics. Life is sacred. To the Hindus who believe in the transmigration of souls there is no moral difference between the killing of a man and that of a beast. The Buddhist and Tau religions also believe this. In the western hemisphere, two contemporary protestant sects—the Bible Christians and the Seventh-Day Adventists—respectfully ask their followers to abstain from flesh eating. They believe that all life has a right to live out the full span of its existence, that no one but God should destroy a life.

Philosophy

Philosophically speaking, many people say that if humans had been intended to eat meat, they would have been constructed more like a carnivore, with claws for catching prey and long teeth for eating it and a gastrointestinal tract that would eliminate animal toxics instead of absorbing them. Many say, therefore, that we should substitute some other product for meat, instead of killing. Gandhi stated, "We err in copying the lower animal world—if we are superior to it."[4]

Aesthetics

For some, the thought of killing animals is repugnant. To many who become vegetarians, aesthetically speaking it is degrading. Jean Mayer stated, "The humane vegetarians believe that just as air bombing, through its remoteness, has 'sanitized' the killing of large numbers of civilians, our assemblyline methods of having animals killed, butchered, and made into steak or salami has made many people forget where their meat comes from."[5] Were others to view the bloody scene of a slaughterhouse, the aesthetic vegetarians believe that they too might join the ranks of vegetarianism.

Economics.

People in the United States consume an incredible amount of flesh yearly—an estimated 1/2 pound of meat per person daily. In other countries, Japan for instance, 1/2 pound per person is a monthly average. In a recent year, the average American devoured 66 times as much meat as did the average Indian.[6] In a world where so many people are starving and an even more overwhelming number are suffering from malnutrition, vegetarians, as well as others, are asking if the economy can stand our foolish consumption of meat.

The agriculturists tell us that plants produce eight of the essential amino acids more efficiently, pound-to-acre, than does meat. For instance, "crops such as soybeans, peas, and beans yield 13 pounds of these amino acids per acre; others, including carrots, potatoes, cauliflower, grown rice, and cabbage, yield approximately 4.2 pounds per acre, whereas the corresponding figure of only 1.6 pounds for poultry, beef, lamb, and pork."[7] The following table compares yields of one acre of land for meat and nonmeat products.

Final Product	Total Weight (in pounds)
Beef	182.5
Mutton	228.0
Wheat	1,680.0
Barley	1,800.0
Beans	1,800.0
Oats	2,300.0
Maize	3,120.0
Rice	4,565.0
Potatoes	20,160.0

From "Meat: Too Dear A Price To Pay?" Today's Health, *October 1974, p. 73.*

The relationships in terms of protein yield are just as disparate. According to the President's Science Advisory Committee, it takes 21.4 pounds of nonanimal protein to produce one pound of beef protein.[8] Considering these statistics and the high prices of meat, many cannot afford a flesh diet. Vegetarianism is economically wise.

Nutrition

Vegetarians feel that animal products are poison to the body. They contain toxins, the wrong nutrients, and infectious bacteria, while foods from the plant kingdom are wholesome, pure, and, above all, health promoting.[9] Some research findings have shown that reliance on plant foods *may* reduce the incidence of obesity, heart disease, cancer, osteoporosis (softening of the bones), hypertension, and some gastrointestinal disorders.[10] However, further studies are needed to clarify and substantiate these studies.

WHAT ARE SOME OF THE FACTS AND FALLACIES?

"Man cannot live by bread alone." Thus spake Jesus on the Mount of Temptation, and truer words were never spoken.

A common fallacy today is that of George Ohsawa, a proponent of macrobiotics, who stated that if man's spirit is right, his body will transmute the one food ingested (brown rice generally) into the elements needed by the body.[11] Louis Kervan and Professor Boranger, of the Polytechnique School in Paris, postulate that if one's thoughts are right, one's body can literally change vegetable to animal matter, carbohydrate to sugar, sugar to protein, etc.[12] This is certainly false—and extremely dangerous to one's health, if followed. The machine that houses a human mind must have certain elements to exist, and if any of these vital ingredients should be omitted, malfunction will ensue. No single food, regardless of its source, can supply all of our vital nutritional needs.

On the other hand, the idea that we must have meat to obtain the adequate nutrition necessary for good health is also a fallacy. True, meat is a complete protein source; however, a diet containing certain combinations of vegetable proteins will supply the needed amount of life-giving proteins to the body. Moreover, there is no substance to the popular belief that vegetable protein is inferior to meat protein. The truth is that we can subsist perfectly well on vegetable proteins. Just to illustrate, during World War I, the British naval blockade made it virtually impossible for the Danish to obtain meat. Those nutritionists who studied the people during this time indicated a meaningful change for the good in their overall health. Following the war, when supplies of meat were again available, a general decrease in good health was recorded.[13]

One of the facts we might consider at this point is that of weight. A vegetarian diet can cause a weight loss. Studies have shown that vegetarians are closer to their correct weight size than nonvegetarians. In fact, one nutritionist stated that she has "never seen a new vegetarian who was overweight. In fact, most weighed a good deal less than average."[14]

WHAT IS A VEGETARIAN DIET?

Not all vegetarians are the same, nor do they all follow the same code of dietary ethics. For classification purposes we will put them into three groups, although there certainly are variations. First are the *strict vegetarians*. They exclude all meat and meat byproducts, such as milk, eggs, cheese, ice cream, etc. Many of the newest dietary fads groups adhere to this rigid pattern. However, some, for no explainable reason, include honey in their diet, even though it is an animal product.

The *lacto-vegetarians* are less strict. Their diet includes milk and other dairy products, but excludes meat and eggs. The final group is the *ovo-lacto-vegetarians.* In this group, meat is still taboo, but eggs, milk, and other dairy products are acceptable.

WHAT ARE SOME OF THE NUTRITIONAL PROBLEMS?

Protein   Protein tends to be a big worry for those considering a vegetarian diet. The thing to remember when considering proteins is that to be useful to humans all eight essential amino acids must be ingested simultaneously, and in right proportion. Incomplete proteins end up as fat or are used as energy, but cannot be used to build muscle or tissue.

Two criteria are used when evaluating protein sources: quality and quantity. *Quality* is expressed on a scale of 0 to 100, measuring the usefulness of protein to the body. The following table gives a protein quality rating for various foods.

WHO PROTEIN QUALITY RATING

Product	Rating
Meat	67
Whole Rice	70
Cheese	70
Fish	80
Milk	82
Eggs	95

Quantity, on the other hand, is the proportion of usable protein to total weight, expressed as a percentage. If a food has a rating of 20 to 30 percent, it means that only 20 to 30 percent of the total weight of that food is usable protein—the rest is water, fat, and trace elements. The following table gives quantity ratings for various products.

WHO PROTEIN QUANTITY RATING

Soybean Flour	40%
Parmesan Cheese	36%
Nuts & Seeds	20–30%
Peas, Lentils and Dried Beans	20–25%
Eggs	13%
Milk	4%

A person can eat proportionally less meat than vegetables to obtain equal amounts of usable protein. Meats are a complete source of protein and are therefore easier to use. However, with careful planning, vegetable proteins can be equally effective.

Meat analogs are simulated meat products made from edible plants and should provide the necessary protein requirements. Soybeans are the most common ingredient used because it provides the highest quality protein. However, analogs often contain egg whites or nonfat dry milk, so they would not be suitable for strict vegetarian diets.

Another concern is that vegetarian diets are often so high in bulk that they may not meet caloric needs. Because of diminished calories, protein is used as an energy source; thus, a protein content equivalent to the recommended daily allowance (RDA) may become marginal.

Calcium

Calcium tends to be the biggest problem in any diet that avoids milk and dairy products, particularly for women and children. A lack of calcium combined with a lack of vitamin D is a major cause of rickets, and a woman who is nursing a child will rob her own bones to produce the calcium not available through her diet. In a lacto- or ovo-lacto-vegetarian diet this is no problem, of course.

There are certain vegetables that are worthwhile sources of calcium, such as collards, dandelion greens, kale, mustard greens and turnip greens. However, not even these are sufficient for mother and child. Many believe that powdered alfalfa and similar uncooked vegetables make excellent sources of milk. This is not true! Cows may be able to produce milk by eating the like, but humans cannot. Milk is the only reliable source of calcium.

Vitamin B$_{12}$

Strict vegetarians who exclude all animal products including milk and eggs risk the danger of a vitamin B$_{12}$ deficiency. Vitamin B$_{12}$ is essential for blood cell formation and normal functioning of the nerves. The Vegans, a popular dietary group, prescribe a diet that frequently causes a degeneration of the spinal cord (now known as Vegan Back), which is usually not detected until the condition is irreversible.[15] No known vegetable source can supply this essential vitamin, so supplement is mandatory.

Iron

Women must consider the fact that they chance a loss of iron in their systems if they are of child-bearing age. This may be obtained through the eating of eggs if these have not been eliminated from the diet.

Iodine

Iodine, though it is not generally a problem, should be mentioned. A lack of this element will cause a goiter or swelling of the thyroid gland. This can be easily prevented through the use of iodized salt.

WHAT ARE SOME GUIDELINES TO A SAFE DIET?

Considering the nutritional requirements for maintaining good health, are there guidelines to be followed in planning a balanced vegetarian diet and what might a sample diet be?

A safe answer would be to simply follow the basic four food plan.

1. *Meats* should be replaced by a variety of legumes, nuts, meat analogs, and textured vegetable protein (TVP).
2. If *milk* is not included in the diet, fortified soybean milk and some kind of vitamin B$_{12}$ supplement should be substituted.

3. *Bread and cereal* intake should be increased, since bread and cereals do supply some protein and necessary vitamins. These will not, however, take the place of the other food groups.
4. *Fruits and vegetables* are usually well represented and are important in the balanced vegetarian diet. Use a variety.[16]

Larger quantities of food must be ingested on a vegetarian diet to secure sufficient amounts of protein and other nutrients. However, this does not bring about an increase in weight, since much of our dietary fat is in meat, and hence is eliminated.

In addition to implementing the above guidelines, one should also make the following dietary changes:

1. Increase the total amount of foods eaten from all four food groups to supply adequate calories.
2. Reduce substantially the intake of "empty calorie" foods (i.e., alcohol, sugar, and nonessential fats).
3. Substitute whole-grain cereals for refined types.
4. Select a wide variety of legumes, nuts, seeds, meat analogs, whole grains, vegetables, and fruits.[17]

Table 11-1 gives some suggested menus for the ovo-lacto-vegetarian and the strict or pure vegetarian.

Table 11-1. One-day Vegetarian Menu

Breakfast	Noon Meal	Evening Meal
4 oz orange juice	2 soy patties with	1 cup vegetable soup
1 cup cooked oatmeal	tomato sauce	(200 grams)
4 oz milk (LV)*	1 baked potato	sandwich
4 oz soymilk (PV)+	1 pat margarine	2 slices whole wheat
1 slice whole wheat	2/3 cup cooked fresh or	bread
toast	frozen peas	garbanzo-egg filling (LV)
1 Tbsp peanut butter	½ cup (scant) shredded	savory garbanzos (PV)
clear hot cereal	carrot salad	½ cup sliced peaches
beverage, if desired	½ Tbsp dressing	4 walnut-stuffed dates
	wheat roll	8 oz milk (LV)
	1 pat margarine	8 oz soymilk (PV)
	3/4 cup strawberries, fresh	
	or frozen without sugar	
	8 oz milk (LV)	
	8 oz soymilk (PV)	

*LV - ovo-lacto-vegetarian.
+PV - pure vegetarian.

Frankle and Heussen state:

> Widely differing dietary practices appear among vegetarians and near-vegetarians. A reasonably chosen plant diet, supplemented with a fair amount of dairy products, with or without eggs, is apparently adequate for every nutritional requirement of all age groups.[18]

CAN VEGETARIANISM BE DANGEROUS?

If vegetarianism is so safe, why do we hear the pitiful cries across the nation from so many adherents to it who suffer malnutrition and even the agony of death? Jean Mayer made an interesting statement. He said, "Vegetarianism can range from a healthy and morally admirable discipline to a misguided and dangerous fanaticism."[19] Too many, unfortunately, have fallen blindly into the latter category.

Vegetarian, contrary to popular belief, does not refer to vegetable, but is derived from the Latin *Vegetus,* meaning "whole, sound, fresh, lively." This is, perhaps, why so many "nutrition seekers" pursue the course of vegetarianism, hoping to enrich their lives with such attributes. According to many young people, dietary control will bring one a sense of physical, mental, and spiritual well-being, and eventually lead to the ultimate (Nirvana). Unfortunately, spiritual well-being is often sought at the price of physical health. Vegetarian diets may be high in bulk but still not meet caloric needs. They may also be protein-deficient, although a combination of legumes and cereal grains can provide an adequate mixture of protein. The risk of other dietary deficiencies is decreased when a large variety of foods is consumed and undue reliance on a single cereal staple is avoided. On the other hand, strict adherence to a more rigid diet, such as the Zen macrobiotic diet, can result in serious deficiencies and disorders. The adequacy of the vegetarian diet, like any other, depends upon individual food selections. Vegetarians can meet the demands of normal growth and development and of pregnancy, as well as provide adequate nutrients for healthy adults.

In order to be safe, a vegetarian diet must contain adequate amounts of essential nutrients, and this requires careful planning and an adequate variety of food intake. Judgment and reason must be used if this is to be a healthy and happy way of life. The decision is yours!

SUMMARY

Vegetarians can be classified according to their acceptance of nonflesh animal products. Ovo-lacto-vegetarians include eggs, milk, and dairy products in their diets. Lacto-vegetarians avoid eggs but partake of milk and dairy products. Pure vegetarians abstain from all foods of animal origin.

Vegetarian diets supplemented with milk or with milk and eggs tend to be nutritionally similar to diets containing meat.

NOTES

1. Daniel Grotta-Kurska, "Before You Say 'Baloney'... Here's What You Should Know About Vegetarianism," *Today's Health,* October 1974, pp. 18-21, 73-74.
2. Ibid.
3. Sanat K. Majumder, "Vegetarianism: Fad, Faith, or Fact?" *American Scientist,* March/April 1972, p. 175.
4. Grotta-Kurska, "Before You Say Baloney," pp. 18-21, 73-74.
5. Jean Mayer, "Can Man Live by Vegetables Alone?" *Family Health,* February 1973, pp. 32-33, 48.
6. Grotta-Kurska, "Before You Say Baloney," pp. 18-21, 73-74.
7. Majumder, "Vegetarianism," pp. 175-179.
8. Grotta-Kurska, "Before You Say Baloney," pp. 18-21, 73-74.
9. Darla Erhard, "The New Vegetarians: Part One—Vegetarianism and Its Medical Consequences," *Nutrition Today,* November/December 1973, pp. 4-12.
10. Clara Lewis, *Vegetarian Diets* (Chapel Hill, N.C.: Health Sciences Consortium, 1978).
11. Darla Erhard, "The New Vegetarians: Part Two—The Zen Macrobiotic Movement and Other Cults Based on Vegetarianism," *Nutrition Today,* January/February 1974, pp. 20-27.
12. Ibid.
13. Grotta-Kurska, "Before You Say Baloney," pp. 18-21, 73-74.
14. Erhard, "The New Vegetarians: Part One," pp. 4-12.
15. Ibid.
16. National Academy of Sciences, Committee on Nutritional Misinformation, "Can a Vegetarian Be Well Nourished?" *Journal of the American Medical Association,* August 1975, p. 898.
17. Lewis, *Vegetarian Diets.*
18. Reva T. Frankle and F. K. Heussenstamm, "Food Zealotry: New Dilemmas for Professionals," *American Journal of Public Health,* January 1974, pp. 11-18.
19. Mayer, "Can Man Live by Vegetables Alone?" p. 32.

12

Nutrition and Disease

Although good nutrition does not promise one a life free from disease, poor nutrition may lead to a greater risk for developing some diseases. Cancer, heart disease, and hypoglycemia may all be caused, at least partially, by the food one eats. Although the development of these diseases is probably a result of a combination of such factors as environment, heredity, and diet, it never hurts to lessen one's risk for them. Unfortunately, many people in the United States are following diets that make them prime candidates for illness and early death.

RISK FACTORS

The majority of dietary factors and non-dietary factors discussed in this chapter are known as risk factors rather than causes. Since we are not entirely sure of what causes cancer or heart disease, we refer to possible factors as risks.

Here is an example of one type of risk factor:

> The tubercle bacillus is accepted as the cause of tuberculosis because the disease does not occur in the absence of the organism. There are, however, other conditions such as poverty and malnutrition which are frequently associated with tuberculosis, but which cannot be regarded as causes of it. Such conditions may be referred to as risk factors, since their presence involves a greater likelihood of the development of the disease, without the implication of a primary causal relationship.[1]

For instance, if you are male, over thirty-five, and your father suffered from heart disease, then you have a good chance of suffering a cardiovascular disorder also. However, that doesn't mean you will. If these were causes of heart disease there would be few left to tell the story. In the same way, if you come from a family where your mother, sisters, or aunts developed breast cancer, your chances of developing the same disease are significantly increased. However, this does not mean that you will develop the disease—it merely refers to an increased risk that you *might* develop breast cancer.

An individual may have more than one risk factor. For instance, one may smoke, have a high serum cholesterol level, and engage in insufficient physical activity. This would, of course, increase susceptibility to heart disease, but there is still no sure way of knowing that you will encounter the disease. Most scientists agree that cancer and heart disease are the result of interaction among different **cofactors**.

CANCER

One of the greatest mysteries in modern medicine is that of cancer. Where does it come from? Why do some get it while others are immune? Does nutrition play an important role in it? These questions and many more are still unanswered and occupy the time and money of many individuals.

To begin with, there are several hundred types of cancer. Some, such as leukemia, may be linked with various viruses. To other kinds, we have affixed the possibilities of certain **carcinogens**. In others we seek a possible link with the environment, including diet. In fact, "it does not seem much to assert that perhaps 80 percent of all cancers are related to one or more factors in the environment."[2]

Studies show that environment and diet have a lot to do with the development of cancer. For example:

> Chinese are highly susceptible to cancer of the nasopharynx so long as they dwell in China. Many thousands of them have migrated to California; by the second or third generation their diet no longer differs from that of other Californians. The incidence of nasopharyngeal cancer then declines.[3]

Chapter 9 discussed lack of fiber in the diet and the possible connection with cancer of the colon. Thus in this chapter we will not discuss fiber further except to note its connection with nutrition and to state that herein may lie the answer to this particular type of cancer. There is also evidence suggesting a connection between dietary fat and cancer of the breast and colon. Testifying before the Select Committee, Dr. Gio Gori, Deputy Director of the National Cancer Institute, said:

> There is a strong correlation between dietary fat intake and incidence of breast cancer and colon cancer. As the dietary intake of fat increases, you have an almost linear increase in the incidence of breast and colon cancer.[4]

Dr. Gori also said:

> Colon cancer has also been shown to correlate highly with the consumption of meat, even though it is not clear whether the meat itself or its fat content is the real correlating factor. Mortality rates from colonic cancer are high in the United States, Scotland, and Canada, which are high meat consuming countries; other populations such as in Japan and Chile, where meat consumption is low, experience a low incidence of colon cancer. Seventh Day Adventists and Mormons have a restricted fat and meat intake when compared to other populations living in the same district and, as indicated, they suffer considerably less from some forms of cancer, notably breast and colon.[5]

Increased amounts of fat in animal diets have also resulted in increased incidence of certain tumors—notably breast tumors—and the tumors have also occurred earlier in the life of the animal.

The possibility exists that dietary composition affects the type of bacteria contained in the intestinal tract. These bacteria may work on a high-fat diet to yield cancer-causing derivatives.

Not only the amount of fat in the diet but also the saturation of the fat tends to influence tumor incidence. Furthermore, animals consuming a diet containing polyunsaturated fat, compared to a group consuming saturated fat, had a lower incidence of colonic tumors. Amino acids, the component parts of protein, have also been noted to influence cancer development in animals. Low levels or even deficiencies of certain amino acids seem to have a therapeutic effect on cancer.[6]

Dr. Gori also points out that the association between diet and certain types of cancer does not mean there is a cause and effect relationship. As in heart diseases, development of cancer is probably a multifactorial problem, which in this case may be a combination of nutritional imbalances, environmental hazards, and individual susceptibility.[7]

Whatever the exact cause, Dr. Ernst L. Wynder, the man who did pioneering work in the link between cigarettes and lung cancer, thinks the main dietary factor in colon cancer is a high consumption of saturated fats and cholesterol. Dr. Wynder indicates that the same diet (low in saturated fats and cholesterol) that is recommended to prevent coronary heart disease may help prevent a variety of cancers, including cancer of the colon, pancreas, or kidney, and the hormone-related cancers of ovaries, uterus, and breast.[8]

With the evidence associating high intakes of animal fat, particularly beef, with certain cancers mounting, wholesale modification of national dietary habits may be premature, but individual reduction in fat and animal protein would be prudent until all the evidence is in.

There are also some studies that indicate vitamin C, vitamin E, and selenium may help prevent experimental cancer in animals.[9] Where these antioxidants occur in the environment, human cancer mortality seems to decrease. A lack of these antioxidants in food (especially beef) may cause a breakdown of unsaturated fat to form a carcinogen, malonaldehyde. Malonaldehyde is formed as a result of uncontrolled oxidations leading to harmful changes in unsaturated fat. Although this has not been totally substantiated in the research literature, there are some researchers who recommend the following precautions:

1. Boil or simmer beef and chicken to steam away the malonaldehyde.
2. If you do not simmer or boil, a cut of about 50 percent in beef and chicken consumption may be advisable. Eating of cheese, milk, and beans should then be increased for extra protein you need.
3. Eat at least one salad and helping of fruit a day. (The fiber may help to soak up harmful substances, and the antioxidants help prevent disease.) In addition, eat at least one cooked vegetable.
4. A tablespoon of bran added to your food every morning or certain cereals rich in selenium would be helpful.
5. Increase your intake of vitamin C and selenium.[10]

The above recommendations are controversial, and their efficacy has not been proven. But for those who are concerned, the recommendations may provide a prudent safeguard.

HYPOGLYCEMIA

Hypoglycemia has become the medical scapegoat for many ailments, from fatigue to dizziness. Yet it is actually a rather infrequent condition caused by the too rapid movement of glucose out of the blood or too little entry of glucose into the blood. It can, but doesn't always, result in sudden fatigue, nervousness, trembling, dizziness, headache, hunger, sweating, and various mental aberrations, including depression and anxiety.

Many feel there is some connection between the extensive ingestion of sugars and starches and the cause of hypoglycemia. However, this point is widely disputed.

Another possibility is that excessive caloric intake may relate to hypoglycemia. Studies have shown that those who eat all of their daily requirement of calories in one meal, as opposed to dividing the intake between three or four meals, are unable to control the glucose tolerance in their bodies and thus have a greater possibility of becoming either diabetic or hypoglycemic.

Diagnosis of this problem should be made by a reliable physician, who may prescribe dietary measures to forestall hypoglycemia reactions.

HEART DISEASE

The Executive Board of the World Health Organization once called heart disease potentially "the greatest epidemic mankind has faced."[11] It is the number one killer in the United States today:

> Of the 866,000 people who die (of causes other than accidents) each year in the United States, more than 165,000 persons under sixty-five succumb to coronary heart disease. Three men die from coronary heart disease for each woman who thus succumbs. To put these depressing statistics another way, one can say that the average apparently healthy man has about one chance in five of experiencing a myocardial infarction before age sixty, one in fifteen of dying from a coronary attack.[12]

The causes or possible causes of this dreaded disease are being argued and researched extensively. Although heart disease is multifactorial in cause, the Intersociety Commission for Heart Disease Resources suggests that the most attention should be paid to diet, hypertension, and cigarette smoking.[13] Improper dietary intake contributes to elevations in serum concentrations of cholesterol and trigylcerides, and to obesity, all known risks to the development of cardiovascular disease. Other factors that may predispose one to the development of heart disease include insufficient physical activity, the presence of *diabetes mellitus,* emotional stress (not documented), a lack of essential trace elements, and the presence of harmful trace materials.

Terms used when discussing heart diseases may become stumbling blocks to the layperson who tries to digest one of the many articles appearing daily in popular periodicals and newspapers. Thus, before we discuss possible causes of this specific disease, it is best to have an understanding of the malady itself.

First of all, the term cardiovascular is an all-inclusive term referring to anything having to do with the heart (*cardio,* from the Greek *kardio,* meaning heart) and with the vessels (*vascular,* from the Latin *vasculum,* meaning vessel). Therefore, anything that is cardiovascular is related in one sense or another to the circulatory system.

Atherosclerosis is a buildup of patches of fatty materials and other substances within and upon the smooth inner walls of the coronary arteries that nourish the heart. It is a form of arteriosclerosis, which is a condition marked by thickening and hardening of the walls of arteries, resulting in loss of elasticity. Arteriosclerosis may occur anywhere in the arterial system.

Atherosclerosis is the underlying **pathology** (the cause of a disease which creates structural and functional changes) in manifest coronary heart disease. The initial thought was that if one eliminated cholesterol and fats from the diet, one could eliminate atherosclerosis and coronary heart disease. But, as we will see, the problem is much more complex, and diet must be viewed as just one part of the entire situation.

For the moment, let's investigate what happens when a person is said to have a heart attack. Coronary arteries afflicted with atherosclerosis may gradually become less elastic and narrowed. This reduces the amount of blood flowing through the vessels, and may eventually bring on a condition known as angina pectoris in which a sudden, vise-like pain occurs in the chest and sometimes radiates into the shoulder and arm. When the blood supply to the heart is severely reduced, or stopped, a heart attack usually occurs.

Complete blockage of an artery may be caused by atherosclerosis or by coronary thrombosis. The latter is the formation of a blood clot in narrowed blood vessels. This may result in insufficient blood supply to the heart, and damage occurs from lack of oxygen—a condition known as **myocardial infarction**. The severity of such an attack varies; sometimes the heart action ceases, and death results.

Coronary thrombosis may be initiated by atherosclerosis. Medical scientists do not know whether coronary thrombosis is caused by atherosclerosis or whether the two processes are entirely separate. Atherosclerosis does not always lead to heart muscle damage.

Coronary heart disease is just one form of cardiovascular disease. Other forms include high blood pressure (hypertension), stroke, rheumatic heart disease, congestive heart failure, and congenital defects. Approximately 66 percent of all deaths due to cardiovascular disease are attributed to coronary heart disease. Diet is only one of many factors associated with the development of atherosclerosis and increased risk of coronary heart disease, but it can be an important one. Scientists are currently evaluating the specific role played by obesity and by different foods and nutrients in increasing or decreasing the risk of atherosclerosis.

Obesity

The advances in food science and technology which increased both the quality and quantity of our dietary protein, minerals, and vitamins have also increased the calories. An increase in calories does not necessarily cause obesity, but an increase combined with a lack of activity does. Everything is now arranged for convenience, and consequently we get less exercise and inconveniently put on weight. It seems that the more advanced a society becomes, the fatter it becomes.

Discussing the importance of **obesity** in heart disease, the Ashley-Kannel reports says:

> The clinical and preventive implications seem clear. Weight gain is accompanied by atherogenic alterations in blood, lipids, blood pressure, uric acid and carbohydrate tolerance. It is uncertain whether the nutrient composition of excess calories, derived largely from saturated calories accompanied by cholesterol and simple carbohydrates, or the positive energy balance per se, is important. But whatever the cause, development of ordinary obesity encountered in the general population is associated with excess development of coronary heart disease.[14]

The same report indicated that each 10-percent reduction in weight in men thirty-five to fifty-five years old would result in about a 20-percent decrease in the incidence of coronary disease. Conversely, each 10-percent increase in weight would result in a 30-percent increase in coronary disease.

Obesity itself may not be a cause of heart disease, but it does occur simultaneously with hypertension, hyperglycemia, or hypercholesterolemia (high serum cholesterol levels) and increases the risk of these diseases. The correction of obesity often results in reduced serum lipid level, lower blood pressure, and improved glucose tolerance, thus reducing the risk factors in these areas. Whatever the mechanism may be, there appears to be little doubt that obesity potentiates the risks of hypertension and increased lipids in the blood, and a combination of these factors markedly increases coronary heart disease.

Further, as has been previously mentioned, people who are overweight are more prone to high blood pressure than are those of normal weight. In fact, for each 10 percent excess in weight, blood pressure rises 6.5 mm Hg. Conversely, lower weights cause a drop in blood pressure.[15]

Fat   It has been recommended by the American Heart Association that the total fat content of the diet be reduced to 35 percent of total calories. The reasons include:

> Avoidance of excessive post prandial hyperlipidemia and its possible adverse effect on coagulation; the desirability of limiting unnecessary calories, particularly in weight control programs; the fact that many foods high in fat are also high in cholesterol and the amount of fat may effect cholesterol absorption; empiric observations that associate a low-fat intake with a low incidence of coronary heart disease.[16]

The Intersociety Commission for Heart Disease Resources recommended that people be encouraged to modify their intake of the major sources of fat: meats, dairy products, eggs, and table and cooking fats. They should use lean cuts of meats, as well as salad oils, cooking oils, and soft margarines low in saturated fats; and they should avoid highly saturated fats, such as butter and certain margarines, and high-cholesterol foods, such as egg yolk, bacon, lard, and suet.[17]

Diets high in fat can lead to above-normal amounts of lipids in the blood, a condition called hyperlipidemia. (Lipids include triglycerides, fatty acids, cholesterol, and other fatlike substances.) A number of studies have clearly shown that elevated concentrations of both cholesterol and triglycerides are related to increased risk of coronary heart disease. One explanation of this relationship states that a high dietary intake of fat leads to an increase in plasma cholesterol and triglycerides, which, in turn, contributes to atherosclerosis and coronary heart disease.

An individual's utilization of fats is affected by many factors:

1. By the food we eat all our lives and our state of nutrition.
2. By our endocrine system—thyroid, adrenal, pituitary, ovarian, pancreatic, and other glands.
3. By how active we are. Exercise increases the oxygen supply to the tissues, improves circulation, and relieves tension.
4. By our emotional characteristics and our reactions to the modern highly industrialized and technological environment.
5. By our aging. Aging means that physiological processes slow down, enzyme mechanisms become unable to keep up with the usual pattern of eating, and some tissues throughout the body become less active.
6. By our heredity. In some individuals a tendency to cardiovascular disease seem to be inherited. This does not mean that the disease is inevitable for those individuals. Neither does it mean that an apparent lack of a hereditary tendency guarantees the absence of the disease.
7. By diseases that may interfere with the absorption and metabolism of fat.

We are also certain that the body's utilization of fat and fat's role in nutrition are affected by food constituents of all kinds and the interactions among them.

Carbohydrates

Generally, when dietary fat is reduced, then dietary carbohydrates must be increased to provide a caloric balance. Carbohydrates should be supplied largely by cereals, breads, fruits, and vegetables. Foods such as candy and soda pop, which are high in calories but have no nutritional value, should be avoided.

The kind of carbohydrate in the diet can be important in lessening the risk of heart disease. A recent study involving the dietary histories of 253 men indicated that higher intakes of protein of vegetable origin, carbohydrates (preferably derived from grains and tubers), starch, and fiber are associated with less atherosclerotic lesions. Even when the diet-lesion relationships were examined on the basis of nutrient-to-calorie ratios, starch and vegetable protein in the diet resulted in less lesions than animal protein and fat.[18]

Some studies have shown that a high sucrose intake can produce elevated blood lipid levels in laboratory animals and humans. Excessive carbohydrate ingestion also seems to increase lipid concentrations by converting glucose into fatty acids, triglycerides, and cholesterol. It is generally thought that sucrose has a more serious and important effect on the formation of these lipids than starch, but further research is needed to settle this question.[19] Some investigators do not think tissue changes resulting from feeding high amounts of sucrose are characteristic of atherosclerosis.

The death rate from heart disease is far greater with a diet high in saturated fatty acids than with one high in dietary sucrose. There are exceptions though, particularly when the country the diet is from has a low energy content, with a small proportion of saturated fatty acids and high sucrose content. In most countries there exists no correlation between high carbohydrate diets and death from heart disease except when there is an increase of sucrose intake, yet the fat intake remains the same.[20] This occurs because of the balance effect between the two. If the proportion of calories from fat in the diet is reduced, the caloric difference will generally be made up by carbohydrates.[21]

Triglycerides

In those population studies in which serum triglyceride concentration (triglycerides in the blood) has been measured, there is a positive correlation between high levels and the death rate from heart disease.[22]

Many physicians consider serum triglycerides to be elevated when they measure 150 to 200 milligrams per 100 milliliters in blood after fasting.

Any increase in serum cholesterol also leads to an increase in triglycerides:

> In general, any change in the diet which leads to an alteration in the serum cholesterol concentration has a quantatively similar effect on the concentration of serum triglycerides. Nevertheless, there is evidence that an alteration in the amount of dietary sucrose has a greater effect on the concentration of serum triglyceride than on that of serum cholesterol. When some of the starch in the diet of a healthy individual is replaced by sucrose the concentration of serum triglyceride rises, but the effect may be only shortlived.[23]

Most people with hypertriglyceridemia are overweight, so weight reduction and exercise are probably the most important aspects of treatment.

Occasionally we find that a person with a high carbohydrate intake of 75 to 90 percent of the total calories develops a form of hypertriglyceridemia, whereas those on a normal intake of 60 to 65 percent carbohydrates do not develop hypertriglyceridemia, if they are not obese.[24]

Cholesterol

Cholesterol is a fat that is essential to all body tissues. It is a building block of cells and hormones and can be synthesized by the body. However, high serum cholesterol concentration is strongly correlated with the death rate from heart disease and therefore, exists as a risk factor.

Insurance studies have found that adults whose serum cholesterol is more than 225 mg have double the chance of a heart attack before fifty compared to those whose blood cholesterol is below 200. The risk triples for 240 mg or more.[25]

To date, studies have not shown convincingly that restriction of dietary cholesterol in the general population reduces the frequency of atherosclerosis. However, persons with atherosclerosis usually have higher blood cholesterol levels than persons without atherosclerosis; and persons with high cholesterol levels develop atherosclerosis more often than those with normal levels.[26]

It is commonly accepted that:

> Dietary cholesterol is a substantial contributor to total body cholesterol, although a major portion is endogenously synthesized. A reduction in the serum cholesterol level can be effected by dietary cholesterol only when its intake is very sharply restricted. Therefore, it is recommended that the average daily intake of cholesterol approximate three hundred milligrams. For persons with severe hypercholesterolemia, an even greater reduction may be warranted.[27]

Studies have shown that proteins of vegetable origin are less hypercholesterolemic than those of animal origin.[28] Diets low in animal products and, therefore, unsaturated fatty acids, cause relatively less cholesterol to be released in the blood.[29] In fact, blood cholesterol concentration is depressed as a result of the intake of a vegetarian diet containing considerable amounts of unsaturated, especially polyunsaturated, fatty acids. Foods of plant origin—such as fruits, vegetables, cereal grains, legumes, and nuts—do not contain cholesterol. They contain plant sterols, which have been shown to reduce blood cholesterol levels.[30] Dietary fiber, largely cellulose, which is high in vegetarian diets, may also play a part in reducing fat by partially interferring with the reabsorption of cholesterol.

> Long-term experimental trials have provided evidence that both in individuals and in groups of people a fall of the serum cholesterol concentration may occur when the amount of dietary fat is reduced or when part of the saturated fatty acid (from either animal or vegetable sources) is replaced by polyunsaturated fatty acid. Reduction of total dietary saturated fatty acid alone has a greater effect on serum cholesterol concentration than the addition of a polyunsaturated fatty acid to the usual diet without a reduction of the intake of saturated fatty acids.[31]

However, new research information indicates that it may not be just the amount of cholesterol that counts but also the type. When there are excessive amounts of cholesterol in the blood (from dietary intake), it circulates through the body by way of lipoproteins (substances that pick up and transport cholesterol through the bloodstream).

> Lipoproteins are classified by density. The beneficial type of cholesterol is contained in high-density lipoproteins (HDLs). The bad type is in low-density lipoproteins (LDLs). At birth, about half the total cholesterol in the blood is contained in HDLs. As we reach adulthood, however, the HDLs decrease and the LDLs increase.
> HDLs and LDLs are a good indicator of risk to coronary disease. Researchers have found that members of families who have enjoyed long, heart disease-free lives have very high levels of HDLs. They also found that if you are over 50 and have high amounts of LDLs, you have a greater chance of developing coronary disease.[32]

Vigorous exercise, reduction of saturated fats and overall calories, along with plenty of fruits and vegetables, helps in the development of good HDLs.

Salt

Thirty million Americans have high blood pressure. It has been found that there is a definite relationship between excess salt intake and an aggravation of high blood pressure, and Americans are taking in two to five times as much salt as they need. Salt elevates blood pressure by causing the retention of fluids in the body.[33] Since many foods are naturally high in salt, physicians worry about foods to which salt is added at the time of preparation and at the time of consumption.

There are ways to curb high salt intake. First, you can stop seasoning with salt at the table and limit the use of salt in cooking. Also, it is helpful to taste food before salting. Many people get in the habit of reaching for the salt shaker before even tasting the food. It is also important to find out which prepared foods are high

Table 12-1. Hints on Sodium Use

Some high-sodium foods to avoid

Food	Portion	Sodium content (milligrams)
Baking soda	1 teaspoon	1,360
Bouillon	1 cup	782
Buttermilk	1 cup	312
Canned soups	1 cup	
Chicken noodle		979
Split pea		922
Vegetable beef		1,025
Canned spaghetti	1 cup	955
Cheeses	1 ounce	
American		210
American (processed)		341
Camembert (domestic)		210
Cheese spread (processed)		488
Roquefort		210
Swiss		213
Chow mein (canned)	½ cup	290
Cold cuts	1 ounce	390
Cookies (homemade)	1	
Chocolate chip		70
Sugar		32
Crab (canned)	¼ cup	400
Crackers	1	
Saltines		33
Soda		72
Doughnuts	1	175
Dried beef	1 ounce	1,290
Frankfurters	1	550
French fries (salted)	½ cup	276
Ham	1 ounce	330
Mustard (regular, prepared)	1 tablespoon	188
Olives	1	165
Pickles (dill)	1 large	714
Pie (fruit)	1 slice	452
Pizza	1 slice	647
Pot pies	1	
Beef		1,024
Turkey		876
Salad dressings	1 tablespoon	
French		205
Italian		314
Roquefort		164
Sardines (canned)	1 ounce	247
Sauerkraut	½ cup	560
Soy sauce	1 tablespoon	1,099
TV dinners: chicken, fish, ham, meat loaf, swiss steak	1	Over 1,000
Vegetable juice	½ cup	240

Three rules from the American Heart Association

1. Use only *half* the salt that you are accustomed to using. Most canned and processed foods are already salted, so do not add to these.

2. Use salt and MSG sparingly.

3. Do not eat foods that are very salty or that are preserved in salt or brine. This rules out commercial bouillon, potato chips, pickles, most cheeses, olives, anchovies, bacon, cold cuts, and soy sauce.

Information that will help you

Sodium compounds to know about

These are the most common sodium compounds added to foods. When listed on labels of foods, they indicate the presence of sodium. The words "soda" or "sodium" or the symbol Na on a label will often help you recognize a product that contains a sodium compound.

Use lightly
Salt (sodium chloride)
Monosodium glutamate (MSG)

Use only in baking
Baking powder
Baking soda (bicarbonate of soda, sodium bicarbonate)

Do not use foods prepared in
Brine (salt and water)

Do not worry about these
Sodium cyclamate and
Sodium saccharin
  (artificial sweeteners)
Disodium phosphate
Sodium alginate
Sodium propionate
Sodium benzoate
Sodium sulfite
Sodium hydroxide

Did you know that

One level teaspoon of salt is about 2,300 milligrams (mg) of sodium.

One level teaspoon of baking soda is about 1,000 mg of sodium.

One level teaspoon of MSG is about 750 mg of sodium.

Brine is used in canning vegetables and in making corned beef, pickles, and sauerkraut.

Sodium cyclamate and sodium saccharin are often used in low-calorie foodstuffs.

Other sodium compounds are used to inhibit mold, to preserve foods, to help cereals cook quickly, or to give a smooth texture to chocolate products.

Seasonings to avoid

Most of these seasonings contain one or more sodium compounds:

Celery salt*
Garlic salt*
Onion salt*
Catsup
Chili sauce
Commercial bouillon in any form

Meat and vegetable extracts
Barbecue sauces
Meat sauces
Meat tenderizers
Soy sauce
Worcestershire sauce

Salt substitutes (unless recommended by your physician)
Olives, pickles, relishes
Cooking wine (salt has been added)

*Unless used lightly

Seasonings to use

Except for the ones listed above, almost every seasoning imaginable can be used. Try some of these flavor ideas.

Beef	Chicken	Lamb	Fish	Veal
Bay leaf	Cranberries	Curry	Bay leaf	Apricots
Mustard	Mushrooms	Garlic	Curry	Bay leaf
Green pepper	Paprika	Mint	Dill	Curry
Grape jelly	Parsley	Rosemary	Mustard	Currant jelly
Sage	Poultry		Green pepper	Garlic
Marjoram	seasoning		Lemon	Ginger
Mushrooms	Thyme	*Pork*	Mushrooms	Marjoram
Nutmeg	Sage	Apples	Onion	Mushrooms
Onion		Applesauce	Paprika	Oregano
Pepper		Garlic	Parsley	Paprika
Thyme		Onion	Tomato	
Tomato		Sage		

Remember that meat and vegetable broths—lightly seasoned with salt and/or MSG—are bouillons that you can use.

Reprinted from "Hypertension and Diet," *Drug Therapy*, February 1979, p. 103.

in salt (foods such as pickles, canned soups, olives, relishes, and frankfurters). Table 12-1 will let you know which foods are high in salt so that you can limit your salt intake and guard against the hazardous effects of high blood pressure.

Water is an essential element in the diet, used both for preparation purposes and as a beverage. Differences in the mineral make-up of various drinking supplies may prove to add additional risk for cardiovascular diseases. Soft water contains less calcium and other essential elements. In recent years, researchers have discovered the ill effects of such deficiencies. The harder the water supply, the lower the death rate from cardiovascular disease.[34]

Trace Minerals

The real cause of differing health relationships with soft and hard water is unknown. Some believe it is because of a lack of vital nutrients; others feel that perhaps there is some substance in hard water that protects against diseases.

One study concluded as follows:

It seems unlikely that the presence or absence of any one element could explain the various findings in different areas. Most of the published work on the subject is concerned with the observation that mortality from cardio-vascular and coronary heart disease appears to be related to the quality of drinking water, the most commonly used criteria being hardness and softness. More data on trace elements in drinking water should be collected in order to determine if a pattern occurs.[35]

As far as trace elements in general go, there is no convincing evidence that the presence or absence of any element in the diet has a measurable negative effect on the cardiovascular system.

SUMMARY

We cannot say that a simple dietary change could possibly solve a problem so complex as that of heart disease or cancer. We would certainly not recommend a sudden and drastic dietary change in all areas, as the implications of such a course require more research.

There are some things we do know, however. First, obesity increases the risk of hypertension, and hypertension in an obese patient increases the risk for heart disease. Second, the level of saturated fat in the diet has been directly linked to excessive levels of cholesterol in the blood and therefore to heart disease.

It appears that the best way to reduce coronary risk is to:

- Adjust caloric intake to maintain optimum weight.
- Exercise regularly.
- Reduce total dietary saturated fats and cholesterol.
- Reduce sugar intake and increase complex carbohydrates (starches).
- Be moderate in salt consumption.
- Eat a balanced diet suitable for one's age and activity.

NOTES

1. G. E. Godber, "Diet and Coronary Heart Disease," *Nutrition Today,* January/February 1975, pp. 16-27.
2. Lauren Ackerman, "Some Thoughts on Food and Cancer," *Nutrition Today,* January/February 1972, pp. 2-9.
3. Ibid.
4. Select Committee on Nutrition and Human Needs, U.S. Senate, *Dietary Goals for the United States* (Washington, D.C.: U.S. Government Printing Office, 1977).
5. Ibid.
6. Gio B. Gori, Statement before Select Committee on Nutrition and Human Needs, U.S. Senate, 1977, pp. 175-91.
7. Gio B. Gori, "Diet and Cancer," *Journal of the American Dietetic Association,* October 1977, p. 377
8. Ernest L. Wynder, "The Dietary Environment and Cancer," *Journal of the American Dietetic Association,* October 1977, pp. 385-391.
9. "Do Vitamins C and E Prevent Cancer of Large Bowel?" *Medical World News,* July 24, 1978, p. 24.
10. Raymond J. Shamberger, "On Your Risk of Stomach Cancer from Untreated Beef." *Executive Health,* September 1978, Vol. 14, No. 12.
11. Louis Goldman, "Same Data and Different Experts = Different Conclusions," *Modern Medicine,* May 1, 1976, pp. 68-70.
12. William B. Kannel, "The Disease of Living," *Nutrition Today,* May/June 1971, pp. 2-11.
13. Goldman, "Same Data = Different Conclusions," pp. 68-70.
14. Select Committee, *Dietary Goals for the U.S.,* pp. 16, 33, 35, 36.
15. Excerpts from Edward D. Frohlich and Alton Ochsner, "Hypertension and Diet," *Drug Therapy,* February 1979, pp. 99-100. Reprinted from *Drug Therapy.*
16. Robert E. Shank, "Status of Nutrition in Cardiovascular Disease," Introductory Statement to John F. Mueller, "A Dietary Approach to Coronary Artery Disease," *Journal of the American Dietetic Association,* Vol. 62, June 1973, pp. 611-616.
17. Goldman, "Same Data = Different Conclusions," pp. 68-70.
18. Margaret C. Moore, "Dietary-Atherosclerosis Study on Deceased Persons," *Journal of the American Dietetic Association,* March 1976, pp. 216-223.
19. John B. Anderson, *Nutrition and Cardiovascular Disease* (Chapel Hill, N.C.: Health Sciences Consortium, 1978).
20. Ibid.
21. "Diet and Coronary Heart Diseases," *Nutrition Today,* May/June 1974, pp. 26-27.
22. Godber, "Diet and Coronary Heart Disease," pp. 16-27.
23. Ibid.
24. William E. Conner, "Diet and Coronary Heart Disease," *Modern Medicine,* November 30, 1970, pp. 85-88.
25. Harris C. Faigel, "The Importance of Screening for Hyperlipidemia," *Medical Opinion,* August 1976, pp. 26-27.
26. Adapted from *Fats in Food and Diet,* U.S. Department of Agriculture, Bulletin No. 361.

27. "Diet and Coronary Heart Disease," pp. 26-7.
28. David Kritchevsky, "Are Dietary Components Risk Factors in Athero-sclerosis?" *Geriatrics,* May 1978, pp. 35-39.
29. K. K. Carroll, "Dietary Protein in Relation to Plasma Cholesterol Levels and Atherosclerosis," *Nutrition Reviews,* Vol. 36, No. 1, January 1978, pp. 1-4.
30. Faigel, "Screening for Hyperlipidemia," pp. 26-27.
31. Godber, "Diet and Coronary Heart Disease," pp. 16-27.
32. Jean Mayer, "The Mysterious Fat Family," *Family Health,* June 1978, pp. 45, 46.
33. Frohlich, "Hypertension and Diet," pp. 99-100.
34. Godber, "Diet and Coronary Heart Disease," pp. 16-27.
35. R. Masironi et al., "Geochemical Environments, Trace Elements, and Cardio-vascular Diseases," pp. 139-150.

13

Nutrition, Learning, and Behavior

In recent years, nutrition has received greater and greater attention throughout the world. In the United States, people are becoming concerned as community surveys indicate that 0.5 to 5 percent of the population under six years of age suffer from severe forms of **malnutrition** and 4 to 40 percent from moderate forms.[1] Those living in low-income areas feel the heaviest weight from this malady, yet even the middle and upper class may feel its pinch. We are sickened as we note how it not only stunts physical growth but may also have a retarding effect on the behavior and mental development of the afflicted. Children who are malnourished tend to be smaller and to be sick more often. They also may be less able to learn.

UNDERSTANDING MALNUTRITION

Types   Dr. Merrill S. Read defines malnutrition as "the state of impaired functional ability or development caused by an inadequate intake of essential nutrients or calories to provide for long-term needs."[2] Thus, malnutrition is a state in which a prolonged lack of one or more nutrients retards physical development or causes specific clinical conditions to appear, as, for example, anemia, goiter, and rickets. Malnutrition prevents children from achieving their full potential and realizing a healthy and satisfying adult life. For developing nations worldwide, where malnourished children may constitute a large percent of the population, malnutrition may constrain the country's future social and economic development.

Severe malnutrition generally is characterized by clinical manifestations that often result in hospitalization. There are two basic types of severe malnutrition: kwashiorkor, in which there is protein deficiency; and marasmus, where there is an overall deficit of food, especially calories. Infantile marasmus is caused most frequently by early cessation of breast feeding, overdilution of bottle-fed formula, or gastrointestinal infection early in life. Marasmus is accompanied by wasting away of tissues and extreme growth retardation. Kwashiorkor generally occurs at or after weaning, when milk which is high in protein is replaced by a starchy staple food providing insufficient protein. A child with kwashiorkor is usually stunted in growth, and has **edema** (accumulation of water), skin sores, and discoloration of dark hair to red or blond.

While only 1 to 2 percent of the world's children have severe malnutrition, up to half may suffer from moderate malnutrition or chronic undernutrition.

How are undernourished children identified? Biochemical and clinical signs of malnutrition are often used, but they are not very precise except in cases of extremely inadequate diets. Chronic undernutrition generally results in stunting of growth; the degree of malnutrition is often proportional to the degree that the child is subnormal in height or weight. Therefore, anthropometric measures (height, weight, and fatness) are the most commonly used indices of undernutrition.

There are two types of moderate malnutrition. One is caused by chronic food restriction (manifested by growth retardation), while the other results from vitamin or mineral deficiency and is accompanied by clinical symptoms such as rickets or pellagra.

Malnourished children are most frequently from families that are poor, have many children closely spaced in age, and do not participate fully in public health programs. They are more likely to come from one-parent households. Parents of malnourished children generally have low-status, unskilled jobs reflecting their lack of education. However, malnutrition is also evident among the "privileged" due to unbalanced diets lacking essential nutrients. It may also be prevalent in obese people who eat poorly.

Determining malnutrition's effects on a given individual is extremely difficult, since many other factors influence human growth and behavioral development, including an individual's innate potential, health status, and environment.

Malnutrition is the world's most pervasive health problem. Probably more than half of the children in developing countries are moderately or severely undernourished. A recent United Nations report estimated that about 400 million people, 1/9 of the world's population, are starving or seriously malnourished. *Prevalence*

Calorie deprivation, not necessarily protein lack, seems to be the primary problem. The shortage of food quantity is so serious in many populations that it masks vitamin and mineral deficiencies.

Three extensive surveys of nutritional status in the United States have been conducted in recent years.[3] They have reached similar conclusions: in the United States, marasmus and kwashiorkor are quite rare, but chronic undernutrition and iron deficiency are surprisingly common.

These studies provided a wealth of information concerning food habits. For instance, almost 20 percent of the children under six consumed less than the recommended daily intake of calories. For low-income families this figure increased to 30 percent. Children from some Southern states and poor black and Hispano-American children were much more likely to have insufficient calorie intakes.

Contrary to the expectations of many, adults and children generally had enough protein in their diets. The study of preschool children found that less than 2 percent did not eat sufficient protein. Protein consumption was closely tied to total calorie consumption. Thus, the children not eating enough protein tended to be those with low calorie intakes. In short, the problem appeared to involve the quantity rather than the nutritional quality of food.

Recommended daily allowances are only gross estimates of nutritional needs and, in fact, are not designed to assess an individual's nutritional status. A more accurate criterion of whether a child is receiving sufficient nutrients is the child's growth record.

The nationwide surveys consistently found a larger-than-expected percentage of children with very low anthropometric indices (measurements of the body, its parts, and functional capacities). Many factors, including the mother's weight and nutritional status during pregnancy as well as the child's history of infection, contribute to the height and weight of a child. Nevertheless, the primary determinant is the adequacy of the child's diet. This suggests that chronic undernutrition is a significant problem in this country.

Many studies have shown that iron deficiency is widespread in the United States. Iron is present in only trace amounts in milk and in most baby foods. Furthermore, iron needs are greater after an infection or blood loss. More than half of the children one to five years old in the United States may have inadequate iron intakes, a deficiency which is not restricted to lower socioeconomic classes. Anemia, the medical consequence of prolonged iron deficit, is common in this age group also, climbing to 30 percent in some low-income groups. Iron deficiency seems to recede in incidence at about age five and reappear as a major nutritional problem in adolescence for both boys and girls.

Finally, except for iron, the national surveys found little dietary or clinical evidence of vitamin or mineral deficiencies among the children in this country.[4]

Malnutrition and Infections

Malnutrition impairs the body's defenses against disease. Consequently, infection, omnipresent in underdeveloped regions of the world because of poor sanitary conditions, occurs more frequently in malnourished children. Just as malnutrition increases susceptibility to disease, certain types of infection, especially gastrointestinal ones (including the widespread diarrheal disease of infancy), heighten vulnerability and aggravate the severity of malnutrition.

To the extent that the poor in the United States live under unsatisfactory health conditions and are without access to medical care, malnutrition and infection interact here also.

NUTRITION AND BRAIN DEVELOPMENT

The brain, like the rest of the body, requires food in order to grow. The human brain approaches its adult size, weight, and cell number by age two. From about the second trimester of pregnancy to six months of age, there is a "brain growth spurt" when brain cells rapidly multiply and grow. To a lesser extent this period of rapid brain growth continues until eighteen to twenty-four months of age.

At birth the brain is already 25 percent of its adult weight, and by six months, 50 percent. In contrast, the human body matures relatively slowly. At birth, it is only 5 percent of its mature weight, and it does not reach 50 percent until about the age of ten.

This brain growth spurt occurs during a very critical period. If the brain does not grow during this time, it will never catch up. Malnutrition may not show its effect on the brain outwardly or immediately, but even milk under-nutrition throughout the whole of the period during which the brain growth spurt is occurring does affect the size, weight, structure, cell number, and chemical composition of the brain. These effects do not seem to be reversible later even if a well-balanced diet is provided. Instead, they persist throughout life. If, on the other hand, animals are well fed during the development period and ill fed later in life, the effects on the brain are slight, and full recovery is possible.[5]

Let us understand one very vital point. Brain growth is *not* psychological development. The relationship between the two is not completely understood. We must rely strongly on animal studies for any knowledge we obtain on this matter. Therefore, statements concerning psychological development and brain growth are not conclusive.

The brain growth spurt may be described as occurring in two general stages. The first stage, concurrent in humans with the second trimester of pregnancy, involves increasing the number of neurons, the basic functional cell of the brain. The second stage extends from the third trimester of pregnancy through the first four to nine months after birth. Throughout this stage the supporting cells of the nervous system (the neuroglia) multiply, and branches (dendrites) from already established neurons grow to form synaptic connections which transmit impulses between neurons.

The two stages overlap considerably, and many neurons are still multiplying even after birth. Of immediate interest is the fact that the processes of dendritic growth and formation of synapses, which occur mainly during the second stage, are probably more important to human mental performance than is neuronal cell number.

Superimposed on the two stages of the growth spurt are regional variations in brain development. Some sections of the brain develop earlier than others, and some develop quickly while others evolve more slowly.

Research findings in animals now indicate that severe malnutrition during this growth spurt can produce brain deficits which cannot be rectified nutritionally. In rats, severe nutritional deprivation during the first phase of the growth spurt leads to a permanent reduction in neuronal cell number. Extremely restricted food intake in the course of the second stage, prior to weaning, creates a brain reduced in diameter (because of stunting of cell growth) and diminished in cell number. A combination of prenatal and early postnatal malnutrition has a cumulatively greater effect than either alone. In lower animals the brain growth spurt is a critical period during which malnutrition leads to permanent behavioral changes.

The unique human brain, however, may not be so vulnerable throughout the growth spurt because: (1) it is so complex and comparatively large that many cells or branches perform similar functions, suggesting that loss of a few cells may not portend behavioral deficit; (2) the brain may be preferentially allocated scarce nutrients, thereby sparing it from developmental deficiencies; and (3) the first stage of the human growth spurt occurs during the second trimester of pregnancy, when the developing brain is relatively protected by the nutrient stores and body processes of the mother.

Nevertheless, the available evidence shows that the human brain, like those of other animals, is probably more vulnerable to malnutrition throughout the growth spurt than at other times. The fetal brain is most likely to be affected in women whose body stores of nutrients are reduced due to a lifetime of undernutrition and an inadequate diet during pregnancy. Since each region is involved in certain brain and behavioral functions, a deficit in one region caused by malnutrition might produce specific behavioral abnormalities.

The period of pregnancy is not time to restrict dietary intake. Studies have shown that such a restriction can cause physical and mental retardation.[6] An amino acid deficiency has proved especially detrimental to the brain.

> Winick distinguished two types of intrauterine growth retardation that can be produced experimentally in laboratory animals. These types are clinically distinguishable and are the result of distinct procedures. In one, the uterine artery is ligated, causing insufficient delivery of nutrients to the developing fetus; in the other, the fetus is affected by undernutrition of the pregnant animal. The first mechanism results in an asymmetrical growth failure that spares the brain. In the second type, in which the mother was malnourished, the growth failure is symmetric, affecting all systems, including the brain. The number of brain cells has been permanently reduced and the effects on the animal progeny are abiding. These effects on the brain occur when malnutrition is operative during the time that the brain is developing rapidly. There is evidence that similar reduction of brain cells occurs during human intrauterine development when the mother is seriously malnourished. Cell number is not affected when the malnutrition occurs in children after birth, although psychological manifestations have been observed frequently in poorly nourished children.[7]

Malnutrition during the period of brain growth spurt can produce profound physical and chemical changes and may lead to a permanent reduction in the number of brain cells, degree of myelination, and brain weight.[8]

However, recent data show that an improved environment may overcome such difficulties. In fact, some researchers now believe that normal development may be possible for children who have suffered malnutrition.

EFFECTS OF MALNUTRITION ON DEVELOPMENT

Severe Malnutrition and Learning

Many studies have been done with humans and animals to determine if severe malnutrition (prolonged calorie or protein deprivation leading to gross clinical symptoms and frequently to hospitalization) results in permanent learning handicaps. A number of important conclusions have been drawn.

Animal studies provide significant leads to human behavior. However, research findings from animals cannot be directly extrapolated for two reasons. First, the rat brain growth spurt takes place almost exclusively after birth, when the rat is quite vulnerable to nutritional insult, whereas human brains undergo much of their development in the comparative security of the womb. Furthermore, nutritional deprivation corresponding to 40-percent reduction in weight gain is necessary before permanent neurological deficits can be induced in the rat. Comparable curtailment of growth in humans is rarely seen, except in cases of severe malnutrition such as marasmus or kwashiorkor or in those low-birth-weight babies who do not grow adequately after birth.[9]

In spite of these differences, severe malnutrition in infancy apparently does significantly alter human behavior. The impact on human behavior is directly related to the severity of malnutrition and its duration during the brain growth spurt period. One investigator has suggested that any malnutrition severe enough to require hospitalization due to growth failure before two years of age will have irreversible adverse results. Another has postulated similar effects from any bout of extreme malnutrition lasting longer than four months during early life.[10]

Early research on malnutrition and behavior tended to use general indices of intelligence, such as the intelligence quotient (IQ), when measuring behavior after infancy. In most of these studies, environmental variables were not taken into account in comparing previously malnourished children to others. Not surprisingly, therefore, these studies asserted that malnutrition had a potent effect on all aspects of intelligence.

Behavioral Effects

Recently, research in the field of malnutrition has become more discerning. Environmental variables that contribute to behavior and intelligence have been more correctly measured and accounted for, so that malnutrition's effects alone could be better approximated. Also, intelligence measures have been refined so that behavioral alterations could be delineated. What has emerged, as animal studies suggested, is a picture of severe malnutrition exerting specific effects on later behavior.

First, there is a permanent effect on motivation, attention span, and arousal. Children who were severely malnourished early in life seem to have short attention spans and consistently perform poorly on tests on concentration ability. On the other hand, long-term memory does not appear to be impaired by malnutrition.

Also, severely malnourished babies tend to develop into children with motor insufficiencies. Many show abnormal difficulties manipulating objects, owing to a lack of fine motor control.

Finally, children malnourished during infancy probably have some as yet undefined retardation in sensory integration. For example, such a child learning to read may have difficulties connecting the visual image of a word with the sound of a word. Obviously, learning would be considerably retarded by impaired sensory integration, but the types of integration that may be affected are not yet fully delineated.

As might be expected, these previously deprived children do poorly in school. They tend to be marked as problem children by their teachers and usually get lower grades.

In sum, very severe malnutrition in infancy, if of long duration and followed by childhood undernutrition, produces irreversible effects on behavior which, in turn, impair a child's ability to learn.

Moderate or chronic undernutrition is more prevalent in the world than severe malnutrition, and occurs even in the United States, as evidenced by poor physical growth and anemia. In spite of this, there are fewer reported studies on undernutrition, and the findings are more confusing. First, the effects, if any, are

Chronic Undernutrition and Learning

probably less serious and therefore harder to measure. Second and equally important, moderate or chronic malnutrition must be viewed in the context of the malnourished child's social and familial environment, which also shapes behavioral development. Thus, studies have been difficult to design and execute and even harder to interpret.

Despite these problems, a number of studies in Mexico, India, Africa, and the Caribbean have shown that chronically undernourished children tend to lag behind their well-nourished counterparts in behavioral development.[11] This retardation probably lasts at least until adolescence. The primary deficits appear to involve motor-integrative performance, reading ability, concentration, and motivation. Even within the same family, those children who were more poorly nourished did less well on behavioral tests and in school than did their better-nourished brothers and sisters.

Nevertheless, not all of the behavioral effects can be attributed to malnutrition. Socioeconomic factors contribute importantly to performance, as was seen when physically comparable children from different social strata were compared.

The best way to determine an individual's nutritional status is to measure what he or she eats over time, and recent studies have undertaken this longitudinal approach. Generally, one group of participants is nutritionally supplemented while another group from the same environment is not. All participants in these projects receive previously unavailable comprehensive medical care.

The largest and most thorough of these studies is presently being conducted in rural Guatemala. The infants, both supplemented and unsupplemented, are being followed throughout childhood, to be tested and measured frequently on nutritional, physical growth, and intellectual parameters. Socioeconomic variables and family interactions are being recorded as well.[12]

Nutritional supplementation has increased birth weight, which tends to be low in these populations. The supplemented children have grown better. By the age of three years, there are significant differences in behavioral test scores between the supplemented and unsupplemented children. The improvements involve motor and manipulative skills rather than cognitive ability per se.

Other intervention studies have shown that nutritional supplementation starting in pregnancy and continuing into early childhood creates more physically active children who demand much more of their parents' time and attention. Conversely, undernourished children are less active and do not participate fully in the surrounding environment. The behavioral development of these latter children is below normal.[13]

Hunger and
Learning
Up to a fourth of American school children arrive at school without having eaten breakfast; many others do not have lunch. Yet relatively few studies have been done on the effects of hunger on the behavior and learning ability of children. Behavior studies have given us a little insight into hunger, learning, and behavior: "Undernourished or hungry children have been reported to exhibit behavioral alterations—including apathy, lethargy, inability to pay attention, and perhaps over-concern about food—so that responses to educational stimulation do not occur. Hyperactivity or hyperirritability may also accompany hunger and contribute to poor learning ability."[14]

However, hunger and malnutrition are not identical. Whereas malnutrition consists of specific physiological symptoms caused by prolonged lack of food, hunger is a physiological and psychological state resulting when immediate food needs are not met. Hunger can be relieved quickly by food, but recovery from malnutrition requires extended rehabilitation.

Hunger is nearly impossible to quantify. Consequently, despite the numerous studies based on school breakfast, snack, or lunch programs (food intervention to relieve hunger), many of the questions about hunger's effects on behavior and growth remain unanswered. The varying results of school food programs in terms of improved growth and nutritional status undoubtedly reflect the varying degree of undernutrition among the children in the programs. Attempts to measure behavioral changes resulting from school feeding programs have been poorly controlled, and many children in the studies were both undernourished and hungry, further obscuring research results.

Nevertheless, the consensus of the studies is that hunger affects behavior. It increases a child's nervousness, irritability, and disinterest in a learning situation. Thus, although hunger probably has neither direct effects on learning nor permanent effects on behavior, it disrupts the learning process. A hungry child's disinterest and inability to concentrate tend to isolate him or her, and when others respond negatively to the child's behavior, isolation is heightened, creating a vicious circle. The child fails to learn for social and psychological rather than biological reasons.[15]

Iron Deficiency and Learning

Iron deficiency, the depletion of iron stores in the body, is the most prevalent nutritional problem in the United States. It can be measured in various ways. Usually, a significant and prolonged deficit in iron intake will cause **anemia**, a condition in which either the hemoglobin concentration or the volume of packed red blood cells (hematocrit) is lower than normal. Many people are iron deficient without manifesting anemia. Since anemia constitutes the most frequent evidence of iron deficit, most of the published studies have used this as the primary variable.

Like other forms of malnutrition, the more severe the anemia, the greater its effect on behavior. Only very severe anemia appears to have any measurable impact on adult performance. Mild anemia, on the other hand, significantly influences behavior in young children. This is probably due to the combined impact of anemia and rapid growth. However, no data as yet suggest that permanent neurological damage results from anemia during either pregnancy or early childhood.

Childhood anemia does not seem to have any direct effects on intelligence, as measured by IQ tests. Rather, selected behaviors appear to be affected. Attentiveness and persistence are decreased in anemic children, while irritability is increased. Chronic undernutrition in conjunction with anemia probably has a more deleterious effect on behavior than anemia alone.

Unlike severe malnutrition, a history of anemia, either in gestation or early infancy, does not impair current performance. The presence of iron deficit at the time of testing is the significant variable.

The impact of iron deficiency on behavior probably is not related to the anemia which so often accompanies it. Iron supplementation will quickly relieve adverse

behavioral consequences. The physiological bases behind the effects of iron depletion are, at this point, unknown, although some have speculated that enzymes
which require iron for activity are sensitive to iron levels in the body.

Whatever the physiological explanation, if a child withdraws from his or her
environment as a result of iron deficiency, he or she fails to learn. By missing one
step in the learning process, the child is less equipped to learn the next. Prolonged
iron deficiency, like chronic undernutrition, could irreparably impair intellectual
development, even if neurological structures remained essentially intact.[16]

*Possibilities for
Rehabilitation*

How much can children who were severely malnourished in infancy be rehabilitated
behaviorally? Two recent reports have shed light on this question.

One intriguing study involved babies with cystic fibrosis, a disease which leads
to a failure of intestinal absorption. These babies were well fed by their middle-class
families, but they failed to grow due to malabsorption. They were therefore judged
to be severely malnourished. After treatment they grew normally. Follow-up tests
on them showed behavioral retardation through the first five years of life. After
that, the retardation gradually disappeared, presumably because the children were
raised in a favorable social environment.[17]

In another study Korean children known to have had severe malnutrition early
in life were adopted by families in the United States. By age seven, the children
were normal in intellectual performance by American standards. Other Korean
children who had never been malnourished and were also adopted by American
families were similarly tested. They were above normal in intelligence. These
observations suggest that the malnourished children, even though they were not
retarded in later life, were never able to achieve their full intellectual potential.[18]

What about rehabilitating the chronically undernourished child? A study of
preschool children in urban Colombia revealed that nutritional supplementation
alone starting at age three had almost no effect on psychological test scores. When
educational stimulation and additional food were combined, however, both
malnourished and normal children from poverty areas improved their performances
markedly on various behavioral indices. Even so, the poor children remained below
upper-class children in intellectual performance, emphasizing again the importance
of the environment.

Also, an investigation of Mexican children showed that up to age seven, intellectual test scores corresponded above all to previous nutriture (determined by
physical growth). By age eleven to twelve, however, performance was more a
function of socioeconomic status and regularity of school attendance than it was of
nutritional history.[19]

These studies suggest that physical rehabilitation from malnutrition is not
enough. Improved health care, nutritional supplementation, and enrichment of the
child's social and cognitive environment must be combined. Comprehensive
interventions will help most malnourished children, except the most severely
malnourished, to achieve close to normal intellectual performance for their
cultures.

How much more could these children have learned and achieved, however, if
they had never been malnourished? Are malnourished children prevented from

reaching their innate intellectual potential even though they may reach normal levels, as was suggested by the studies on adopted Korean children? A comprehensive answer to this question lies in the realm of future research.

LEARNING BEHAVIOR AND OTHER NUTRITIONAL DISORDERS

Not all nutritional disorders that have an effect on the brain development and growth of an individual are due to a deprivation in either quantity intake or quality, but rather may be caused by a metabolic disorder. Many of these are inherited as recessive traits of the parents. These can generally be detected shortly after birth, and treatment given to prohibit damage. Tay-Sachs disease, which results in progressive, uncontrollable deterioration of the brain, blindness, and death, is probably the most dangerous of these disorders. Other inherited metabolic disorders that affect protein metabolism are phenylketonuria (PKU) and maple syrup urine disease (so called because of the characteristic odor of the newborn's urine). Both may result in mental retardation and neurological dysfunction. However, maple syrup urine disease is the more serious, as it prevents three or perhaps four amino acids from completely metabolizing.

Caelic syndrome, in which malnutrition occurs, is a result of faulty absorption and assimilation of nutrients. In Caelic syndrome, the body fails to absorb complex fats and sugars so growth is unavoidably stunted. There is presently no cure for cystic fibrosis of the pancreas, which is a more serious malabsorption syndrome.

Some diseases may be endemic (occurring in certain areas only), such as cretinism, a nongenetic metabolic disorder which produces a lack of thyroxine and can stunt both physical and mental growth. Cretinism, although sometimes congenital, is endemic in areas distant from the sea where people lack iodine in their diets. Without this element, the thyroid gland cannot produce thyroxine. The ill effects of this problem can be prevented in certain regions by the addition of iodine to the salt, or using thyroxine.

THE CYCLE OF MALNUTRITION

As is apparent from the previous sections, malnutrition and environment are intimately intertwined. This interaction often creates a cycle wherein poor environment leads to malnutrition, which in turn shapes behavior to perpetuate poverty, intellectual disability, and malnutrition.

Women who have been undernourished throughout life differ from well-nourished mothers in at least three significant ways. First, they tend to give birth to babies who are undernourished and underweight. Second, if they are undernourished during pregnancy, the quantity of their breast milk and the duration of breastfeeding are reduced, even though the quality of the milk is probably unaffected. Finally, the undernourished mother plays less with her new child since she is considerably less active than a normal mother.

From birth until weaning the infant receives most of his or her nourishment and environmental stimulation from mother. The breastfed child is probably fairly well fed throughout early life because of low nutritional needs. But, by six months of age (or even earlier if the mother is very malnourished), the amount of maternal milk begins to limit growth.

As the infant's needs begin to surpass the undernourished mother's ability to fulfill them, the infant tends to become less active, conserving food energy. The energy needs for physical growth take precedence over energy for activity and play.

Not surprisingly, at about six months of age, the undernourished infant becomes visibly distinguishable from normal infants. According to a longitudinal study done in rural Mexico, this infant sleeps more and plays and explores his or her environment considerably less.[20] The less active malnourished young child elicits less stimulation and attention from parents, siblings, and later from peers. The mother leaves the baby in the cradle for longer periods of time. The net effect is that the malnourished infant tends to develop into a passive, apathetic child.

Furthermore, an infant undernourished before weaning is apt to become more malnourished. This is due to his or her lack of activity and demands on the mother. In addition, the child's sucking behavior may be both less effective and less frequent. Thus, this baby probably receives less milk because he or she is already undernourished.

At weaning the infant more fully enters the outside world. During the post-weaning period, the malnourished child's developmental deficits may be multiplied. The normally active infant plays more and more with parents and brothers and sisters at this stage. Well-nourished children are spoken to more frequently, praised and rewarded more often. The undernourished infant, on the other hand, does not advance in developmental level, probably because he or she is timid and passive, exploring and demanding little. This child has become accustomed to meager food supplies and has assumed a conservative mode of living consistent with available energy. He or she cannot develop satisfactorily because development requires physical activity which he or she cannot, over the long run, afford.

Thus a picture has emerged of a chronically undernourished child developmentally disadvantaged in many ways. What happens when this child interacts with peers and goes to school?

By the time a child enters school, he or she has developed a self-concept based on how parents and others respond to him or her. Up until this time, the malnourished child has probably had great difficulty concentrating and was spoken to and praised infrequently. The child most likely thinks of himself or herself as less able, a picture which will be confirmed when the child tries to concentrate on learning tasks in school. Activity is harder for him or her, and attention is often interrupted by concern for food. What results is a discouraged child whose future prospects in school are gloomy at best.

Early malnutrition then has come full circle, helping to create a child with learning difficulties. It is important to understand that a continuum exists extending from one end, where prolonged severe malnutrition causes an infant to be very passive throughout early life, to the other end, where a transitory episode of hunger may induce an infant to be less active for a while. Obviously, the longer and more profound the passivity, the greater the effect on overall intellectual development.[21]

SUMMARY

Prolonged severe malnutrition during gestation or early infancy, when the brain is rapidly growing, can lead to permanent behavioral handicaps. Such severe malnutrition is quite infrequent in the United States.

The effects of moderate or chronic malnutrition are not as clearly understood. We live in a complex environment where nutrition, health, family, and social factors interact to shape behavioral development. Adverse behavioral consequences of chronic undernutrition seem to lie in the areas of attentiveness, curiosity, activity, and social responsiveness rather than in learning itself.

Furthermore, the consequences of iron deficiency, the most common nutritional problem in the United States, are likely to be in these same areas. Iron deficiency probably has no permanent effects on brain structure and function. Even so, the temporary changes in behavior it induces interfere with learning.

The incidence of hunger among children is nearly impossible to measure. A hungry child is listless, nervous, and disruptive. Consequently, even though hunger does not permanently affect the brain, it probably adversely affects learning.

Although all the research has not yet been completed on malnutrition and learning, corrective policies should be started now. These must include ensuring preventive health care, beginning with the pregnant mother and extending through childhood, assuring nutritionally adequate food supplies over the same period, and providing suitable social stimulation and education for children.[22] Merrill S. Read suggests that:

> Carefully designed studies will be required to clarify the role of parents and of the social and environmental factors that accompany malnutrition. Because research cannot at this time give an unequivocal or complete answer to the question of what effect malnutrition has on intellectual development is not reason to delay programs for improving the nutritional status and eating practices of mothers and infants.[23]

NOTES

1. "Malnutrition and Mental Development," *WHO Chronicle,* 1974, pp. 95–102.
2. Merrill Read, "Malnutrition and Learning I: Malnutrition, Hunger, and Behavior," *Journal of the American Dietetic Association* Vol. 63, October 1973, pp. 379–385.
3. *Preliminary Findings of the First Health and Nutrition Examination Survey, U.S., 1971–1972: Dietary Intake and Biochemical Findings.* DHEW Publication No. (HRA) 74-1219-1, 1974.
4. Adapted from *Malnutrition, Learning, and Behavior,* National Institute of Child Health and Human Development, DHEW Publication No. (NIH) 76-1036.
5. Jack Tizard, "After Childhood Malnutrition: Can the Brain Catch Up?," *World Health.*
6. Myron Winick, "Preventing Growth-Retarded Children," *Current Prescribing,* July 1976, pp. 43–47.

7. Joseph H. Dileo, "Effects of Early Malnutrition and Structure and Function: The Case for Secondary Prevention," *Handbook of Learning Disabilities* Englewood Cliffs, N.J.: Prentice-Hall, pp. 63–71.

8. Myron Winick, "Early Malnutrition Starves the Mind—If You Let It," *Modern Medicine,* May 15, 1978, pp. 57-59.

9. Adapted from *Malnutrition, Learning, and Behavior,* (NIH) 76-1036.

10. John Dobbing, "The Later Development of the Brain and Its Vulnerability," from John A. Davis and John Dobbing (eds.), *Scientific Foundations of Pediatrics* (Philadelphia: W. B. Saunders, 1974).

11. Read, "Malnutrition and Learning I," pp. 379–385.

12. Nathan J. Smith and Ernesto Rios, "Iron Metabolism and Iron Deficiency and Childhood," *Advanced Pediatrics,* Vol. 21, 1974, pp. 239–280.

13. Adapted from *Malnutrition, Learning, and Behavior,* (NIH) 76-1036.

14. "Present Knowledge of the Relationship of Nutrition to Brain Development and Behavior," *Nutrition Reviews,* Vol. 32, No. 8, August 1973, pp. 242–246.

15. Adapted from *Malnutrition, Learning, and Behavior,* (NIH) 76-1036.

16. Ibid.

17. Ibid.

18. Ibid.

19. Ibid.

20. David J. Kallen, "Nutrition and the Community," *Nutrition, Development, and Social Behavior,* DHEW Publication No. (NIH) 73-242, 1973, pp. 35–50.

21. Adapted from *Malnutrition, Learning, and Behavior,* (NIH) 76-1036.

22. Ibid.

23. Merrill S. Read, "Malnutrition and Learning," *American Education,* December 1969.

14

Facts About Food Additives

Did you realize that Columbus ended up in America as a result of his search for food additives? Well, chances are you never quite thought of it in that way.

Few people understand what food additives are and why they are used so extensively in the food industry. First of all, not all food additives are of synthetic origin. Many of them are natural or at least come from natural sources. According to the Food Protection Committee of the National Academy of Science–National Research Council, a food additive is "a substance or a mixture of substances other than a basic food stuff, which is present in food as a result of any aspect of production processing, storage, or packaging,"[1]

Using this description, spices, even those that led to the discovery of America, are considered food additives. Sugar too is included under that definition. In fact, sucrose is the most widely used of all food additives; the average North American consumes up to 128 pounds per year. Sodium chloride, or table salt, is the second most widely used additive, with corn syrup coming in third. The remaining additives together, more than 2,000, only account for about ten pounds of a person's food consumption per year.[2]

It should be understood that the hazards posed by food additives are at the lower end of the danger scale. Without any question, the food hazard that is most important to the public in terms of illness, and certainly in terms of food-related cause of death, is microbiological foodborne disease. Second on the scale are nutritional hazards (health risks from food intake)—in terms of contributing to early death, they may well be more important than microbiological hazards. The other hazards are environmental and naturally occurring toxic materials and contaminants in foods, and pesticide residues. The least important hazard, then, is food additives.[3] Although there certainly are risks involved in the indiscriminate use of food additives, instances of human harm caused by food additives are rare.

THE USES OF FOOD ADDITIVES

Many additives perform important functions. We know more about most additives (which make up less than 1 percent of our diet) then we do about the chemistry of many foods.

Food additives are used for four general purposes. They maintain or improve the nutritional value of many foods. Foods that are **fortified** (such as milk) or foods that are enriched (such as flour) are examples of foods that use additives for this purpose. Other food additives maintain the freshness of foods. Preservatives and

antioxidants are often added to food to maintain freshness. When food processors want to add body and texture to food, evenly distribute particles of one liquid in another, affect the cooking or baking results of foods, control acidity or alkalinity of food, retain moisture, prevent lumping or caking, they may add elements such as emulsifiers, thickeners, humectants, or leavening agents. Food additives also help make food more appealing to the consumer. Coloring agents, natural and synthetic flavors, flavor enhancers, and sweeteners are often added for this purpose.[4]

Preservatives

With an increase in population and urbanization, food producers and manufacturers had to discover more efficient ways of getting food to the people. Preservatives allow us to have what we want, when we want it. Unlike most other food additives, preservatives also have some nutritional value, since they allow us a wider variety of foods, year round. Some preservatives are effective with certain kinds of foods, others with particular spoilage organisms. They are called antioxidants, inhibitors, and fungicides.

Some chemical additives protect against spoilage through the actions of microorganisms. These include sugar, salt, and vinegar. Other such additives used for decades are benzoic acid, sulfur dioxide, boric acid, borox, and hydrogen peroxide. These types of additives can prolong the useful life of dried, frozen, heated, fermented, cured, and refrigerated foods.

Antioxidants inhibit the oxidation of foods during storage. Foods generally susceptible to oxidation are fatty foods, i.e., lard, crackers, potato chips, margarine, some precooked meals containing meat, pie fillings, cake mixes, and sausage. The most widely used commercial antioxidants are butylated hydroxytoluene (BHT) and butylated hydroxyanisole (BHA). Also used are the natural antioxidants ascorbic acid (vitamin C) and the tocopherols (vitamin E). BHT and BHA also help keep bread from getting moldy.

Nutrition Supplements

Nutrition supplements are often added to foods to replace those nutrients lost during processing. Others are added as a result of government concern over the physical well-being of the American people. In 1924, iodine was first added to salt to prevent simple goiter. By 1941, goiter had become a thing of the past.[5]

Other programs of enrichment have been developed in recent years. In 1940, iron was added to breads and cereal. Today we find milk enriched with vitamin D. Vitamin A is added to margarine and vitamin C in fruit drinks. Other common foods that often have nutritive value added include bread, breakfast cereals, macaroni, and noodle products.

Emulsifiers, Stabilizers, and Thickeners

Emulsifiers are most often used in margarine and bakery products. They prevent water and oil from separating and thereby improve the uniformity, fineness of grain, and smoothness of body.

Stabilizing agents, such as gum, arabic, guar gum, sodium carboxymethylcellulose, and gelatin, serve to give ice cream its consistency. Chocolate milk, soda pop, beer, bread doughs, puddings, and cheese spreads remain constant and won't separate or settle as a result of these and thickening agents. Thus stabilizers and thickeners function to give smooth uniform textures and flavors as well as desired consistency to certain foods.

Flavors and flavoring agents constitute the largest and most diverse group of food additives. They come from two main sources, natural (oil and extracts) and artificial. It has been estimated that there are as many as 1,100 such flavor agents. They pose the largest problem in connection with government regulations, because of their number and our lack of knowledge. Since most of them have been used for centuries, many people feel time and money could be used more wisely studying other chemicals that present a more obvious danger.

Flavors and Flavoring Agents

Without flavoring agents, there would be no such foods as spice cake, gingerbread, sausage, and some ice creams and fruit-flavored gelatins.

Flavor enhancers do not add flavor to food, but bring out the flavor that is already present. Monosodium glutamate (MSG) is perhaps the best known of these. MSG was first used in Japan to season food. It is still associated with oriental cooking and is the cause of "Chinese Restaurant Syndrome." "Chinese Restaurant Syndrome" occurs when susceptible individuals eat Chinese food containing large amounts of MSG. These hypersensitive individuals complain of numbness in the neck (which gradually radiates down into both arms and the back), generalized weakness, and palpitations of the heart. In 1969, MSG was removed from baby foods, following some studies which proved it induced brain lesions in mammal babies. The enhancer was really of no benefit to the babies anyway, but merely made the food more appealing to the mothers.[6]

When flour has been freshly milled, it is yellow and lacks the ability to become elastic, a quality that is necessary for good bread. However, time works a wonder on it—oxidation and maturing processes result in the white flour we know. In 1915, it was discovered that bleaching agents and maturing agents can work the same wonder in less time. These same chemicals are also used to whiten certain cheeses, such as blue and gorgonzola. In flour, these agents modify the **gluten** characteristics and improve baking results.

Bleaching Agents and Maturing Agents

The acid/alkali content of many foods affects texture, flavor, and cooking results. The tart taste of soft drinks is caused by certain acids. Other uses of these additives are in chocolate, processed cheese, and baked goods. These agents are important as chemical leavening agents in the baking industry. They also make fruits and tubers easier to peel (for canning); neutralize sour cream for butter-making; and help control the texture of candy.

Acids and Alkalies

It has been said that "we taste with our eyes." Not many of us would eat a green orange, even if it was ripe. Nor would we savor the taste of brown noodles. Thus, the food industries have made a practice of adding dyes to many foods. Many of the dyes used in foods come from natural sources such as caramel color, beet juice, paprika, saffron, etc.

Coloring Agents

Government regulations, however, do not sanction the use of such coloring merely as a cover-up for bad products. No chemical now can be added to the vast list of coloring agents without proof of its harmlessness in quantities proposed. The FDA recently banned the use of Red Dye No. 2, Red Dye No. 4, and carbon black coloring agents that have been used in food. These coloring agents were withdrawn after research studies showed some relationship between their use and cancers in laboratory animals.[7]

Improving Agents

The last group, improving agents, is the catch-all for remaining food additives. The agents in this group perform many, many tasks essential to the modern food industry. Sequestrants, for example, are added to remove minerals from solution or set them aside. They inactivate trace metals which may cause flavors and colors in food to deteriorate. Sodium citrate, for example, is commonly used in soft drinks as a sequestrant. Surfactants are agents that prevent the separation of one substance from another—for example, the oil from the peanuts in peanut butter.

Artificial sweeteners, for those who must or desire to reduce their intake of natural sugars, would also come under this heading. Humectants help keep moisture in products. Curing agents preserve meats. Other uses of improving agents include hardening, drying, leavening, antifoaming, firming, crisping, antisticking, whipping, creaming, clarifying, and sterilizing. Without such agents, the grocery store shelves would be nearly bare, and we would not have the great foods we enjoy today. Foods that commonly include these types of additives include coconut, table salt, frankfurters, dietetic foods, and marshmallows.

Table 14-1 gives an alphabetical list of some substances commonly added to foods. You will recognize the properties of the additives from the previous discussion.

Table 14-1. Food Additives

Acetic acid	pH control	Calcium propionate	preservative
Acetone peroxide	mat-bleach-condit	Calcium silicate	anti-caking
Adipic acid	pH control	Calcium sorbate	preservative
Ammonium alginate	stabil-thick-tex	Canthaxanthin	color
Annatto extract	color	Caramel	color
Arabinogalactan	stabil-thick-tex	Carob bean gum	stabil-thick-tex
Ascorbic acid	nutrient	Carrageenan	emulsifier
	preservative		stabil-thick-tex
	antioxidant	Carrot oil	color
Azodicarbonamide	mat-bleach-condit	Cellulose	stabil-thick-tex
Benzoic acid	preservative	Citric acid	preservative
Benzoyl peroxide	mat-bleach-condit		antioxidant
Beta-apo-8′ carotenal	color		pH control
Beta carotene	nutrient	Citrus Red No. 2	color
	color	Cochineal extract	color
BHA (butylated	antioxidant	Corn endosperm	color
hydroxyanisole)		Corn syrup	sweetener
BHT (butylated	antioxidant	Dehydrated beets	color
hydroxytoluene)		Dextrose	sweetener
Butylparaben	preservative	Diglycerides	emulsifier
Calcium alginate	stabil-thick-tex	Dioctyl sodium	emulsifier
Calcium bromate	mat-bleach-condit	sulfosuccinate	
Calcium lactate	preservative	Disodium guanylate	flavor enhancer
Calcium phosphate	leavening	Disodium inosinate	flavor enhancer

Dried algae meal	color
EDTA (ethylenediamine-tetraacetic acid)	antioxidant
FD&C Colors:	
Blue No. 1	color
Red No. 3	color
Red No. 40	color
Yellow No. 5	color
Fructose	sweetener
Gelatin	stabil-thick-tex
Glucose	sweetener
Glycerine	humectant
Glycerol monostearate	humectant
Grape skin extract	color
Guar gum	stabil-thick-tex
Gum arabic	stabil-thick-tex
Gum ghatti	stabil-thick-tex
Heptylparaben	preservative
Hydrogen peroxide	mat-bleach-condit
Hydrolyzed vegetable protein	flavor enhancer
Invert sugar	sweetener
Iodine	nutrient
Iron	nutrient
Iron-ammonium citrate	anti-caking
Iron oxide	color
Karaya gum	stabil-thick-tex
Lactic acid	pH control
	preservative
Larch gum	stabil-thick-tex
Lecithin	emulsifier
Locust bean gum	stabil-thick-tex
Mannitol	sweetener
	anti-caking
	stabil-thick-tex
Methylparaben	preservative
Modified food starch	stabil-thick-tex
Monoglycerides	emulsifier
MSG (monosodium glutamate)	flavor enhancer
Niacinamide	nutrient
Paprika (and oleoresin)	flavor
	color
Pectin	stabil-thick-tex
Phosphates	pH control
Phosphoric acid	pH control
Polysorbates	emulsifiers
Potassium alginate	stabil-thick-tex
Potassium bromate	mat-bleach-condit
Potassium iodide	nutrient

Potassium propionate	preservative
Potassium sorbate	preservative
Propionic acid	preservative
Propyl gallate	antioxidant
Propylene glycol	stabil-thick-tex
	humectant
Propylparaben	preservative
Riboflavin	nutrient
	color
Saccharin	sweetener
Saffron	color
Silicon dioxide	anti-caking
Sodium acetate	pH control
Sodium alginate	stabil-thick-tex
Sodium aluminum sulfate	leavening
Sodium benzoate	preservative
Sodium bicarbonate	leavening
Sodium calcium alginate	stabil-thick-tex
Sodium citrate	pH control
Sodium diacetate	preservative
Sodium erythorbate	preservative
Sodium nitrate	preservative
Sodium nitrite	preservative
Sodium propionate	preservative
Sodium sorbate	preservative
Sodium stearyl fumarate	mat-bleach-condit
Sorbic acid	preservative
Sorbitan monostearate	emulsifier
Sorbitol	humectant
	sweetener
Spices	flavor
Sucrose (table sugar)	sweetener
Tagetes (Aztec Marigold)	color
Tartaric acid	pH control
TBHQ (tertiary butyl hydroquinone)	antioxidant
Thiamine	nutrient
Titanium dioxide	color
Toasted, partially defatted cooked cottonseed flour	color
Tocopherols (vitamin E)	nutrient
	antioxidant
Tragacanth gum	stabil-thick-tex
Tumeric (oleoresin)	flavor color
Ultramarine blue	color
Vanilla, vanillin	flavor
Vitamin A	nutrient
Vitamin C (ascorbic acid)	nutrient
	preservative
	antioxidant

Vitamin D (D^2, D_3)	nutrient	Yeast-malt sprout extract	flavor enhancer
Vitamin E (tocopherols)	nutrient	Yellow prussiate of soda	anti-caking

Key to Abbreviations: stabil-thick-tex = stabilizers-thickeners-texturizers; leavening = leavening agents; pH control = pH control agents; mat-bleach-condit = maturing and bleaching agents, dough conditioners; anti-caking = anti-caking agents. From *FDA Consumer,* April 1979, pp. 14–16.

HISTORY OF FOOD ADDITIVES: LEGISLATION FOR SAFETY

Food additives existed even before Columbus "sailed the ocean blue." Prehistoric people used salt to preserve their meat and fish. Spices were employed to give foods a more appealing taste. Later, when people raised and processed their own food, they used available additives—vegetable and fruit juices, salt, spices, smoke, etc.

Following World War I, rural people flocked to the cities to work in factories; they now needed food that was grown and processed by someone else. An array of food manufacturers appeared. However, rapid, inexpensive methods of food preservation that picked up production and profit were of prime import for the manufacturers. Food purity did not matter. The science of food and nutrition was practically nonexistent.

Dangerous food adulteration existed everywhere. The problem of additives was especially acute. Chemicals were used without restraint either to preserve food just until it reached the consumers or merely to disguise smell and spoilage. Something had to be done for the health of the American nation.

Right after the turn of the century, people became aware of problems existing with food production. Upton Sinclair, after spending months with the mid-European immigrants who were working in Chicago's packinghouses, wrote his book *The Jungle* which lashed out at the poor conditions and dangerous filth which accompanied the production of meat and meat products. He stated later, "I aimed at the public's heart and by accident I hit it in the stomach." His book disgusted and angered the public and helped bring popular demand for a pure food and drugs act and meat inspection laws.[8]

About the same time, Dr. Harvey Washington Wiley, chief chemist for the U.S. Department of Agriculture in Washington, D.C., became aware of the hazards and stated that the American people were steadily being poisoned by the foods that were being consumed. To prove his point, in 1902 he formed what became known as "Dr. Wiley's Poison Squad." It consisted of twelve healthy, robust men who volunteered not to eat anything except what was fed them by Dr. Wiley.

Dr. Wiley explained later: "I wanted young, robust fellows, with a maximum resistance to deleterious effects of adulterated foods. If they should show signs of injury after they were fed with such substances for a period of time, the deduction would naturally follow that children and older persons, more susceptible than they, would be greater sufferers from similar causes."[9]

Over a period of five years, the Poison Squad was fed numerous kinds of commonly used food additives. Dr. Wiley was not only able to determine their effects, but was also able to arouse the public interest. He, along with Sinclair and other concerned consumers, convinced President Theodore Roosevelt to sign the Food and Drugs Act on June 30, 1906.

Under the Act of 1906, adulterated foods were those containing "any added poisonous or other added deleterious ingredient which may render such article injurious to health." This kept many toxic materials out of foods. However, it did not effectively restrict pesticide residues, for the act provided that the government had to prove in each case that the residues were harmful.

One of the major problems was lead arsenate, which was used to kill the coddling moth on apples. In efforts to enforce an "informal FDA tolerance", many seizures of the poison were made. This only led to feelings of hostilities on the part of many apple growers who lost their apple crops.

Finally, in 1938, the New Food, Drug and Cosmetic Act was passed. It prohibited the addition of poisonous or deleterious substances to food, but provided for exemptions and safe tolerances for substances that were necessary in production or unavoidable. However, the act did not require that the user prove the safety of a substance to the FDA before it was used in the food supply. As a result, enforcement of this act soon became untenable.

With thousands of new chemicals being used in food production and processing, the problem was completely out of hand. New substances could be proven harmful if taken to court, but that did not account for a host of unsafe substances presently on the market.

After almost ten years of hassle, a committee was formed and the "Delaney Hearings" got underway. The committee discussed with experts in all fields of nutrition what should be done about the chemicals-in-food problem. Out of these hearings came the Pesticide Chemicals Act of 1954, the Food Additives Amendment of 1958, and the Color Additive Amendment of 1960. These new laws put the responsibility directly on the manufacturers, who had to scientifically prove to the FDA the safety of a substance.

As far as Congress is now concerned, under the Delaney Clause, a part of the 1958 Amendment, no degree of risk is acceptable. No food additive will be approved if it is found to induce cancer when digested by either humans or animals, regardless of the amount to be consumed over a lifetime. Some feel the Delaney Clause should be modified because it sets an unreasonable standard of safety—one that we demand for no other food products, practices, or services. But until we have more facts, the Delaney Clause remains an essential safeguard to the general powers of the Food, Drug, and Cosmetic Act.

GRAS Substances

Certain substances which had been recognized as safe under the conditions of their intended use were not considered "food additives" under the Act of 1958. Instead, they were classified as "generally recognized as safe" (GRAS) and were exempt from premarketing procedures. Table 14-2 lists GRAS ingredients in common foods, while Table 14-3 classifies GRAS substances by their effects.

Presently, many of these GRAS chemicals are under fire by those who feel that these substances may not be safe.

Table 14-2.   GRAS Ingredients in Common Foods

Breads	Soft Drinks	Cheeses
Bleaching Agents	Acids	Acids
Nutrients	Antioxidants	Coloring Agents
Preservatives	Coloring Agents	Preservatives
Sequestrants	Flavoring Agents	Sequestrants
Surfactants	Non-nutritive Sweeteners	Thickeners
	Nutrients	
	Preservatives	
	Sequestrants	
	Thickeners	

Cake Mixes	Canned Fruits/Vegetables
Acids	Alkalies
Antioxidants	Antioxidants
Bleaching Agents	Coloring Agents
Coloring Agents	Non-nutritive Sweeteners
Flavoring Agents	Thickeners
Non-nutritive Sweeteners	
Sequestrants	
Surfactants	
Thickeners	

From "The Subtraction of Additives" by George Haber, *The Sciences,* June 1974, p. 22. © 1974 by The New York Academy of Sciences.

A group of scientists is well past the halfway mark in a major study, conducted under contract to the FDA, on the use and safety of over 400 food ingredients. About two-thirds of the group of GRAS food ingredients are being studied.

In its reports issued so far, the committee has found that most GRAS substances present no hazard to health from current uses or predictable future uses. For about 6 percent of the substances reported on, the scientific group has expressed various reservations or concerns. Some of these are occasioned by data showing adverse effects on test animals exposed to the substances; others arise from the lack of significant scientific data on safety. In either instance the committee usually has suggested that studies be undertaken. Many of these studies are underway.[10]

Among the more commonly used GRAS substances about which the committee has raised questions or made comments are caffeine, monosodium glutamate, protein hydrolysates, licorice, sucrose, some spices, and some coloring agents.

Caffeine.   The committee studied the use of caffeine as an additive in cola-type beverages and in other soda water beverages. It did not consider caffeine that occurs naturally in beverages such as coffee and tea.

In a tentative report, the committee said there have been no studies showing harmful effects from caffeine at current levels of use, but the group was unable to arrive at a unanimous judgment about caffeine's potential as a health hazard. Some members believe it is prudent to assume a potential hazard may exist for some parts of the population exposed to daily doses, particularly children, and believe the evidence on caffeine is inadequate to make a finding that there are no adverse effects. Others think the cause for concern is considerably reduced by the absence of significant biological effects and the lack of adverse reports from tests involving people who consumed high levels of caffeine.

The committee said additional long-term studies in animals with corroboration in human adults and children, are needed to check for any behavior or birth defect problems that might be caused by caffeine. In addition, the committee said more data is needed about the 10 percent of the population that consumes cola beverages in the greatest amounts.

Monosodium glutamate. The committee found no evidence of a hazard to adults at present levels of use of MSG as a flavor enhancer, although a small percentage of people have been shown to suffer "Chinese restaurant syndrome" from eating foods containing MSG. Additional studies are required on some uses, including the possible hazard to infants from MSG in baby food. Food containing MSG should not be given to infants under twelve months of age, the committee said. United States baby food manufacturers no longer use the substance in their products.

Protein hydrolysates. Protein hydrolysates are vegetable- and animal-based proteins that have been chemically broken down (hydrolyzed) into the amino acids of which they are composed. The committee found that casein (principal protein in milk) that has been hydrolyzed by enzymes is safe when used as a protein supplement in food for infants or adults. For other protein hydrolysates (used primarily as flavor enhancers), the committee found no evidence of hazard to adults at present levels of use, but recommended further studies to resolve safety concerns and also recommended that these ingredients no longer be added to commercial infant formulas, strained baby food, or junior food.

Licorice, licorice extracts, and *ammoniated glycyrrhizin.* There is no evidence of hazard with normal use of licorice, its extracts, and ammoniated glycyrrhizin, but overindulgence can cause temporary high blood pressure symptoms.

Sugars. Sucrose (cane and beet sugar products) and dextrose (corn sugar products) also were studied. The committee found no evidence of harmful effects other than tooth decay but said additional studies would be needed to determine if significantly increased consumption would be hazardous to health.

Spices. Nutmeg, mace, and their essential oils, used as flavors, were not found to be hazardous, but they require further study to clear up uncertainties.

Color Agents. The committee recommended setting limits on certain trace compounds, created in **processing,** which appear in caramels used as coloring agents.

Table 14-3.   Classification of GRAS Substances by Technical Effect

Technical Effect Code	Technical Effect Group
01	**Anticaking agents, free-flow agents,** such as calcium stearate, which keeps garlic salt from turning into a solid chunk during damp weather.
02	**Antioxidants** include substances which keep fat from turning rancid and others, such as ascorbic acid (Vitamin C), which prevent cut fruits and vegetables from turning brown.
03	**Colors, coloring adjuncts** (including color stabilizers, color fixatives, color-retention agents, etc.) consist of synthetic colors (including the so-called FD&C colors), synthesized colors which also occur naturally, such as beta-carotene; the pigment of many of our yellow vegetables, and other colors from natural sources, such as the yellow from turmeric.
04	**Curing, pickling agents** include particularly such things as the nitrites and nitrates used in curing meats.
05	**Dough conditioners** (including yeast foods) are both simple chemicals, such as phosphates or sulfates, or enzymes (see enzymes) which modify the protein and cellulose in such a way as to reduce the "toughness" or "springiness" of dough and make it both easier to handle and more appealing to consume.
06	**Drying agents** are intended to absorb moisture from other food components. Specially dried corn starch is often used for this purpose.
07	**Emulsifiers** are an important group of substances used to obtain stable mixtures of liquids which otherwise would not mix. Lecithin is an example. It is what permits egg yolk to make the emulsion in mayonnaise.
08	**Enzymes** are complex proteins which promote almost all of the chemical reactions that occur in all living things. Some of these can be adapted to specific processing needs.
09	**Firming agents** produce desirable crispness or texture as alum does in pickles.
10	**Flavor enhancers** do not themselves contribute significant flavor, but increase the effect of certain kinds of other flavors. MSG does this for meat and protein flavors.
11	**Flavoring agents** are the ingredients, both naturally occurring and added, which give the characteristic flavor to almost all of the foods in our diet. Diacetyl, for example, is important in foods as different as butter, chicken, and pineapple, to mention only a few. Flavor adjuvants are substances not themselves flavors, which improve the usefulness of flavors, such as solvents and fixatives.
12	**Flour-treating agents** (including bleaching and maturing agents) usually both bleach and "mature" the flour; i.e., they provide the same effect as increased age. They oxidize some of the proteins and lead to better handling characteristics and larger loaf volume.
13	**Formulation aids** cover a hodgepodge of substances which simply allow foods to be put together in a commercially useful way. Among them are carriers for flavors or other substances used in small amounts and binders, such as starch, to hold things together.

14	**Fumigants,** such as methyl bromide or ethylene oxide, kill undesirable organisms.
15	**Humectants, moisture retention agents, and antidusting agents** are substances, such as sorbitol, which keeps candy fresher, or propylene glycol, which keeps coconut from drying out.
16	**Leavening agents,** such as yeast and baking powder ingredients, produce light, fluffy baked goods.
17	**Lubricants, release agents** allow the extrusion of foods and permit rapid, economical production of bread by permitting it to come cleanly out of the baking pan.
18	**Non-nutritive sweeteners,** such as saccharin, replace sugar or corn syrup in dietetic foods.
19	**Nutrient supplements,** such as the vitamins and minerals, restore values lost in processing or storage or insure higher nutritional value than nature may have provided.
20	**pH Control agents** (including buffers, acids, alkalies, neutralizing agents) reduce or increase the acidity or sourness of a food. The vinegar in pickles does this.
21	**Preservatives** prevent bacteriological spoilage. The sodium benzoate in beverages and the calcium propionate in bread serve in this way.
22	**Processing aids** are added not for the continuing effect they exert on the food, but to help make it better in the first place. They assist in filtering or removing unwanted color.
23	**Propellants, aerating agents, gases** push the whipped cream topping from the can and make it fluffy or exclude oxygen and prolong the shelf life and nutritional value of a packaged food.
24	**Sequestrants** combine chemically with traces of metals present naturally in all foods and which, if uncombined, would promote instability and off flavors.
25	**Solvents and vehicles,** such as alcohol or glycerine, permit us to use flavors, colors, and many other ingredients in an easy-to-use form.
26	**Stabilizers, thickeners,** such as starch or gums, give desirable viscosity and ''mouth feel,'' prevent emulsions from separating, and prevent a pudding from being ''sloppy.''
27	**Surface-active agents** are related to the emulsifiers and permit rapid wetting of dry ingredients, better whipping of toppings, and promote foam where it is wanted or prevent it where it is not wanted.
28	**Surface-finishing agents** include ordinary waxes, as well as more complex substances. They are used on fruits, candies, and baked goods both for protection and appearance.
29	**Synergists** is a catch-all category of substances which produce no particular effect in themselves, but assist in the operation of other additives.
30	**Texturizers** contribute or preserve desirable appearance or mouth-feel; e.g., a smooth, slick sauce or pudding produced with normal starch is often less attractive than one with a somewhat pulpy appearance and feel produced by modified starches.

"Food Additives" by Richard L. Hall, *Nutrition Today,* July/August 1973, pp. 24–25. Reproduced with permission of *Nutrition Today* Magazine, 703 Giddings Avenue, Annapolis, Maryland 21404. © July/August 1973.

The committee's findings are being used by the FDA to help it decide whether a given substance is safe enough to permit its continuance in the GRAS classification with or without restrictions, or whether more drastic restriction is called for, such as limiting use while studies are conducted or prohibiting use of the ingredient.

TESTING OF FOOD ADDITIVES

The requirements for approving new food additives are becoming more difficult. The manufacturer must file a petition with the FDA with the following information:

1. The name and all pertinent information, including, when available, the chemical identity and composition.
2. A statement of the conditions of the proposed use of such an additive.
3. All relevant data on the effect the additive is intended to produce and the quantity required.
4. A description of a practical method for the determination of the presence of the additive in or on food.
5. Full reports of investigations (using animal and human research findings) made with respect to the safety of use of the additive.[11]

If, after investigation of information and reports received, the FDA can see no hazards or harmful effects, a regulation is established permitting use of the substance. However, a tolerance level is often placed on it too. Though an attempt is made to adjust the tolerances to take into consideration multiple chemical ingestions (i.e., food additives, air pollution, drugs, cigarette smoke), many question the safety levels of these tolerances.

Testing Procedures   We cannot test for absolute safety; we can only test for the presence of known hazards. If no hazards are discovered, an additive is assumed to be safe. If, on the other hand, a new hazard is uncovered, and this has happened many times, the tests are repeated.

A typical testing sequence involves two animal species. Humans cannot be used as was Dr. Wiley's Poison Squad because there are too many chemicals to test and it is very dangerous. So the FDA feels two separate species can best give a representation of humans. In addition, animals can be tested over several generations in a short period of time.

After all this testing, the FDA still uses a precautionary measuring stick which might be called the philosophy of the minimum. It goes something like this:

- A tolerance or limitation will not exceed the smallest amount needed, even though the higher tolerance may be safe.
- After determining the maximum amount that will not produce an undesirable effect on the test animals used, .01 of that amount is normally the maximum allowed for use by humans. If it is proven that even a smaller amount than .01 will do the job, the smaller amount will be used instead.

- It is quite natural to think of desired safety—in anything—in the realm of 100 percent only. Such perfection is impossible.[12]

We should realize here that the risks are generally small while the benefits (more wholesome and better protected food) are usually very desirable, and in many cases essential, for the maintenance of an adequate, nutritious, and safe food supply.

DANGEROUS ADDITIVES

We do know that some additives are more hazardous than others. Nitrates, or nitrites, have been used to prevent botulism in meats such as bacon. However, nitrites may combine with certain amines present in the meats, fish, and poultry being processed and form substances called nitrosamines, some of which have been shown to cause cancer in laboratory animals. The government's immediate objective is to eliminate any uses in which nitrosamines may be formed in the processing of a food product or in its preparation (such as cooking) before it is eaten. Nitrates or nitrites might possibly combine with amines that are present in the human body and form nitrosamines after the food is eaten; investigations on this question continue. There is also concern about excessive use of nitrites, which in heavy doses impair the capability of the blood to carry oxygen.

Nitrates are far less toxic than nitrites and occur naturally in water, vegetables, and other parts of the environment. This being the case, the ingestion by humans of nitrates—and, to a much lesser extent, nitrites—is not confined to what they consume in cured meats, fish, and poultry. The nitrates used as food additives account for only a fraction of the total nitrates ingested by the average person.

Even with that knowledge, the FDA for many years allowed nitrites in carefully monitored low doses because the benefits appeared to outweigh the risk. The assumed benefit was the protection of some meats, such as bacon and sausages, from the deadly botulism toxin (nitrates and nitrites inhibit or prevent growth of the bacteria that cause botulism); the threat of botulism poisoning was considered far greater than the risk of cancer from nitrates.[13]

Then, in 1978 the U.S. Department of Agriculture (USDA) announced two actions designed to eliminate cancer-causing nitrosamines from fried bacon and to reduce the total level of nitrite in bacon.[14]

First, the Department issued a proposed regulation that would lower to 10 parts-per-million (ppm) the level of sodium nitrite allowed to be used in curing bacon. The sodium nitrite (or an equivalent amount of potassium nitrite) would be used in combination with 0.26 percent by weight of potassium sorbate. Data indicate that this formula would provide protection against botulism equal or superior to that of formulas now in use, and eliminate confirmable levels of cancer-causing nitrosamines.

The proposed regulation would reduce by at least two-thirds the amount of nitrite presently used by most meat packers. At the time of this writing there is a moratorium on this proposed legislation. Indications are that nitrite will be phased out only if alternative forms of protection against botulism can be developed for implementation on a commercial basis. So, at the present time, there is a race on to collect and evaluate as much information as possible about the uses and risks of nitrite and of alternatives.

Although the ban would be implemented cautiously, it would have a major impact on both the meat industry and consumers, who eat more than 10 billion pounds of nitrite-treated products a year.

Meanwhile results from a new study conducted by Paul Newberne at the Massachusetts Institute of Technology show that 13 percent of about 1,300 rats that had been fed nitrite developed cancer of the lymphatic system, compared with 8 percent of a control group.[15]

The difference is significant, say health officials. It suggests that a person eating six pieces of bacon or two slices of bologna a day has a 1-in-7,400 chance of developing cancer from this source alone.[16]

FOOD ADDITIVES AND HYPERACTIVE CHILDREN

Dr. Benjamin Feingold suggests that synthetic colors and flavors used in food cause some children to be unusually active and interfere with their ability to learn. He claims that putting **hyperkinetic** children on an "elimination" diet (free of all foods containing additives, dyes of any type, or compounds containing salicylates) can help control or cure their problem. This would mean no soft drinks, ice cream, bakery goods, candies, hot dogs and many other foods, and no toothpaste or aspirin.[17]

Recently an advisory committee of distinguished pediatricians, nutritionists, psychologists, and other professionals concluded that no controlled studies have demonstrated that hyperkinesis is related to the ingestion of food additives. The American Academy of Pediatrics urges parents not to use the elimination diet on any long-term basis simply because no one yet knows its long-term effects.[18]

SAFETY OF PESTICIDES

It is evident that pesticides have brought tremendous benefits to human health by controlling insect-borne disease and improving the production of food and fiber. At the same time, an increased public health and environmental hazard has been associated with the use of insecticides on fruits and vegetables. Some pesticides persist in the environment for very long periods and can move up the food chain through a process called biological magnification.

Acute poisoning in humans is rare and usually involves young children who have accidentally swallowed DDT or one of its derivatives. The symptoms of acute poisoning include vomiting, diarrhea, dizziness, rapid heart rate, shallow rapid breathing, difficult breathing, abdominal swelling, unconsciousness, and convulsions.

Long-term exposure to small or moderate amounts of pesticides results in little evidence of illness. Insecticide is rapidly stored in fat and is thus removed from the remainder of body tissues. The potential danger arises, however, when fat is used for energy and the insecticide is released again. Signs of poisoning may be observed if the amounts released are large enough.

In humans the amount of insecticides found in fatty tissues is rising; the average yearly intake of DDT and its derivatives is reported to be about 50 milligrams, 90 percent of which comes from food. However, this level is not dangerous, and samples of fruits and vegetables rarely have insecticide residues that exceed safe levels.[19] Studies of 1975 levels show there is little risk of poisoning of the average population.

The greatest danger is for those groups involved in spraying orchards and crops or handling sprayed materials. These people do harbor high fat levels of insecticide, but no adverse effects are observed unless illness, surgery, stress, or dieting uses up the body fat and releases the chemical. Female agricultural workers and the wives of farmers would be in the most danger during pregnancy, because the insecticide might be liberated from fat and transferred to the unborn baby, as well as appear in the mother's milk, to the ultimate handicap of the child.[20] The greatest danger to the general public is probably improper use of insecticides and pesticides in and around the house.

THE TRUTH ABOUT NATURAL FOODS

With the saccharin scare and the banning of cyclamates people joined the ranks of this health food diet and that, hoping to avoid contamination by additives. In general, natural substances are readily metabolized by the body and are probably safer than the synthetic ones. However, natural foods do have problems of their own.

Natural foods can prove more hazardous than the so-called "poisons" put into foods by the various food industries. For example, potatoes contain an alkaloid called solonine which blocks off the transmission of nerve impulses. Solonine poisoning is a frequent occurrence and in some outbreaks has involved hundreds of people, occasionally causing death.[21] This usually occurs when parts other than the tuber are eaten.

Tapioca, almonds, and lima beans are among substances that produce cyanide during digestion. One particular strain of lima beans has been responsible for many human poisonings.

And cyanide is not the only potentially dangerous natural substance in foods. "Evidence is now conclusive for the presence in vegetables of the potent carcinogens 3,4–benzpyrene, 1,2,–benzanthracene, and other polynuclear aromatic hydrocarbons, as normal products of plant biosynthesis rather than from contamination."[22]

There are other examples of naturally occurring carcinogens, such as **aflatoxins**, and some mushrooms that are highly toxic. Aflatoxins, a group of naturally occurring mold-produced chemicals, have been the subject of much study because under some conditions they may get into our food. Animal studies have shown that short-term exposure to certain levels of aflatoxins can result in poisoning, and that chronic low-level exposure can cause liver cancer. When tested in sensitive strains of some experimental animals, one of the aflatoxins, called B_1, revealed itself to be the most potent cancer-causing agent known (although there are other animal strains that are resistant to these effects).

How susceptible humans are to the toxic effects of aflatoxins is unknown. There is no direct evidence on the subject because such toxic substances cannot be tested in humans. But there is good reason to believe that there is some risk to humans when they are inadvertently exposed to aflatoxins. Studies of people in certain areas of Africa and Southeast Asia have demonstrated an association between the level of aflatoxins that occurs naturally in the diet and the incidence of liver cancer. A direct cause-effect relationship has not been established, however.

Despite scientific uncertainty about the health effects of aflatoxins, most scientists would exclude them from our food supply if they had a choice. And if aflatoxins were present in food because they were intentionally added (that is, if they were direct food additives), it is clear that FDA would prohibit them. Unfortunately, it is not that easy to rid the food supply of aflatoxins.

Although consumers have become more aware of aflatoxins in recent years, particularly because of animals deaths from aflatoxin contamination, there seem to be widespread misconceptions about the problem. Consumers should keep in mind that it is not possible to definitively determine by visual inspection whether aflatoxins are present in any food or feed.[23] The presence of visible mold growth on a food does not mean there is aflatoxin present. The mold may not be the type that produces aflatoxin. And even if it is an aflatoxin-producing mold, it does not always procduce the toxins. Chemical analysis (which destroys the product) is necessary. And, because aflatoxin contamination may be unevenly distributed in food, the results of analysis of one portion of a lot do not necessarily apply to portions of the product that are not analyzed. Thus, there is almost always some uncertainty regarding the aflatoxin content of specific units of food that are not analyzed, even when the lot from which the units are prepared has been analyzed. For this reason, manufacturers must set their quality control limits at an aflatoxin level below the guideline set by FDA. For example, to comply with the proposed 15-ppb guideline, manufacturers of peanut products have to set their limits at a maximum of 5 to 7 ppb.

It is impossible to draw conclusions about the extent to which the entire output of a specific manufacturer complies with FDA guidelines. For example, when analysis of one sample (or even a series of samples) of one brand of peanut butter shows aflatoxins, this does not mean consumers need assume that this particular brand is always contaminated. Likewise, when analysis shows no detectable aflatoxin, consumers should not assume this brand is always aflatoxin-free.

Consumers can contribute to their own protection by examining foods carefully before consuming them. Molds that do not produce aflatoxins may produce other chemicals. Some of these other chemicals have been found in various foods, and the FDA is now conducting extensive toxicity studies to determine whether any constitute a serious health risk. Heavily molded foods should be returned to the supermarket or discarded. Partially molded foods should be well-trimmed before use. Peanuts and tree nuts in the shell should be examined before consumption, and moldy, badly damaged, or shriveled nuts should be discarded. Small children probably cannot practice this kind of discrimination without help from adults. Also, do not toss moldy food to your pet.

QUANTITY AND SAFETY

We must conclude that nothing is entirely safe. Quantity is usually the ruling factor. As the Renaissance physician Paracelsus once said, "Sole dosis facit venenum," or in other words, "Only the dose makes the poison."

> We must recognize that safety is a pathway between hazards, some of which are visible and measures, others indistinct, other unknown. Sometimes the path is wide, and the margins of safety are large. At times, as with Vitamin D or solanine, the path is narrow. There is no escape from all risk, no matter how remote. There are only choices among risks. Safety lies in staying on the path—through balance and moderation—rather than indulgence in dietary extremes."[24]

The amount of any one additive may be small, perhaps insignificant. But there are scores of others in our foods, not to mention the chemicals taken in from medications and polluted air and water. Since the effects may be cumulative or interacting, many people think it is sensible to minimize the intake of all unnecessary chemicals. The idea is to make sure that the benefit of additives outweigh the risks; and to reduce the risks to a minimum. There will probably always be some doubt concerning the safety of eating small amounts of additives over an entire lifetime.

The key to food safety is three simple words: sanitation, variety, and moderation.[25]

SUMMARY

Food additives, in one form or another, have been present in foods since before the time of Columbus. They may be synthetic, such as BHT and BHA, which are added to many foods as preservatives. Or they may be natural, such as spices.

Food additives have various functions—they enhance food, make it more colorful or palatable, and make it last longer. The major categories of additives are preservatives; nutritional supplements; emulsifiers, stabilizers, and thickeners; flavors and flavoring agents; bleaching agents and maturing agents; acids and alkalies; coloring agents; and improving agents.

The controversy over the safeness of these agents has raged for years. Right after the turn of the century, Upton Sinclair and Dr. Harvey Washington Wiley led the opposition to a number of potentially hazardous substances that had been added to food. Their campaigning led to legislation designed to control the use of dangerous substances that had previously been indiscriminately added to foods.

The government has tested numerous substances that scientists felt might be hazardous to health. Many of the substances were not withdrawn from foods, because they were found to present no significant hazard to health. Others that were found to present some hazard were either limited in use or excluded entirely from the market.

It has been suggested that the use of food additives contributes to and aggravates hyperactivity in children. As of yet, there has been no conclusive evidence that this is the case, but the research in this area continues.

Another subject of current research is pesticides. Indiscriminate use of pesticides to control insects and diseases in growing plants could contaminate the food that eventually ends up on the tables of America. However, pesticides do bring tremendous benefits to the food industry, and acute poisoning in humans is rare.

Whatever one's view concerning the use of food additives, the fact remains that many of the foods we enjoy would not be available in their present form without food additives. For those who are concerned, the best policy would be to give up foods made up largely of additives, and, to demand thorough testing of food, and accurate labeling. The health hazard can be taken out of food technology, but only with constant vigilance by everyone concerned.

NOTES

1. Richard A. Ahrens, "The Question of Food Additives," *School Health Review,* November 1970, pp. 19-23.
2. Richard L. Hall, "Food Additives," *Nutrition Today,* July/August 1973, pp. 20-28.
3. Richard L. Hall, "Food Additives: An Industry View," *FDA Consumer,* January/February 1978, pp. 6-11.
4. Phyllis Lehmann, "More Than You Ever Thought You Would Know About Food Additives," *FDA Consumer,* April 1979, pp. 10-11.
5. Ahrens, "The Question of Food Additives," pp. 19-23.
6. Ibid.
7. Harold Hopkins, "Countdown of Color Additives," *FDA Consumer,* November 1976, p. 5.
8. Edward G. Damon, "Primer on Food Additives," *FDA Consumer,* May 1973, pp. 10-16.
9. Ibid.
10. Harold Hopkins, "The GRAS List Revisted," *FDA Consumer,* May 1978, pp. 13-15.
11. "The Use of Chemicals in Food Production, Processing, Storage, and Distribution," *National Review,* Vol. 31, No. 6, July 1973, pp. 191-198.
12. Damon, "Primer on Additives," pp. 10-16.
13. Jean Mayer, "Let's Subtract Additives," *Family Health/Today's Health,* December 1977, pp. 42-43.
14. "Update," *FDA Consumer,* June 1978, p. 3.
15. "Nitrite Danger," *U.S. News and World Report,* August 28, 1978.
16. Ibid.
17. F. J. Stare and E. M. Whelan, "Food Additives and Health," *Food and Nutrition,* Vol. 1, No. 4, 1975, pp. 2-5.
18. Timothy Larkin, "Food Additives and Hyperactive Children," *FDA Consumer,* March 1977, pp. 9-11.

19. David Pimentel et al., "Pesticides, Insects in Foods and Cosmetic Standards," *BioScience,* March 1977, pp. 178-184.
20. D. J. Ecobichon, "Chlorinated Hydrocarbon Insecticides: Recent Animal Data of Potential Significance for Man," *Journal of the Canadian Medical Association,* October 10, 1970, pp. 711-716.
21. "Naturally Occurring Toxicants, Food Additives, and Cosmetics," *Chemicals and Health* (report of the Panel on Chemicals and Health of the President's Science Advisory Committee), September 1973, pp. 63-76.
22. Ibid.
23. Joseph V. Rodricks, "Aflatoxins," *FDA Consumer,* May 1978, pp. 16, 18.
24. "Naturally Occurring Toxicants, Food Additives, and Cosmetics," pp. 63-76.
25. Richard L. Hall, "Safe at the Plate," *Nutrition Today,* November/December 1977, p. 7.

15

Nutrition Labeling: Read and Heed

Senator Richard Schweiker (R-Penn.) once stated, "We are on the threshold of a nutrition revolution. I liken the nutrition situation today to where we were fifteen years ago environmentally, before Rachel Carson's *Silent Spring*. Once people begin to understand the relationship between sound nutrition and good health, they will demand nutritional labeling and education, just as they demand responsible environmental policy today."[1]

In 1973 the Food and Drug Administration brought forth new regulations pertaining to the use of uniform and informative nutrition labeling. The regulations require manufacturers to use nutrition labeling when they add any nutrient to the food or when they make some nutritional claim for it on the label or in advertising, such as "enriched" or "fortified." Diet foods must also exhibit complete nutritional information.

Some companies provide a nutritional rundown on their labels even if they're not required to. Several bills have been introduced in Congress to make nutritional and ingredient labeling mandatory. Eventually, 90 to 100 percent of all food products will carry nutritional labeling.

The basic premise of nutrition labeling is that consumers have a right to information about the minimum levels of protein, vitamins, and minerals, and the maximum levels of calories, fats, and carbohydrates in foods. It can be assumed that nutrition labeling will increase consumer awareness and knowledge of nutrition. With the availability of nutrition information, consumers should be able to do a better job of selecting, comparing, and substituting foods.

NUTRITIONAL LABELING

Certain information must be on all food labels: the name of the product, the net contents or net weight (the net weight on canned food includes the liquid in which the product is packed, such as water in canned vegetables and syrup in canned fruit), the name and place of business of the manufacturer, packer, or distributor.

On most foods, the ingredients must be listed on the label. The ingredient present in the largest amount, by weight, must be listed first, followed in descending order of weight by the other ingredients. Any additives used in the product must be listed, but colors and flavors do not have to be listed by name. The list of ingredients may simply say artificial color or artificial flavor or natural flavor. If the flavors are artificial, this fact must be stated. Butter, cheese, and ice cream, however, are not required to state the presence of artificial color.

The only foods not required to list all ingredients are so-called standardized foods. The FDA has set "standards of identity" for some foods. These standards require that all foods called by a particular name (such as catsup or mayonnaise) contain certain mandatory ingredients. Under the law, these mandatory ingredients need not be listed on the label. Manufacturers may add optional ingredients, however, and the FDA is revising the food standards to require that optional ingredients in standardized foods be listed on the product label.

Whenever nutritional labeling is used, it must follow the specified format of the FDA. Except when space is not available, labels must appear directly to the right of the main display panel. In this way, consumers do not have to spend their shopping time searching for nutrition information.

As shown in Table 15-1, the FDA has designed the nutrition labels to be as easily understood as possible. The first line of the label gives the size of a serving, which the FDA has defined as a reasonable amount usually eaten by an adult male engaged in light physical activity. If this food is to be used as an ingredient in the preparation of some other food—for example, tomato paste—the quantity may be expressed in terms of a portion. The next line of the nutrition information panel tells how many servings or portions are in the container.

Table 15-1. Sample Nutrition Label for Frozen Main Dish

NUTRITION INFORMATION
(per serving)
SERVING SIZE = 8 OZ.
SERVINGS PER CONTAINER = 1

CALORIES	560	FAT (percent of calories 53%)	33 g
PROTEIN	23 g	*Polyunsaturated	2 g
CARBOHYDRATE	43 g	Saturated	9 g
		*CHOLESTEROL (20 mg/100 g)	45 mg
		SODIUM (300 mg/100 g)	680 mg

PERCENTAGE OF U.S. RECOMMENDED
DAILY ALLOWANCES (U.S. RDA)

PROTEIN	35%	RIBOFLAVIN (VITAMIN B_2)	15%
VITAMIN A	35%	NIACIN	25%
VITAMIN C (ASCORBIC ACID)	10%	CALCIUM	2%
THIAMINE (VITAMIN B_1)	15%	IRON	25%

*Information on fat and cholesterol content is provided for individuals who, on the advice of a physician, are modifying their total dietary intake of fat and cholesterol.

Food and Drug Administration.

Immediately after the serving and package contents information comes a breakdown of calories, protein, carbohydrates, and fat. (Protein is also listed later as a percentage of the U.S. Recommended Daily Allowances.) Calories are expressed in 2-calorie increments up to 20 calories, in 5-calorie increments from 20 to 50 calories, and in 10-calorie increments above 50 calories. Quantities of protein, carbohydrates, and fats are expressed to the nearest gram. Nutrition labels show amounts in grams rather than ounces because grams are a smaller unit of measurement and many food components are present in very small amounts. Here is a guide to help you read nutrition labels:

$$1 \text{ pound (lb)} = 454 \text{ grams (g)}$$
$$1 \text{ ounce (oz)} = 28 \text{ grams (g)}$$
$$1 \text{ gram (g)} = 1{,}000 \text{ milligrams (mg)}$$
$$1 \text{ milligram (mg)} = 1{,}000 \text{ micrograms (mcg)}$$

The fat content statement must also give the percentage of calories from fat. Statement of the amounts of polyunsaturated and saturated fats (to the nearest gram) is optional if the food contains 10 percent or more total fat on a dry-weight basis and not less than two grams of fat in a serving.

Next, the manufacturer may state cholesterol content (expressed to the nearest 5-milligram increment per serving). When the cholesterol content or fat content is stated, this statement must appear on the label: "Information on cholesterol (and/or fat) content is provided for individuals who, on the advice of a physician, are modifying their total dietary intake of cholesterol (and/or fat)."[2]

Next on the nutrition information panel will come the statement of protein, vitamin, and mineral content in percentages of the U.S. RDA for each. This list includes two groups of nutrients. The first is a group of eight, consisting of protein, vitamin A, vitamin C, thiamine, riboflavin, niacin, calcium, and iron.

The FDA feels that a person who eats foods containing all of the nutrients in the first group is likely to obtain the necessary amounts of the twelve other essential vitamins and minerals in the second group: vitamin D, vitamin E, vitamin B_1, folic acid, vitamin B_{12}, phosphorus, iodine, magnesium, zinc, copper, biotin, and pantothenic acid. Listing any of these in part or in total is optional. However, if any of them are added to the food, they must be listed.

See Figures 15-1 and 15-2 for an overview of labeling information.

In all cases, the quantities of the protein, vitamins, and minerals are given as percentages of the U.S. RDA rather than as absolute amounts. Thus, consumers do not have to memorize or constantly refer to a table of the U.S. RDA to know if they are getting enough of any given nutrient; instead, they can simply add the percentages for all the foods they have eaten that day.

The FDA is concerned about those overzealous food manufacturers who, in hopes of selling more products, are adding excessive amounts of vitamins and minerals. So under the new ruling, any food that is fortified with 50 percent more vitamins and minerals than the RDA is considered a dietary supplement; if it contains more than 150 percent more vitamins and minerals, it is no longer classified as a food, but becomes a drug and must be handled as are all other over-the-counter drugs.

OTHER LABEL INFORMATION

Some foods are labeled as "imitations" of other foods. Under an FDA regulation, the word imitation must be used on the label when the product is not as nutritious as the product which it resembles and for which it is a substitute. If a product is similar to an existing one and is just as nutritious, a new name can be given to it rather than calling it imitation. For example, eggless products which are nutritionally equivalent to eggs have been given names such as Eggbeaters and Scramblers.

Imitation

Some foods may look from the label as though they are one thing and actually be another. To prevent deception of consumers, the FDA has ruled that such foods must have a "common or usual" name which gives the consumer accurate information about what is in the package or container.

Common or Usual Names

For example, a beverage that looks like orange juice but actually contains very little orange juice must use a name such as "diluted orange juice drink." The product also may be required to state the percentage of the characterizing ingredient it contains. In this case, the label might say, "Diluted orange juice beverage, contains 10 percent orange juice."

A noncarbonated beverage that appears to contain a fruit or vegetable juice but does not contain any juice must state on the label that it contains no fruit or vegetable juice.

Another special labeling requirement concerns packaged foods in which the main ingredient or component of a recipe is not included, as in the case of some "main dishes" or "dinners." On such foods, the common or usual name consists of the following:

- The common name of each ingredient in descending order by weight—for example, "noodles and tomato sauce."
- Identification of the food to be prepared from the package—for example, "for preparation of chicken casserole."
- A statement of ingredients that must be added to complete the recipe—for example, "you must add chicken to complete the recipe."

Some food products carry a grade on the label, such as "U.S. Grade A." Grades are set by the U.S. Department of Agriculture, based on the quality levels inherent in a product—its taste, texture, and appearance. U.S. Department of Agriculture grades are not based on nutritional content.

Grades

Milk and milk products in most states carry a "Grade A" label. This grade is based on the FDA-recommended sanitary standards for the production and processing of milk and milk products, which are regulated by the states. Although the grade is not based on nutritional values, the FDA has established standards for milk which require certain levels of vitamins A and D when these vitamins are added to milk.

Calories

A calorie is a unit of measurement that tells you how much energy you get from food. The body needs energy for activity and even at rest. Eating foods day after day that have fewer total calories than you use up will help you lose weight. If you eat foods that have more total calories than you need, the extra energy is stored as fat and you can gain weight. All foods provide calories.

On labels, the calorie content is shown to the nearest 2 calories (2, 4, 6, etc.) up to 20 calories; to the nearest 5 calories (20, 25, 30, etc.) up to 50 calories; and to the nearest 10 calories (50, 60, 70, etc.) above 50 calories.

Protein

Protein is the basic part of every cell in your body. The kind of protein that best meets the body's needs comes from animal foods—meat, fish, poultry, eggs, and milk. Protein from legumes, especially soybeans and chickpeas, is almost as good. Protein from cereals and vegetables performs best when these foods are used with a little meat, egg, milk, or cheese in the meal.

Carbohydrate

Foods contain three types of carbohydrate—starch, sugar, and cellulose. Starch and sugar give energy. You get starch from grain products (cereal, flour, breads, pastas), potatoes, and dry beans and peas. Concentrated sugar comes from such sources as cane and beet sugar, jellies, candy, honey, molasses, and syrup. Cellulose, important for bulk or roughage in the diet, is found in fruits, vegetables, and whole-grain cereals.

Fat

Fat is a concentrated source of energy. (A gram of fat provides roughly twice as much energy as a gram of protein or carbohydrate.) Fat in food digests slowly and helps keep you from feeling hungry. Fat carries the fat-soluble vitamins—A, D, E, and K.

Some foods are high in fat; for example, butter, margarine, shortening, cooking and salad oils, cream, nuts, and bacon. Meat, whole milk, and eggs also have some fat. Many popular snacks, baked goods, pastries, and desserts contain substantial amounts of fat.

Figure 15-1. Nutrition Information. From *Nutrition Labeling*, U.S. Department of Agriculture Information Bulletin No. 382, pp. 2–5.

Nutrition Information

Information must be given for a specified serving of the product as found in the container. This label shows information for a serving of potato flakes. Additional information may be listed for the product in combination with other ingredients—flakes prepared with butter, milk, salt, and water, for example.

Serving (portion) size

The amount of food for which nutrition information is given. It might not be the same as the amount you eat.

NUTRITION INFORMATION
(PER SERVING)
SERVING SIZE = 1 CUP*
SERVINGS PER CONTAINER = 24

	FLAKES	FLAKES+BUTTER, MILK, WATER, SALT*
CALORIES	140	280
PROTEIN, GRAMS	4	6
CARBOHYDRATE, GRAMS	30	32
FAT, GRAMS	0	14

PERCENTAGE OF U.S. RECOMMENDED DAILY ALLOWANCES (U.S. RDA)

PROTEIN	4	8
VITAMIN A	2	10
VITAMIN C	80	80
THIAMIN	10	15
RIBOFLAVIN	2	8
NIACIN	10	10
CALCIUM	2	4
IRON	4	4

*PREPARED ACCORDING TO RECIPE ON BACK OF PACKAGE.

Grams

Grams are units of weight. They are used on the label to express amounts of protein, fat and carbohydrate. A gram is a much smaller unit of weight than an ounce (1 ounce = 28 grams). A paper clip weighs about 1 gram.

Servings per container

The number of servings of the size shown that are in the container. This number may help you visualize the size of the serving. For example, if there are four servings in the container, you know that one serving is equal to one-fourth of the amount in the container.

To find the cost of a serving, divide the price for the container by the number of servings per container.

US. Recommended Daily Allowances

The U.S. Recommended Daily Allowances (U.S. RDA's) are the amounts of protein, vitamins, and minerals used as standards in nutrition labeling.

These allowances were derived from the Recommended Dietary Allowances (RDA's) set by the Food and Nutrition Board of the National Research Council. The RDA's are judged by the National Research Council to be adequate for nearly all healthy persons and generous for most persons.

The U.S. RDA for most nutrients is the highest RDA of all sex-age categories. Therefore, a diet that furnishes the U.S. RDA for a nutrient will furnish the RDA for most people and more than the RDA for many.

Special U.S. RDA's for infants and young children may be used for baby and junior-type food.

Vitamin A

Vitamin A is needed for normal growth and for normal vision in dim light. It also helps maintain the skin and the inner linings of the body. Some foods you can get it from are liver, eggs, butter, margarine, whole milk, and some kinds of cheese. You get carotene, which the body can change to vitamin A, from some vegetables and fruits, particularly dark-green and deep-yellow vegetables and some deep-yellow fruits.

Vitamin C

Vitamin C, or ascorbic acid, helps to keep blood vessels strong and to develop connective tissues. It has a number of other roles, from tooth and bone formation to wound healing. You can get the amount of vitamin C you need in a day from a serving of a rich food source such as citrus fruit or juice, or strawberries. Other important sources include melons, tomatoes, cabbage, certain dark-green leafy vegetables, and potatoes and sweetpotatoes, especially when cooked in the jacket.

Calcium

Calcium is the most abundant mineral element in the body. Teamed up with phosphorus, it is largely responsible for the hardness of bones and teeth. Milk is an outstanding source of calcium. Cheese, ice cream, and certain dark-green leafy vegetables also contribute valuable amounts of calcium to the diet.

Figure 15-2. Nutrition Information. From *Nutrition Labeling*, U.S. Department of Agriculture Information Bulletin No. 382, pp. 2–5.

Percentage

The amounts of protein, vitamins, and minerals in a serving are shown on the nutrition information panel as percentages of the U.S. Recommended Dietary Allowances (U.S. RDA's).

Percentages of the U.S. RDA are given in increments of 2 percent (2, 4, 6, etc.) up to 10 percent; of 5 percent (10, 15, 20, etc.) up to 50 percent; and of 10 percent (50, 60, 70, etc.) above 50 percent.

NUTRITION INFORMATION
(PER SERVING)
SERVING SIZE=1 CUP✱
SERVINGS PER CONTAINER=24

	FLAKES	FLAKES+BUTTER, MILK, WATER, SALT*
CALORIES	140	280
PROTEIN, GRAMS	4	6
CARBOHYDRATE, GRAMS	30	32
FAT, GRAMS	0	14

PERCENTAGE OF U.S. RECOMMENDED DAILY ALLOWANCES (U.S. RDA)

	FLAKES	FLAKES+BUTTER, MILK, WATER, SALT*
PROTEIN	4	8
VITAMIN A	2	10
VITAMIN C	80	80
THIAMIN	10	15
RIBOFLAVIN	2	8
NIACIN	10	10
CALCIUM	2	4
IRON	4	4

*PREPARED ACCORDING TO RECIPE ON BACK OF PACKAGE.

Iron

The body requires iron for making hemoglobin, the red part of blood that carries oxygen to the cells and carbon dioxide away from them. Iron also helps the cells get energy from food. Only a few foods are good sources of iron: lean meats, liver, and other organ meats, shellfish, dry beans and peas, dark-green vegetables, dried fruit, egg yolk, and molasses are some of them. Whole-grain and enriched breads and cereals contain small amounts, but are important sources when eaten frequently.

Thiamin, riboflavin, niacin

These B vitamins play a central role in the release of energy from food. They also help with proper functioning of nerves, normal appetite, good digestion, and healthy skin. Generally, foods in the meat group are leading sources of these vitamins. Whole-grain and enriched breads and cereals supply smaller, but important, amounts. A few foods are outstanding sources—milk for riboflavin, lean pork for thiamin, and organ meats for all three.

Open Dating   To help consumers obtain food that is fresh and wholesome, many manufacturers date their product. Open dating, as this practice is often called, is not regulated by the FDA.

To benefit from open dating, the consumer needs to know what kind of dating is used on the individual product and what it means. Four kinds of open dating are commonly used.

- Pack Date. This is the day the food was manufactured or processed or packaged. In other words, it tells how old the food is when you buy it. The importance of this information to consumers depends on how quickly the particular food normally spoils. Most canned and packaged foods have a long shelf life when stored under dry, cool conditions.
- Pull or Sell Date. This is the last date the product should be sold, assuming it has been stored and handled properly. The pull date allows for some storage time in the home refrigerator. Cold cuts, ice cream, milk, and refrigerated fresh dough products are examples of foods with pull dates.
- Expiration Date. This is the last date the food should be eaten or used. Baby formulas and yeast are examples of products that may carry expiration dates.
- Freshness Date. This is similar to the expiration date but may allow for normal home storage. Some bakery products that have a freshness date are sold at a reduced price for a short time after the expiration date.

Code Dating   Many companies use code dating on products that have a long shelf life. This is usually for the company's information, rather than for the consumer's benefit. The code gives the manufacturer and the store precise information about where and when the product was packaged, so if a recall should be required for any reason the product can be identified quickly and withdrawn from the market.

Universal Product Code   Many food labels now include a small block of parallel lines of various widths, with accompanying numbers. This is the Universal Product Code (UPC). The code on a label is unique to that product. Some stores are equipped with computerized checkout equipment that can read the code and automatically ring up the sale. In addition to making it possible for stores to automate part of their checkout work, the UPC, when used in conjunction with a computer, also can function as an automated inventory system. The computer can tell management how much of a specific item is on hand, how fast it is being sold, and when and how much to order.

Symbols   The symbol "R" on a label signifies that the trademark used on the label is registered with the U.S. Patent Office.

The symbol "C" indicates that the literary and artistic content of the label is protected against infringement under the copyright laws of the United States. Copies of such labels have been filed with the Copyright Office of the Library of Congress.

The symbol that consists of the letter "U" inside the letter "O" is the one whose use is authorized by the Union of Orthodox Jewish Congregations of

America, more familiarly known as the Orthodox Union, on foods that comply with Jewish dietary laws. Detailed information regarding the significance and use of this symbol may be obtained from the headquarters of that organization at 116 E. 27th Street, New York, NY 10016.

The symbol that consists of the letter "K" inside the letter "O" is also used to indicate that the food is "Kosher," that is, it complies with the Jewish dietary laws, and its processing has been under the direction of a rabbi.

None of the symbols referred to above are required by, or are under the authority of, any of the acts enforced by the Food and Drug Administration.

PROHIBITED CLAIMS

The FDA is trying to do two things with nutrition labeling regulation: provide the public with more information about the nutrients in food, and protect the public from misinformation. Thus regulations not only spell out what is to appear on nutrition labels, they expressly forbid certain claims about nutrition and diet. The FDA has long been concerned with misleading claims made to promote the sale of some foods and dietary supplements.

Under the regulations, a label is not allowed to say or even imply:

1. That a food can prevent, cure, mitigate, or treat any disease or symptom;
2. That a balanced diet of ordinary foods cannot supply adequate amounts of nutrients;
3. That a lack of optimal nutritive quality of a food, because of the soil on which that food was grown, is or may be responsible for an inadequacy or deficiency in the daily diet;
4. That storage, transportation, processing, or cooking of a food is, or may be, responsible for an inadequacy or deficiency in the daily diet;
5. That a natural vitamin is superior to an added or synthetic vitamin;
6. That a food contains certain nutrients when such substances are of no known need or significant value in human nutrition.[3]

The FDA states that these prohibitions are intended to stop unsupported generalization and fraudulent statements. However, if a manufacturer has adequate scientific data proving that a product has a higher nutrient retention than a competitor's, he or she may make that claim. However, the burden of proof does rest with the manufacturer.

NEW TERMINOLOGY

Many foods today are manufactured into products that are different from traditional foods. Some classes of these foods include frozen dinners, breakfast cereals, meal replacements, noncarbonated breakfast beverages fortified with vitamin C, and main dishes such as macaroni and cheese, pizzas, stews, and casseroles.

The FDA is establishing voluntary nutritional guidelines for such foods so consumers can be assured of getting a proper level and range of nutrients when using them. A product that complies with an FDA nutritional quality guideline may include on its label a statement that it meets the U.S. nutritional quality guideline for that particular class of food.

With our food supply changing so rapidly, it's difficult to keep all the food terminology straight. If you're having trouble distinguishing between formulated and fabricated or natural and organic, the following definitions will help you out.

Conventional Foods. Traditional foods are those primarily single-entity foods identified as dietary staples.

Formulated Foods. Mixtures of two or more foodstuffs or ingredients other than seasonings, processed or blended together, are called formulated foods. Examples may be "convenience foods" which resemble standard recipes but require little or no preparation in the home; i.e., frozen dinners, meal replacers such as liquid meals and prepared breakfast cereals, and snack foods.

Fabricated Foods. Prepared principally from ingredients specifically designed to achieve a particular function not possible with common food ingredients, fabricated foods may or may not closely resemble existing foods. An example is imitation orange juice, or foods derived from textured vegetable proteins. It is important that nutrient requirements be carefully evaluated, especially when a fabricated food is designed to replace a traditional food in the diet.

Processed Food. Processed foods are already prepared by commercial companies for quick consumer use.

Fast Foods. Fast foods, most often served in drive-in shops, can be reconstituted fast, served fast, and eaten fast. Examples are hamburgers, shakes, chicken, or pizza.

Natural Foods. Natural foods are as unrefined as possible and free from additives such as preservatives, emulsifiers, artifical colors, and flavors. They are not necessarily organically grown. Some examples are whole-wheat flour, undegermed cornmeal, certified raw milk, brown (unpolished) rice, honey, and molasses. They are no more nutritious or safe to eat than regular food. They may be more expensive, however.

Health Foods. The use of the word "health" in connection with foods constitutes a misbranding under the Food and Drug Act. The use of this word implies that these products have health-giving or curative properties, when in general they merely possess some of the nutritive qualities to be expected in any wholesome food product. The label claims on these products are such that the consumer is led to believe that our ordinary diet is sorely deficient in such vital substances as vitamins and minerals, and that these so-called health foods are absolutely necessary to conserve life and health.

However, other types of health foods are geared to special diets and may be called dietetic. Sometimes they're sugarless for the diabetic, though not necessarily lower in calories. They may be salt-free for those on a low-sodium regime. Or they may be low-cholesterol or low-saturated fat for those concerned about blood cholesterol and heart condition. They may be wheat-free or chocolate-free for those with allergy problems. They are not more healthy than other foods regularly found in grocery stores; they are merely specially designed for persons with special health problems and dietetic requirements.

Organic Foods. The term "organically grown food" means food that has not been subjected to pesticides or artificial fertilizers and that has been grown in soil in which the humus content has been increased by the addition of organic matter.

The term "organically processed food" means organically grown food that in its processing has not been treated with preservatives, hormones, antibiotics, or synthetic additives of any kind.

Organic is a misnomer. Plants use only inorganic elements to support growth. In most commercial crops, these elements are supplied by fertilizers. So-called organic crops are supported by soil in which microorganisms consistently transform organic matter into inorganic elements which are used by plants.

Organic foods are likely to cost considerably more than the same items produced and marketed by regular commercial methods. Producing organically grown and processed foods and natural foods does not lend itself to the mass production methods used to supply most of our food. Also organic and natural foods cannot be stored as long as regular foods, and may vary greatly in quality.

Anyone who chooses to use organic, natural, or health foods should be aware that:

- You must find markets where you can feel sure that the foods come from ethical suppliers and are what they claim to be.
- You must be willing to pay more for this food than if you were buying regular foods in usual markets.
- You must not expect the higher cost to buy additional nutritive value.
- You must not neglect total nutritional needs for good health by restricting food choices to only a limited variety of organic foods.[4]

The following are terms that also might be confusing to the average shopper.

Enrichment. Enrichment is the addition of more than one nutrient in conformity with a standard developed by the government. It applies to cereal products (flours, macaroni, noodles, etc.) in which federally prescribed levels of four nutrients—thiamine, riboflavin, niacin, and iron—are met. This does not mean other nutrients lost in the milling process have been replaced.

Restoration.   Restoration is the addition of nutrients to conventional foods in order to restore those nutrients that are present naturally, but have been destroyed or lost in processing.

Fortification.   Fortification is the addition of one or more nutrients that were not present or were present in small amounts in foods before processing. Examples include the vitamin D added to milk or the iodine to salt. Many cereals are fortified.

Nutrient Improvement.   Foods are sometimes enriched or fortified to improve the nutritive value of widely used foods in order to provide good nutrition without the necessity of extensive efforts to change food consumption patterns of the people, an effort which is usually not effective.

Food Supplements.   Food supplements include vitamins, minerals, and special foods such as dried liver protein tablets and brewer's yeast that are taken like medicine rather than eaten as part of a meal. Food supplements are necessary only for those with diagnosed nutrient deficiencies.

Dietary Supplements.   Products supplemented with 50 percent to 150 percent of the U.S. RDA are considered dietary supplements. These foods are taken by well and healthy individuals to increase their total nutrient intakes. This does not cover the use or promotion of vitamins or minerals for the treatment of any disease or medical condition. Fortified cereals, some baby foods, and fortified drinks are all dietary supplements.

SUMMARY

Nutritional labeling is for you, the consumer. It can help you to get more nutrition for less money. It can also aid those with certain shopping needs. For instance, if you are watching your weight, counting calories is a cinch with nutritional labeling. You just look on the label. If you are on a doctor's prescribed diet, labeling lets you know cholesterol and fat content, sodium and sugar levels. Consumers have a right to information about the substances that are in the foods they eat, and about the levels of protein, vitamins, minerals, calories, fats, and carbohydrates.

There are certain facts that the government requires on every food label, such as the name of the product, the net contents or net weight of the product, the name and place of business of the manufacturer, packer, or distributor. Then certain products must carry a list of the ingredients present (the largest, by weight, is listed first), additives, artificial colors or flavors, etc. The FDA has specified that labels with this nutritional material must be placed to the right of the main display appearing on the product. These labels should be as easily understandable as possible.

Nowadays other information often appears on labels as well, such as whether or not the product is imitation, the grade of the product, the date by which the product should be used, the trademark of the product, copyrights on the label, and dietary information for ethnic groups. Once consumers learn more about nutrition and the effect it has on health, and how to buy with nutrition in mind, "We—the best-fed nation in the world—may become the best-nourished."[5]

NOTES

1. "Time to Bone Up on Nutrition Labeling," *FDA Consumer,* February 1975, pp. 22-23.
2. Arletta Beloian, "Nutrition Labels: A Great Leap Forward," *FDA Consumer,* September 1973, pp. 14-17.
3. Ibid., pp. 10-16.
4. Marilyn Stephenson, "The Confusing World of Health Foods," pp. 19-22.
5. Marion McGill, "Nutrition Labeling," *Family Health,* November 1973, pp. 35-38.

UNIT 3

OVERWEIGHT AND OBESITY

16

Overweight — A Twentieth-Century Health Problem

Prior to the twentieth century, adiposity (excess weight) was valued as a mark of affluence, beauty, and health. However, we no longer regard obesity with benevolence. Overeating and consequent overweight is now often regarded as a behavior maladjustment. Insurance companies contend that **overweight** clients are higher risk because obesity is associated with a shortened life expectancy and an increased susceptibility to numerous diseases.

In the United States, a third of the population is overweight and another third is struggling to keep its weight stable. Even 10 percent of school children are overweight. Government surveys show that in nearly all age groups, adults are putting on weight. (See Table 16-1.)

Table 16-1. Adult Weight Gain over the Years

| By Age | Average adult man tipped the scales at— | | | Average adult woman tipped the scales at— | | |
	Early 1960s 166 lb.	Latest 172 lb.	Change + 6 lb.	Early 1960s 140 lb.	Latest 143 lb.	Change +3 lb.
18-24	158 lb.	165 lb.	+7 lb.	127 lb.	132 lb.	+5 lb.
25-34	169 lb.	176 lb.	+7 lb.	134 lb.	140 lb.	+6 lb.
35-44	170 lb.	178 lb.	+8 lb.	142 lb.	148 lb.	+6 lb.
45-54	170 lb.	175 lb.	+5 lb.	145 lb.	149 lb.	+4 lb.
55-64	164 lb.	171 lb.	+7 lb.	150 lb.	149 lb.	−1 lb.
65 and over	158 lb.	164 lb.	+6 lb.	144 lb.	146 lb.	+2 lb.

Department of Health, Education, and Welfare, U.S. Public Health Service.

FAT, OVERWEIGHT, AND OBESITY

Fat synthesis and storage (called lipogenesis) is a normal function of adipose (fatty) tissue in the body. (See Figure 16-1.) Generally speaking, when total energy input (calories) into the body exceeds the total energy output, the excess energy is stored as fat. In an average person, 90 percent of available stored energy is in the form of fat, enough to last one through two months of total starvation.

Fat Distribution

Fat is not stored in the same manner in all people. The mechanisms for fat distribution are unknown, although some anthropologists have formulated an association between body type, degree of ponderosity, and climatic conditions in which people reside. For example, lean, agile people tend to be found in the tropics; large, ponderous people are found in cool climates; short-statured people in cold places; and people with long extremities in warm places. It is theorized that these differences in body build are adaptations to optimize radiant loss of energy from body surfaces. Notably, localized fat on the buttocks (steatopygia) found in some women (such as the Hottentots of southern Africa) resembles the local deposition of stored fat in the camel, in several fat-tailed sheep strains, and in the humped camel. Species with localized fat deposits usually inhabit dry, hot places where food is highly seasonal, giving energy storage a large survival value.

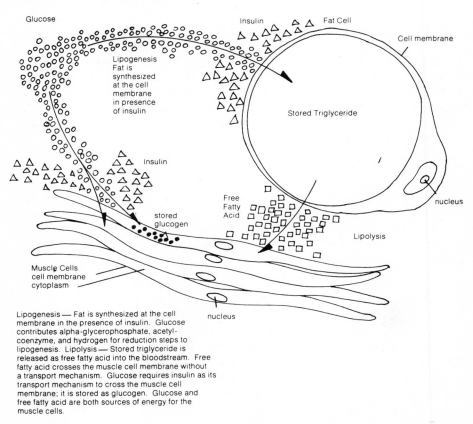

Lipogenesis — Fat is synthesized at the cell membrane in the presence of insulin. Glucose contributes alpha-glycerophosphate, acetyl-coenzyme, and hydrogen for reduction steps to lipogenesis. Lipolysis — Stored triglyceride is released as free fatty acid into the bloodstream. Free fatty acid crosses the muscle cell membrane without a transport mechanism. Glucose requires insulin as its transport mechanism to cross the muscle cell membrane; it is stored as glucogen. Glucose and free fatty acid are both sources of energy for the muscle cells.

Figure 16-1. Lipogenesis (Fat Synthesis and Storage). From George Schauf, "All Calories Don't Count ... Perhaps," *Nutrition Today,* September/October 1971, p. 21. Reproduced with permission of *Nutrition Today* Magazine, 101 Ridgely Avenue, Annapolis, Maryland 21204. © September/October 1971.

Obese persons differ from nonobese individuals in morphologic (external structure and form) characteristics other than quantity of fatty tissue. Several studies suggest that obese persons tend to have a typical somatotype (a particular build or body type), being more endomorphic, somewhat more mesomorphic, and markedly less ectomorphic than the general population. (See Figure 16-2.)

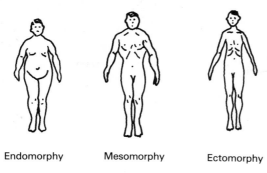

Endomorphy   Mesomorphy   Ectomorphy

Figure 16-2. Human Somatotypes

The problem with fat storage is in determining when the quantity of stored fat becomes excessive and perhaps dangerous to health. "Overweight" and "obesity" are both terms used in describing excess weight, but they are not synonymous. Obesity refers to excessive fat tissue only. Overweight refers to an increase in weight of the total body compartments, which include essential vital tissue (muscle, liver, kidney, blood, glands, joints), water, and fat.

Overweight versus Obesity

Excess weight (overweight) does not necessarily mean obesity. In some people, excess weight may be the result of heavy muscle development and not excessive fat. According to standard height-weight charts many athletes may be considered overweight, but they are rarely obese. There is no evidence that a heavy muscular body is unhealthy. Health problems are associated with an excess accumulation of fat. On the other hand, a sedentary person with poorly developed muscles and an excessive proportion of fat to total body weight can be obese without being overweight according to the chart.

MEASURING OBESITY

Since fat storage is normal **adipose** tissue function, it is difficult to determine when the quantity of stored fat becomes excessive. As a general rule, obesity is defined when the proportion of fatty tissue to total body weight exceeds 20 to 25 percent in males and 25 to 28 percent in females. From nine years of age on, women have a higher percentage of body weight in fat than do men. Young women have over 2½ times as much fat as comparable young men; older women have not quite 1½ times as much fat as men of the same age. Body fatness increases with age in both sexes, but at a faster rate in males. Women increase 55 percent in body fatness from the third to seventh decade of life, while men increase 87 percent over approximately the same age span. Body fat represents approximately 28.7 percent of total body weight for twenty-year-old women and 11 percent of total weight of twenty-year-old men. Body fat has increased to 41.9 percent for women by about age sixty and to 25.8 percent for men aged fifty-and-a-half years.[1]

Most people depend on height-weight charts (such as Tables 16-2 and 16-3) to determine proper body weight. Research indicates that in many cases this type of measure is inadequate. For example, the so-called ideal weight within any one

Height-Weight Charts

category on these tables can vary by as much as 22 pounds, and it is not unusual for a person to meet the criteria in the height-weight tables while actually carrying from 15 to 30 pounds of excess fat. Many height-weight tables provide a range of values for three different sizes of body frames. Unfortunately, no accepted method has been devised for determining which type of frame an individual has. Furthermore, an increase in weight may represent muscle development rather than increased fat.

Table 16-2.   Desirable Weights for Men of Ages 25 and Over

Height (Shoes on 1" heels)	Small Frame	Medium Frame	Large Frame
5'2"	112-120	118-129	126-141
5'3"	115-123	121-133	129-144
5'4"	118-126	124-136	132-148
5'5"	121-129	127-139	135-152
5'6"	124-133	130-143	138-156
5'7"	128-137	134-147	142-161
5'8"	132-141	138-152	147-166
5'9"	136-145	142-156	151-170
5'10"	140-150	146-160	155-174
5'11"	144-154	150-165	159-179
6'0"	148-158	154-170	164-184
6'1"	152-162	158-175	168-189
6'2"	156-167	162-180	173-194
6'3"	160-171	167-185	178-199
6'4"	164-175	172-190	182-204

Courtesy of Metropolitan Life Insurance Company.

Table 16-3.   Desirable Weights for Women of Ages 25 and Over

Height (Shoes on 2" heels)	Small Frame	Medium Frame	Large Frame
4'10"	92-98	96-107	104-119
4'11"	94-101	98-110	106-122
5'0"	96-104	101-113	109-125
5'1"	99-107	104-116	112-128
5'2"	102-110	107-119	115-131
5'3"	105-113	110-122	118-134
5'4"	108-116	113-126	121-138
5'5"	111-119	116-130	125-142
5'6"	114-123	120-135	129-146
5'7"	118-127	124-139	133-150
5'8"	122-131	128-143	137-154
5'9"	126-135	132-147	141-158
5'10"	130-140	136-151	145-163
5'11"	134-144	140-155	149-168
6'0"	138-148	144-159	153-173

Courtesy of Metropolitan Life Insurance Company.

A more accurate estimate of an individual's ideal weight can be made by assessing body composition to determine lean body weight and the weight of body fat.

Obviously, the optimal weight and percentage fat for an individual is that which is most conducive to health. Unfortunately, however, scientists are not yet able to predict for a given individual what these optimal values are. Certainly it is undesirable to weigh a great deal more or less than the average weight of the population, but between high and low extremes, there is a fairly wide range of desirable weights. An estimate of from 10 to 15 percent body fat for men and from 15 to 20 percent body fat for women may be used as a general desirable goal.

Methods for evaluating total body fat include measurement of body density (weight per unit of volume), measurement of body water content (hydrometry), and total body radiopotassium content using whole-body scintillation counters.

Densimetry. Densimetric techniques are based on the fact that fat has the lowest density of any body constituent. The density of fat is 0.90, a value somewhat less than that of water (1.0); the density of the lean body mass (muscle tissue and bone together) is 1.10.

Body density is usually determined by application of Archimedes' principle of underwater weighting. The fat of the body, with its low specific gravity, contributes to the buoyancy of people in water; bones and muscle, being heavier than water, tend to sink. Therefore, a person with a large percentage of body fat will have a specific gravity value approaching 0.90. A very muscular individual with little fat will have a specific gravity close to 1.1. Total body water is related to body fat, presuming fat to be anhydrous (containing no water) and water to be a relatively constant proportion of lean body mass. Because of the difference in water content between fat tissue and lean body mass (muscle tissue), it is possible to determine body fat content by measuring body density.

Hydrometry. Hydrometry is a measure of fatness that is accomplished by injecting deuterium (an isotope of hydrogen) into the body. After it has had time to circulate, a blood sample is taken. By measuring the dilution of the deuterium oxide in the blood, calculations can be made to determine the amount of fat in the body.

Potassium Content. Total body potassium correlates with lean body mass, because potassium is present in only trace amounts in fat. Body composition is determined by counting the gamma rays that are constantly being given off by the potassium. Thus, a high potassium count is indicative of little fat tissue.

Anthropometric Measurements. Measurement of skinfold thickness by a caliper appears the simplest method for evaluation of obesity. Measurement of skinfold thickness provides a reproducible measurement of **subcutaneous** fat (about 50 percent of total fat) and an index of total body fat. The relation of skinfold thickness to body fat content is practically independent of height. A simple pinch skinfold test is done by trained technicians who use the thumb and index finger to pinch skin and fat away from the body at several sites—at the back of the upper arm, beneath the shoulder blade, or over the abdomen. The thickness of the skinfold is measured with special calipers. (See Figure 16-3.)

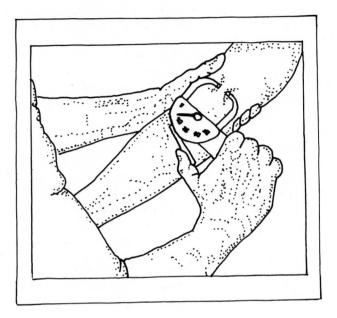

Figure 16-3.   Calipers Provide an Accurate Assessment of Body Fatness

Caliper measurements may help follow the course of obesity therapy and boost the patient's morale during periods when weight loss does not appear on the scale but skinfold measurements show a change in subcutaneous fat deposits. Skinfold measurements should be taken by the same technician throughout therapy.

CAUSES OF OBESITY

Obesity is the visible sign of the consequences of the ingestion of more calories than are being utilized. There are various causes in various people, but they all have the same final manifestation—the increased storage of fat. Obesity most often stems from excess caloric intake combined with inadequate activity. Other contributing factors include metabolic and genetic differences; psychological, social and environmental problems; and sometimes disease. In pinpointing the cause of all obesity, it is probably more accurate to describe a combination of factors, since obesity is not one homogeneous entity.

Fat accumulates in the body when **adipocytes** (fat cells) store excess triglyceride. Adipocytes have an extraordinary ability to expand to an almost unlimited size. Obesity may occur through enlargement of existing fat cells (**hypertrophy**) or through an increase in the total number of adipocytes (**hyperplasia**). All obese persons exhibit some enlargement of fat cells, but individuals with marked obesity also usually have more cells. An average nonobese individual has 25 to 30 x 10^9 adipocytes; obese persons may have 3 to 5 times that number.[2]

Type and Onset

Fundamental characteristics of adipose tissue are determined during the last months of gestation, throughout infancy, and during adolescence. Overnutrition during these critical times may produce a highly cellular adipose tissue (hyperplasia). Adipose tissue loses its ability to grow by cellular hyperlasia with age, and by adult life, any increase in body fat is accomplished by an increase in cell size, not by an increase in cell number. Adipocyte number remains fixed in the adult, and loss in body fat results entirely from decrease in size of cells and not from a decrease in the number.

Metabolism of fat tissues appears to be the same in both obese and nonobese persons. However, juvenile-onset obesity (hyperplasia) is more resistant to treatment than adult-onset (hypertrophy) because of the double burden of an increased number and an increased size of fat cells. Hypertrophic obesity is theoretically relieved simply by emptying the adipocytes of their excess lipid content. Achieving a similar weight loss in the hyperplastic individual, however, may require decreasing the fat content of the excessive number of cells to an abnormally low concentration. We are not yet certain whether long-term maintenance of a reduced body weight can bring about a reduction in number of fat cells.[3]

Calories do count in gaining and losing weight, as the following equations indicate:

Caloric Expenditures and Weight Gain

$$500 \text{ kilocalories deficit/day} = 3500 \text{ kilocalories deficit/week}$$
$$= \text{loss of 1 lb body weight/week}$$
$$= \text{loss of 52 lb body weight/year}$$

$$250 \text{ kilocalories excess/day} = 3500 \text{ kilocalories excess/2 weeks}$$
$$= \text{gain of 1 lb body weight/2 weeks}$$
$$= \text{gain 26 lb body weight/year}$$
$$= \text{gain 100 lb body weight/4 years}$$

Every calorie absorbed by the body must be used as energy or stored as fat. Table 16-4 shows how much weight gain one can expect when eating single portions of a food above daily maintenance requirements for varying periods.

There appears to be a significant difference between the fundamental nature of the problems of moderately and grossly obese individuals. The grossly obese individual is often a voracious overeater who puts on several hundred pounds in his or her teens or early twenties. The average middle-aged American is more likely to gain pounds over several years, because his or her caloric intake has remained high but his or her life style has become more sedentary.

Table 16-4. Body Weight-Gain Equivalent of Food (expressed in days or weeks of eating single portions above daily maintenance requirements to gain specified weight)

food (one portion)	weight	energy	body weight-gain			
			1 lb.	25 lb.	1 kg.	25 kg.
	gm.	kcal	days	weeks	days	weeks
apple, medium (3/lb., 2½″ diam.)	150	87	34	121	75	267
bacon, 2 strips	15	90	33	117	72	258
banana, medium	150	127	23	83	51	183
beef roast, 1 slice (4″ × 2½ × ½″)	53	150	20	70	43	155
beef, hamburger patty, 3″ diam. × 1″	85	224	13	47	29	104
beer, 8 fl. oz.	240	115	26	92	56	202
biscuit, 2″ diam.; 1 pat butter	40	166	18	63	39	140
brandy, cognac, 1 brandy pony	30	75	39	140	87	310
bread (28 slices/loaf), 1 slice; 1 pat butter	28	96	31	110	68	242
bread, peanut butter, and jam: 1 slice; 1 Tbsp.; 1 tsp.	38	195	15	54	33	119
brownie with nuts (2″ × 2″ × ¾″)	30	146	20	72	44	159
cake, plain, à la mode 1/12 of 9″: 1 dip (½ c.) ice cream	110	301	10	35	22	77
candy, hard, 1 oz.	30	110	27	96	59	211
caramel, 1 oz.	30	118	25	89	55	197
carrot, large	100	42	70	251	155	553
cereals, dry, ¾ cup; milk, 4 oz: + sugar, 1 tsp.	153	212	14	50	31	110
cheese, American, 1-oz. slice	30	112	26	94	58	207
cheese, cottage, 1/3 c.	75	80	37	132	81	290
chicken, breast, fried, ½ breast	96	232	12	44	27	97
chicken leg, fried, 1 medium	38	90	33	117	72	258
chocolate mint (45/lb.), 4 small	40	160	18	66	41	145
cola beverages, 8 fl. oz.	240	105	28	100	62	221
cookies, chocolate chip (43/lb.), 2	22	100	30	105	65	232
cookies, vanilla wafers, 4	13	60	49	176	108	387
crackers, saltines, 2	6	28	105	376	232	829
cracker, Graham	7	30	98	351	217	774
cupcake, 2½″ diam.	36	130	23	81	50	179
daiquiri, 3½ fl. oz.	100	125	24	84	52	186
doughnut, cake-type, icing	37	150	20	70	43	155
dressing, salad, 1 Tbsp.	14	75	39	140	67	310
egg, boiled or poached	48	78	38	135	83	298
egg, fried or scrambled	53	108	27	98	60	215

food (one portion)	weight	energy	body weight-gain			
			1 lb.	25 lb.	1 kg.	25 kg.
	gm.	*kcal*	*days*	*weeks*	*days*	*weeks*
French fries, 10 pieces	50	140	21	75	46	166
ginger ale, 8 fl. oz.	240	80	37	132	81	290
high ball, 8 fl. oz.	240	165	18	64	39	141
ice cream cone, 1 dip (½ c.)	72	160	18	66	41	145
martini, 3½ fl. oz.	100	140	21	75	46	166
milk whole, 8 fl. oz.	240	160	18	66	41	145
milk, skim, 8 fl. oz.	240	88	34	120	74	264
milk shake, 12 fl. oz.	345	420	7	25	15	55
orange, medium (2⅝″ diam.)	148	70	42	150	93	332
orange juice, 4 fl. oz.	120	54	55	195	120	430
pancake, with butter, sirup: 4½″ diam.; 1 pat: 2 Tbsp.	90	240	12	44	27	97
peanuts, 1 oz.	30	170	17	61	38	136
pie, apple, 1/6 of 9″ pie	160	400	7	25	16	58
pie, fruit, à la mode, 1/6, 1 dip ice cream	232	560	5	18	12	41
pizza, ⅛ of 14″ diam. pie	75	190	16	55	34	122
potato chips, 10 pieces	20	115	26	92	56	202
pretzels, 3-ring, 4	12	48	61	220	135	484
sandwiches (one each)						
bacon, lettuce, tomato	148	282	10	37	23	82
"Big Mac"	184	557	5	19	12	42
bologna with mayonnaise; 1 slice; 1 tsp.	68	220	13	48	30	106
cheese, toasted: 1 slice, 1 oz.	85	286	10	37	23	81
cheeseburger: 3″ diam. patty, 1-oz. slice cheese	180	462	6	23	14	50
hamburger, 3″ diam. × 1″	150	350	8	30	19	66
frankfurter	110	258	11	41	25	90
peanut butter, 1 round Tbsp.	83	328	9	32	20	71
roast pork, hot with gravy: 2½ oz. slice, 3 Tbsp. gravy	180	503	6	21	13	46
tuna fish salad	105	278	11	38	23	84
wine, champagne, 4 fl. oz.	120	85	35	124	76	273

Inactivity   Activity decreases as the mechanization of work and of transportation increases. Mayer describes obesity as a "disease of civilization." Many people today are sedentary enough to store rather than use the calories eaten.[5]

Sometimes a change in lifestyle produces a change in energy needs. Athletes often suddenly become obese when they stop training but maintain a high caloric intake. It is difficult for them to regulate food intake at low levels of energy expenditure.

Another problem is that the basal metabolism rate declines with age. Obesity and overweight can be produced in subjects of normal weight as they grow older if they do not change exercise or eating habits. At thirty, a person's basic need is 10 percent less than that of a fifteen-year-old. After thirty, one will need 7 percent less food for each decade of life. Because decreased caloric requirements can produce weight gain despite some decrease in caloric intake, daily exercise, in addition to decreasing food consumption, becomes important as a measure to counterbalance the decrease in basal requirements.

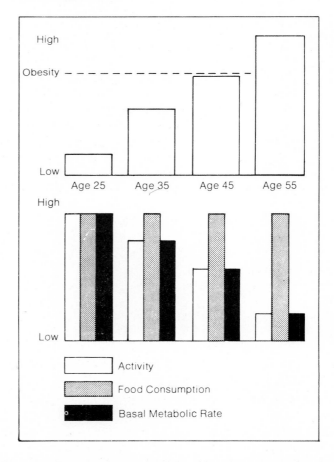

Figure 16-4.   Percentage of Body Fat. From U.S. Department of Agriculture.

Figure 16-4 shows the correlation between diet, activity, basal metabolic rate (amount of energy or calories needed to maintain body functions exclusive of activity and digestive processes), and rising obesity.

It has not yet been determined whether the obese gain weight because they don't exercise or whether they don't exercise because they are obese. At any rate, inactivity is definitely a major factor in making obesity self-perpetuating.

The tendency to be inactive and overweight appears early in life. Studies of infants reveal that fat babies tend to be inactive babies with very moderate appetites, while active babies eat more but are thinner and lighter.[6] Mayer reported a study conducted on high school girls:

> Inactivity is indeed the major factor in perpetuating obesity in many, if not most, overweight youngsters. Examination of the dietary intake and of the schedule of equal groups of overweight and normal weight girls, matched for age and height, showed that the obese students fell into two groups. One group, and by far the larger, contained girls who ate no more than the normal weight girls but who exercised considerably less. All the "sitting" activities were emphasized at the expense of walking and active sports. Television-watching consumed four times as many hours in this group as it did in the normal weight group. The second group (the existence of which emphasized that fact that there is more than one cause of obesity) ate more than the normal and exercised normally. These were of the red-cheeked, cheerful type, and while "overweight," they appeared less "overfat" than the inactive group. Other studies indicate that the same situation prevails with boys as well.[7]

Basal metabolism is the energy needed by each person to sustain vital life processes, including the functioning of vital organs and glands, breathing, metabolism in cells, blood circulation, and maintenance of body temperature. Basal metabolism is unique for each individual, and an accurate measurement of energy caloric requirements would usually be done by a physician or researcher. However, a rough estimate can be obtained by using the formula shown in Table 16-5.

Basal Metabolism and Activity Needs

Table 16-5. Sample Calculation of Basal Metabolism

Surface area of person 5 feet 3 inches tall, weighing 110 pounds	= 1.5 square meters
Basal metabolism standard for female— age 18	= 35.8 kilocalories/square meter/hour
Hours in day	= 24
35.8×1.5	= 53.70 = hourly caloric need
53.70×24	= 1288.80 kilocalories needed daily for basal metabolism

From *Living Nutrition* by Frederick Stare and Margaret McWilliams, 1973, p. 97 (John Wiley and Sons, Inc., New York).

Use Figure 16-5 to determine your own body surface area. Draw a line between your exact height (left column) and weight (right column) to derive the surface area. Multiply the number of square meters of surface area by the correct caloric value from Table 16-6 to determine hourly caloric needs for basal metabolism.

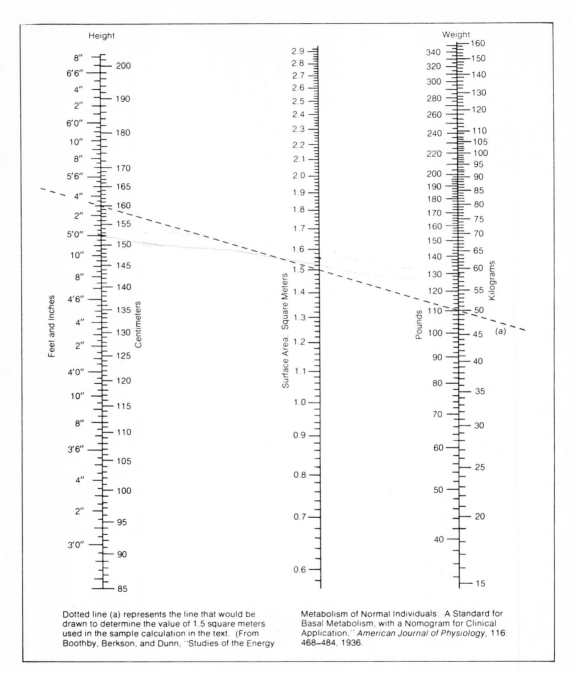

Dotted line (a) represents the line that would be drawn to determine the value of 1.5 square meters used in the sample calculation in the text. (From Boothby, Berkson, and Dunn, "Studies of the Energy Metabolism of Normal Individuals: A Standard for Basal Metabolism, with a Nomogram for Clinical Application," *American Journal of Physiology*, 116: 468–484, 1936.

Figure 16-5.   Chart for Determining Surface Area. From Boothby, Berkson, and Dunn, "Studies of the Energy Metabolism of Normal Individuals: A Standard for Basal Metabolism, with a Nomogram for Clinical Application," *American Journal of Physiology*, Vol. 116, 1936, pp. 468–484.

Table 16-6.   Basal Metabolism Standards

Age (yrs)	Males (cal per sq m per hr)	Females (cal per sq m per hr)
3	60.1	54.5
4	57.9	53.9
5	56.3	53.0
6	54.0	51.2
7	52.3	49.7
8	50.8	48.0
9	49.5	46.2
10	47.7	44.9
11	46.5	43.5
12	45.3	42.0
13	44.5	40.5
14	43.8	39.2
15	42.9	38.3
16	42.0	37.2
17	41.5	36.4
18	40.8	35.8
19	40.5	35.4
20	39.9	35.3
21	39.5	35.2
22	39.2	35.2
23	39.0	35.2
24	38.7	35.1
25	38.4	35.1
26	38.2	35.0
27	38.0	35.0
28	37.8	35.0
29	37.7	35.0
30	37.6	35.0
31	37.4	35.0
32	37.2	34.9
33	37.1	34.9
34	37.0	34.9
35	36.9	34.8
36	36.8	34.7
37	36.7	34.6
38	36.7	34.5
39	36.6	34.4
40-44	36.4	34.1
45-49	36.2	33.3
50-54	35.8	33.1
55-59	35.1	32.8
60-64	34.5	32.0
65-69	33.5	31.6
70-74	32.7	31.1
75+	31.8	

These values are smoothed means of basal calories per sq m per hr from the three largest and most authoritative sets of standards. The British standards (Robertson and Reid) are based on 937 males and 1323 females; the Mayo Foundation standards (Boothby, Berkson, and Dunn) are based on 639 males and 823 females; the Carnegie Nutrition Laboratory standards (Harris and Benedict) are based on 136 males and 103 females.

Reproduced with permission of the Federation of American Societies for Experimental Biology.

Multiply the hourly caloric needs by 24 to calculate the daily need. Total energy needs (basal metabolism + activities) can be determined by assessing basal metabolism plus energy (calories) needed for each activity performed during the day. Table 16-7 provides an example of the total energy requirements of an eighteen-year-old woman. A list of activities for your own use is found in Table 16-8 or Table 16-9 which has BMR included in the activity energy needs.

The specific dynamic action indicated in Table 16-10 allows for the energy costs required to convert and transport food from the form in which it is eaten to the many individual nutrients needed by the cells throughout the body. These energy costs need to be included in computing total caloric requirements.

Table 16-7. Estimated Daily Calorie Requirement for a Female Eighteen Years Old (body surface = 1.5 square meters, wt. 50 kilograms)

Calculations					kcal (24 hrs)
Basal metabolism					
35.8 ×.15 × 24 = 1289					1289
kcal/sq m/hr) age 18 female = 35.8[a]					
Surface area (5'3") = 1.5[b]					
Hours = 24					
Activity[c]					
	Time (hrs)	kcal/ hr	(kg)	kcal[d]	
Dressing	1	× 0.7	× 50	= 35	
Eating	1	× 0.4	× 50	= 20	
Driving	2	× 0.9	× 50	= 90	
Studying	8	× 0.4	× 50	= 160	
Walking	2	× 2.0	× 50	= 200	
Watching TV	2	× 0.4	× 50	= 40	
Sleeping	8			—	
	24			545	545
Specific dynamic action					
Basal metabolism	1289				
Activity	545				
	1834				
1834 × 10% = 183					183
				Total	2017

a. From "Basal Metabolism Standards"
b. From "Chart for Determining Surface Areas"
c. From "Calories Needed to Sustain Various Activities."
d. Time × kcal/hr × (kg) = kcal required.

From *Living Nutrition* by Frederick Stare and Margaret McWilliams, 1973, p. 108 (John Wiley and Sons, Inc., New York).

Table 16-8. Calories Needed to Sustain Various Activities

Activity	cal. per kg per hr	Activity	cal. per kg per hr
Bicycling (century run)	7.6	Piano playing (Beethoven's *Appassionata*)	1.4
Bicycling (moderate speed)	2.5		
Bookbinding	0.8	Piano playing (Liszt's *Tarantella*)	2.0
Boxing	11.4		
Carpentry (heavy)	2.3	Reading aloud	0.4
Cello playing	1.3	Rowing in race	16.0
Crocheting	0.4	Running	7.0
Dancing, foxtrot	3.8	Sawing wood	5.7
Dancing, waltz	3.0	Sewing, hand	0.4
Dishwashing	1.0	Sewing, motor driven machine	0.4
Dressing and undressing	0.7	Shoemaking	1.0
Driving automobile	0.9	Singing in loud voice	0.8
Eating	0.4	Sitting quietly	0.4
Exercise		Skating	3.5
Very light	0.9	Skiing (moderate speed)	10.3
Light	1.4	Standing relaxed	0.5
Moderate	3.1	Stone masonry	4.7
Severe	5.4	Sweeping with broom, bare floor	1.4
Very severe	7.6	Sweeping with carpet sweeper	1.6
Fencing	7.3	Sweeping with vacuum sweeper	2.7
Horseback riding, walk	1.4	Swimming (2 mph)	7.9
Horseback riding, trot	4.3	Tailoring	0.9
Horseback riding, gallop	6.7	Typewriting rapidly	
Ironing (5 lb iron)	1.0	(standard typewriter)	1.0
Knitting sweater	0.7	(electric typewriter)	0.5
Laundry, light	1.3	Violin playing	0.6
Lying still, awake	0.1	Walking (3 mph)	2.0
Organ playing (1/3 hand work)	1.5	Walking rapidly (4 mph)	3.4
Painting furniture	1.5	Walking at high speed (5.3 mph)	8.3
Paring potatoes	0.6	Walking down stairs	b
Playing ping pong	4.4	Walking up stairs	c
Piano playing (Mendelssohn's *Song without Words*)	0.8	Washing floors	1.2
		Writing	0.4

    [b] Allow 0.012 calorie per kilogram for an ordinary staircase with 15 steps, without regard to time.

    [c] Allow 0.036 calorie per kilogram for an ordinary staircase with 15 steps, without regard to time.

Adopted with permission of The Macmillan Company from *Foundations of Nutrition*, 6th ed., by Taylor and Pye. © The Macmillan Company, 1967.

Table 16-9. Energy Used for Some Routine Daily Activities

Activity	Calories per lb per hour[b]	120	140	160	180	200	220
		Weight (lb)[a] Calories Used per Hour					
Sleeping	0.4	48	56	64	72	80	88
Awake, lying still	0.5	60	70	80	90	100	110
Sitting quietly (TV)	0.6	72	84	96	108	120	132
Eating	0.7	84	98	112	126	140	154
Writing	0.7	84	98	112	126	140	154
Standing relaxed	0.8	96	112	128	144	160	176
Dressing and undressing	0.9	108	126	144	162	180	198
Driving automobile	1.0	120	140	160	180	200	220
Dishwashing	1.0	120	140	160	180	200	220
Ironing	1.0	120	140	160	180	200	220
Typing rapidly	1.0	120	140	160	180	200	220
Light laundry	1.1	132	154	176	198	220	242
Walking (3 mph)	1.5	180	210	240	270	300	330
Sweeping with vacuum cleaner	1.9	228	266	304	342	380	418

[a] For those of different weights than those listed, multiply actual weight in pounds by the calories per pound per hour for each activity (e.g., 154 lb × 0.4 = 62 calories per hour for sleeping). This chart may be used to calculate approximate daily caloric expenditure if approximate amounts of time for each activity are tabulated for an average 24-hour day.
[b] Calculated to include basal metabolic needs.

From *Living Nutrition,* by Frederick Stare and Margaret McWilliams, 1973, pp. 87–113 (John Wiley and Sons, Inc., New York).

Table 16-10. Estimated Daily Caloric Requirement Using Figures That Include Basal Needs in the Activity Value

Activity	kcal/lb/hr[b]	Hr spent	kcal
Dressing/undressing	0.9	1	110
Walking (3 mph)	1.5	2	330
Eating	0.7	1	77
Studying and class	0.7	8	616
Driving car	1.0	2	220
Sitting quietly	0.6	2	132
Sleeping	0.4	8	352
Total		24	1837

Specific dynamic action = 1837 × 10% = 184 kcal
Total needs for day = 1837 + 184 = 2021 kcal
[a] Subject used is 110 lb (50 kg) girl.

From *Living Nutrition,* by Frederick Stare and Margaret McWilliams, 1973, pp. 87–113 (John Wiley and Sons, Inc., New York).

Misconceptions about exercise may influence some to avoid activity and its sub-sequent benefits. Many believe, for example, that increased activity also increases appetite and therefore encourages weight gain. Actually, exercise tends to stimulate the regulatory mechanism to control appetite within limits that help maintain normal weight. Prolonged exercise even diminishes eating below normal weight maintenance. *Activity Myths*

When rats were exercised for one to five hours daily, food intake rose to keep body weight constant. But when they were exercised less than one hour per day, food intake did not decline but actually rose, producing an increase in body weight. It has also been shown that restriction in activity will lead to gross obesity in experimental animals.[8] Inactivity does not reduce appetite and thus control weight gain. In fact, inactivity seems to have just the opposite effect.

Another common misconception is that physical activity does not use many calories. Anyone who has carefully perused a table of caloric requirements would understand the importance of exercise. Table 16-11 gives correlations between food and activity. Jean Mayer elucidates:

> The daily caloric allowance for men recommended by the National Research Council varies from 2,400 calories for "sedentary" men to 4,500 calories for "very active" men. The latter figure does not represent an upper limit. Laborers, soldiers, and athletes are advised by the NRC that they may require up to (and occasionally more than) 6,000 calories. Surely a factor which can more than double daily energy expenditure is not one to be casually ruled out as of no great importance in determining caloric balance! In fact, the cost of walking (in terms of caloric expenditure over the cost of sitting) varies from 200 to 350 calories per hour, depending on the speed, for a 150-pound man; swimming will consume twice as much. The peaks reached in athletic competition may approach 1,200 calories per hour, a rate that untrained persons would not reach and which even trained athletes could not maintain. Forgetting such extremes, a caloric expenditure rate of the order of 500 to 600 calories per hour represents a degree of physical activity which can be comfortably endured for at least half an hour by an average healthy adult, even if he is out of condition. A trained man should feel all the better after a full hour or more of such exercise. For those for whom translation into foods means more than caloric counts, the expenditure corresponding to 30 minutes of this type of exercise is equivalent to an average size piece of apple pie decorated by a standard scoop of ice cream. You can eat your cake and not have it with you always, if you substitute regular exercise for regular food deprivation.
>
> Even more important, it has already been noted that the cost of activity is dependent on the subject's size. In exercises where no heavy object outside the body is moved, the cost of exercise increases proportionately to body weight. If excess body weight is such that it impairs body movement, the caloric cost of exercise will actually increase faster than does body weight. An overweight person will thus burn a greater amount of body fat for the same amount of exercise than will a person of normal weight.

The **hypothalamus,** a gland in the body, houses the feeding and satiety centers which control the desire to eat. Responding to the amount of glucose circulating in the blood, it signals the gastrointestinal tract, probably through a hormone system, to produce hunger and satiety sensations to regulate food intake. Both animals and humans can regulate their food intake to match their energy needs. The regulation *Regulation of Food Intake* of food intake is subject to many possible influences, including temperature, osmotic pressure, gastric filling, and conditioning. Damage to the hypothalamus can alter normal food intake regulation and trigger uncurbed food ingestion leading to obesity.

Mayer explains his glucostatic theory of regulation of food intake (the mechanism thought to operate in glucose utilization) as follows:

> . . . there are in the hypothalamus receptors with a special affinity for glucose, which are activated by this blood component in the measure that they utilize it. The concept was based at the start on the fact that glucose is the almost exclusive fuel of the central nervous system. Its availability in turn determines the rate at which fat and protein are utilized; it therefore plays a central role in the economy of the body. It is stored (as glycogen) in small amounts and the stores are depleted within a few hours, faster in the cold or when the subject is exercised. The utilization is influenced by various hormones, and is drastically decreased when insulin is lacking as in diabetics. [The hypothesis included the postulate that the hypothalamic receptors, unlike the rest of the brain, would be found to be influenced by the concentration of insulin.] [10]

Metabolic and Glandular Disorders

A defect in the adipose tissue can cause abnormal amounts of fat to be produced. A person with this type of metabolic condition possesses abnormal amounts of fat in relation to protein tissue. For this person food turns to fat more quickly than for someone with normal metabolism who eats the same amount of food and uses the same amount of energy.

Much obesity has been blamed on glandular or endocrine imbalance. Abnormal endocrine function may encourage increased food intake or decreased energy output and in this way contribute to weight gain. However, only about 2 to 5 percent of all obesity results directly from endocrine problems.

One of the most familiar problems is that of thyroid gland malfunction, in which either too much or too little thyroxine is secreted. Too little thyroxine (hypothyroidism) and the metabolism slows, leading to fat accumulation. Too much thyroxine (hyperthyroidism) and the reverse is true.

It is important to consider the possibility of endocrine abnormalities in every patient, since many of these diseases can be treated.

Effects of Heredity and Genetics

Seventy-five percent of overweight children have at least one overweight parent. Many have thought that this is due to environmental conditioning, and that the child learns eating patterns which cause him or her to overeat and become obese. Supporting this theory are studies of identical twins separated at birth which showed that the twin reared by overweight parents who pushed food on him usually was overweight, while the identical brother or sister reared by normal-weight parents was of normal weight.[11] However, the fact that children adopted at birth do not always show an association with the weight of their foster parents indicates that the genetic component is involved.[12] The implication is that it's possible to counteract genetic tendency to fatness with careful eating habits.

It may be that hyperplasticity in obese children is genetically as well as nutritionally acquired.

Table 16-11.

How much exercise is needed to burn off a given number of calories.* For example, it would take 19 minutes of walking (at 3.5 mph) or 5 minutes of running to burn off the calories contained in an apple.		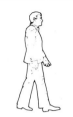 Walking (3.5 mph) 5.2 calories per min.	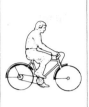 Bike Riding 8.2 calories per min.	Swimming 11.2 calories per min.	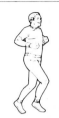 Running 19.4 calories per min.
Food	**Calories**	**Minutes of Activity**			
Apple, large	101	19	12	9	5
Bacon, 2 strips	96	18	12	9	5
Banana, small	88	17	11	8	4
Beer, 1 glass	114	22	14	10	6
Bread and butter	78	15	10	7	4
Cake, 2-layer, 1/12	356	68	43	32	18
Carbonated beverage, 1 glass	106	20	13	9	5
Carrot, raw	42	8	5	4	2
Cereal, dry, 1/2 c. with milk, sugar	200	38	24	18	10
Chicken, fried, 1/2 breast	232	45	28	21	12
Cookie, plain	15	3	2	1	1
Egg, fried	110	21	13	10	6
Ham, 2 slices	167	32	20	15	9
Ice Cream, 1/6 qt.	193	37	24	17	10
Malted milk shake	502	97	61	45	26
Milk, 1 glass	166	32	20	15	9
Milk, skim, 1 glass	81	16	10	7	4
Orange juice, 1 glass	120	23	15	11	6
Pancake with syrup	124	24	15	11	6
Peach, medium	46	9	6	4	2
Pie, apple, 1/6	377	73	46	34	19
Pizza, cheese, 1/8	180	35	22	16	9
Pork chop, loin	314	60	38	28	16
Club sandwich	590	113	72	53	30
Hamburger sandwich	350	67	43	31	18
Shrimp, French fried	180	35	22	16	9
Spaghetti, 1 serving	396	76	48	35	20
Steak, T-bone	235	45	29	21	12
Strawberry shortcake	400	77	49	36	21

*This chart is based on an individual weighing 150 lb.

Adapted from F. J. Konishi, *J. Am. Dietetic Assn.* 46:186, 1965. Copyright The American Dietetic Association. Reprinted by permission from *Journal of the American Dietetic Association*.

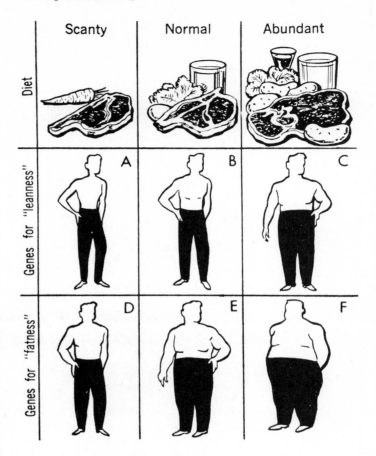

Figure 16-6. Gene Environment Interaction. From "Controversies in Medicine—Nature and Nuture in Human Obesity," by C. S. Chlourerakis, *Obesity/Bariatric Medicine,* Vol. 3, No. 1, 1974, p. 28. Adapted from Theodosius Dobzhansky, *Mankind Evolving* (Yale University Press, 1962) p. 45.

Obesity and Body Build. Chlourerakis suggests that heredity is influential in determining how obese an individual may become in a given set of environmental conditions:

> Two individuals, one having inherited "genes for leanness" and the other "genes for fatness" are subjected to three different environmental settings consisting of scanty, normal, and abundant food. [See Figure 16-6.] The influence of the environment is obvious, as the degree of obesity increases with increasing food. Thus individual C possessing "genes for leanness' but exposed to abundant food is fatter than individual D having "genes for fatness" but exposed to scanty amounts of food. The influence of heredity is also obvious in that each of the three environmental settings the individual with "genes for fatness" is fatter than the individual with "genes for leanness." Awareness of this predisposition to obesity should prevent individual D

from becoming F, by appropriately modifying his own response to his environment. The crucial question is whether the goal of individual F should be to become D or A. In this context, the data of life insurance companies, indicating a more or less continuous falling of mortality rates as obesity decreases, would suggest that the goal of every individual would be to be as thin as possible. The data of insurance companies may be inapplicable in answering this question as they do not take into account the concept of a genetically determined minimum of body fat. This minimum could also be regarded as a physiologic minimum. Assuming that obesity per se is indeed associated with increased mortality, then it would not constitute a conceptual leap to consider this physiologic minimum as representing the ideal body weight of the individual.[13]

Genetic influence is difficult to pinpoint in obesity. As with diabetes, the basic defect is unknown and the disorder may have multiple causes and conditions.

OBESITY AND HEALTH

Aside from social, psychological, and aesthetic problems, obesity complicates and may predispose a number of serious health problems including diabetes, diseases of the digestive system, cerebral hemorrhage, difficulty in breathing, angina pectoris, circulatory collapse, varicose veins, hypertension, and dermatologic problems that develop between the legs and buttocks and other body friction areas.[14] Some research designates obesity as a disease itself because there are distinct metabolic differences between obese and normal-weight persons; others contend that obesity is merely a symptom of disease.

According to a Metropolitan Life study of 50,000 people (see Table 16-12), the death rate of obese men is 42 percent higher for men 30 percent overweight than for men of normal weight. It is unlikely that obesity in itself causes death, but it does contribute to other unhealthy conditions which cause death, and it complicates diseases which could be more successfully managed if the individual were of desirable weight. (See Table 16-13.)

Table 16-12.   Overweight and Excess Mortality

Overweight (Percent)	Excess Mortality* (Percent)	
	Men	Women
10	13	9
20	25	21
30	42	30

*Compared with mortality of standard risks (mortality ratio of standard risks equals 100 percent).

Courtesy of Metropolitan Life Insurance Company. Derived from data of the Build and Blood Pressure Study, Society of Actuaries, 1959.

Table 16-13. Overweight and Excess Mortality from Some Major Diseases

Disease	Excess Mortality* (Percent)	
	Men	Women
Heart disease	43	51
Cerebral hemorrhage	53	29
Malignant cancers	16	13
Diabetes	133	83
Digestive system diseases (gallstones, cirrhosis, etc.)	68	39

*Compared with mortality of standard risks (mortality ratio of standard risks equals 100 percent). These data apply to people about 20 percent or more overweight.

Courtesy of Metropolitan Life Insurance Company. Derived from data of the Build and Blood Pressure Study, Society of Actuaries, 1959.

Respiration

The process of breathing is more difficult for an obese person because of the added weight on the chest wall. Thick pads of fat in the abdomen also restrict breathing. It takes more work to supply oxygen to the blood so it in turn can supply oxygen to the brain and extra tissue. In gross obesity, breathing decreases, resulting in less oxygen taken into the blood stream. Carbon dioxide builds up and the person becomes sluggish and lethargic. In overweight people, an increased body volume must be supplied with oxygen by lungs that have not correspondingly increased their size. Anaesthetic risk is increased in overweight patients, and being overweight is a special problem for asthmatics.

Arthritis

An obese arthritic is likely to suffer more than a thin one. As joints stiffen, any additional weight or strain naturally increases wear on affected joints. While weight reduction can not cure arthritis, it can lessen the discomfort.

A vicious cycle is set up in overweight persons with arthritis of the hip, knees, or feet or in those who suffer from a ruptured intervertebral disc. Increased weight leads to greater wear and tear on these joints, which may become more irritated and painful. The increased discomfort forces the person to become less and less active, thereby favoring further weight gain.[15]

High Blood Pressure

High blood pressure (hypertension) is more common among the obese. Hypertension can result in varying degrees of damage to the brain (stroke) and kidneys (degeneration), as well as the heart. It is not known exactly how obesity contributes to high blood pressure. Weight reduction will lower blood pressure, but no data have yet shown that this improves the health outlook of obese patients. James

K. Alexander suggests that obesity places a hydraulic load on the heart by increasing the amount of tissue that must be perfused.[16] Weight loss should lesson this load.

Blood pressure is better correlated with body weight than with body fat. A study in Framingham, Massachusetts, showed that high blood pressure developed ten times more often in persons 20 percent or more overweight.[17] Men who kept their weights nearly constant over a twenty-year period of adult life had only 1/5 as much high blood pressure in middle life. Initially, more diabetes, cerebrovascular incidence, and coronary heart disease developed in obese persons during the twelve-year observation period. This is not to say a program of weight reduction would cure or prevent the problems, but it is strongly recommended that hypertensive overweight persons lose weight.

Cerebrovascular and Coronary Heart Disease

The relationship between cerebrovascular disease and obesity is more definite. Some studies show that excessive weight gain after the age of twenty is associated with cerebrovascular disease. Men overweight at the age of twenty and gaining weight (30 pounds or more) thereafter had three times more cerebrovascular disease than did men who did not gain.[18] George Mann indicates that the excessive intake of food necessarily promotes glyceride synthesis and transport.[19] Current theory argues that cardiovascular disease is promoted by increased fat production and elevated levels of the low-density lipoproteins that carry these lipids from the sites of synthesis to the adipocytes (fat cells), resulting in deposits and narrowing of blood vessels.

Atherosclerosis is the deposit of fatty material in the lining of the arterial wall. It can result in rupture of the blood vessel or in narrowing of these vessels, which may lead to stroke or heart attack. Studies show that there is a marked increase in the occurrence of atherosclerosis in overweight people.[20]

The contribution of obesity to coronary heart disease appears to be small so no predictive value of body fatness for coronary heart disease has been shown. Only angina pectoris and sudden death have been predicted, and the rate of correlation varies with age.[21] However, as one gains weight, the heart must work harder to supply nutrients to all tissues of the body. The greater the body mass, the greater the strain on the heart and, many feel, the greater the potential for heart disease.

In a contrary vein, Ancel Keys suggests that "No measure of relative weight or obesity made a significant contribution to future coronary heart disease, when factors of age, blood pressure, serum cholesterol, and smoking were comparable."[22] He argues that dietary influence has greater influence than body fat in coronary heart disease.

A similar opinion is voiced by John Gofman, who believes that overweight does not contribute to coronary heart diseases other than by increasing diastolic blood pressure and serum lipoprotein levels.[23]

While research continues to explore this issue, many insurance companies still operate premium control based on the claim that the prevention and treatment of obesity is an effective deterrent to the development of coronary heart disease.

Whether excess fat is or is not a direct cause of coronary heart disease, the National Institute of Health concludes that:

1. More hypertension exists among the obese than among the non-obese.
2. The obese person with high blood pressure experiences a greater risk of coronary heart disease and heart attacks than the non-obese person with high blood pressure.
3. Death rates for obese persons with high blood pressure are higher than those for persons who are only obese or for those with high blood pressure, without the complicating obesity.[24]

Diabetes,
Gall Bladder,
Hernia

Diabetes is more common in overweight individuals than in those of normal weight. Most patients with mature-onset diabetes are or have been obese. In one group of studies, 70 to 85 percent of diabetics had a history of obesity.[25] There is evidence that excess accumulation of fat in adipose cells somehow leads to insulin resistance and impaired glucose tolerance. When an overweight diabetic loses weight, the diabetes often improves.

The incidence of gall bladder disease is also significantly higher in overweight people as compared to those of normal weight. In one study, 88 percent of the 215 patients operated on for gallstones were found to be overweight.[26]

Some types of hernias also seem to be more common in overweight individuals, particularly those involving displacement of the stomach into the chest cavity.

Premature Aging

When overweight turns to obesity, the body physiology changes, as well as outward appearance. Neil Soloman found in a study of obese patients in their thirties, some as much as twice their normal weight, that the psycho-physiological profiles were startlingly similar to those of healthy seventy-one-year-old men who had been observed at the Gerontology Center of the National Institute of Health located at Baltimore City Hospital.[27] The average life expectancy of obese persons, similar to those studied, is approximately 15 years less than that of their normal age group. From the standpoint of lost years, obesity may be regarded as a form of premature aging.

There is scanty evidence relating childhood obesity with subsequent health problems in adult life. S. Abraham examined the adult health status of a group of school children classified as obese and indicated that being 20 percent or more over desirable weight is associated with a real increase in diabetes, arteriosclerotic heart disease, high blood pressure and cardiovascular renal disease. However, the increase in susceptibility among these extreme overweights was not impressive, except in the case of diabetes.[28]

Sexual Response

Sexual drives diminish in a grossly overweight individual. Obesity can present aesthetic and purely physical barriers to normal sexual relations. In addition, obese women more frequently develop menstrual irregularity than do their slim counterparts.

Pregnancy

There is a high correlation between maternal weight gain and the infant's birth weight. Too little weight gain during pregnancy is a common cause of small, premature, and high-risk babies. Data available for western women indicates that the optimal weight gain during pregnancy is about 24 to 27.5 pounds.[29]

Excess weight gain can also be detrimental to the mother and baby, however. Overweight can be a factor in producing difficult and prolonged labor due to abnormal positioning of the fetus. This can cause fetal distress, which in turn may complicate labor and delivery. Stillbirths occur more frequently.

In addition, severely overweight women have more difficult pregnancies and an increased occurrence of maternal and infant deaths. Other complications for the mother include high blood pressure, serious water retention, and kidney failure.[30] Furthermore, weight gained in pregnancy is often not entirely lost afterward, especially if the baby is not nursed.

SUMMARY

Obesity is clearly a multifaceted problem involving physiological, psychological, and cultural factors, all of which are extremely resistant to current therapeutic efforts. "Obesity" is the precise term to use in referring to gain of excess fat tissue. "Overweight" is a more general term referring to increased weight gain in all body tissues and compartments. The obese person is overweight, but the overweight person is not necessarily obese, and being overweight is not always undesirable.

Obesity may occur in two ways: existing adipocytes (fat cells) may enlarge or "hypertrophy"; or the number of fat cells may increase in a process called "hyperplasia." All obese individuals experience hypertrophy, but not all have abnormal amounts of fat cells. Hyperplastic obesity is also called "juvenile-onset" because development of extra adipocytes occurs during early or late childhood. Adult-onset obesity is strictly hypertrophic. Once hyperplastic obesity has developed, weight can be lost from the cells, but the number of cells is not reduced.

The exact mechanism that causes obesity is not known, but the main factor appears to be overeating combined with inadequate levels of activity. Metabolic and glandular disorders account for only 2 to 5 percent of all obesity. Heredity, basal metabolic rate, and body type all influence obesity development.

Obesity has not been shown to cause disease, but it may predispose and complicate numerous serious health problems, including diabetes, digestive diseases, arthritis, cerebral hemorrhage, difficult in breathing, angina pectoris, circulatory collapse, varicose veins, hypertension, and dermatologic problems. Obesity lowers sexual drives and is connected with complications of pregnancy and premature aging.

NOTES

1. *The Health Letter,* Vol. 9, No. 5, March 11, 1977, Communications, Inc.
2. Jules Hirsch, "Can We Modify the Number of Adipose Cells?" *Postgraduate Medicine,* May 1972, pp. 83–86.

3. George A. Bray, Henry A. Jordan, and Ethan A. Sims, "Evaluation of the Obese Patient," *Journal of the American Medical Association,* Vol. 235, No. 14, March 1976, pp. 49–60.

4. "The Endless Fight Against Fat," *Current Prescribing,* March 1976, pp. 49–60.

5. Hearings before the Select Committee on Nutrition and Human Needs of the U.S. Senate, *Nutrition and Disease – 1974, Part 4,* February 26, 1974, pp. 431–435, as submitted by Dr. George A. Bray.

6. Jean Mayer, "Hidden Bonds," *World Health,* February/March 1974, pp. 21–27.

7. Ibid.

8. George A. Bray, "Types of Human Obesity—A System of Classification," *Obesity/Bariatric Medicine,* Vol. 2, No. 5, 1973.

9. Mayer, "Hidden Bonds," pp. 21–27.

10. Jean Mayer, *Overweight* (Englewood Cliffs, N.J.: Prentice-Hall, 1968), pp. 20–21.

11. Thomas J. Coates and Carl C. Thoresen, "Treating Obesity in Children and Adolescents, A Review," *American Journal of Public Health,* February 1978, Vol. 68, No. 2, p. 145.

12. Mayer, "Hidden Bonds," pp. 21–27.

13. C. S. Chlourerakis, "Controversies in Medicine—Nature and Nurture in Human Obesity," *Obesity/Bariatric Medicine,* May/June 1974, pp. 28–31.

14. Jerome L. Knittle and Fredda Ginsberg-Fellner, "Can Obesity Be Prevented?" *Pediatric Annals,* May 1975, pp. 28–31, 34, 36, 38.

15. Sandoz Laboratories, "Overweight Can Hurt More Than Just Your Looks," Wall Chart, 1974.

16. George V. Mann, "The Influence of Obesity on Health," *The New England Journal of Medicine,* July, 25, 1974.

17. Ibid.

18. Ibid.

19. Ibid.

20. Sandoz Laboratories, "Overweight Can Hurt More Than Just Your Looks."

21. Mann, "The Influence of Obesity on Health."

22. Richard Gubner, "Overweight and Health: Prognostic Realities and Therapeutic Possibilities," in Louis Lasagna, (ed.), *Obesity: Causes, Consequences and Treatment* (New York: Medcom Press, 1974), pp. 7–25.

23. Ibid.

24. Neil Soloman, "Health Hazards of Obesity," *Obesity and Bariatric Medicine,* Vol. 1, No. 1, May/June 1972.

25. Sandoz Laboratories, "Overweight Can Hurt More Than Just Your Looks."

26. Ibid.

27. Soloman, "Health Hazards of Obesity."

28. Mann, "The Influence of Obesity on Health."

29. Sandoz Laboratories, "Overweight Can Hurt More Than Just Your Looks."

30. Soloman, "Health Hazards of Obesity."

17

Weight Control Fads and Fallacies

Considering the possibility of taking off a few pounds? Never fear, the weight reduction industry will gladly step in with pills, diets, and painless plans designed especially for you. People in the United States spend over $100 million a year buying dietetic foods, appetite suppressants, and exercise devices and attending reducing clinics.

Many people do need to slim down and are right to want to reduce. Yet, despite the money and time invested in reducing programs and gimmicks, no nationwide decrease in obesity has been reported. Studies on the long-range effects of dieting show that within a year, about 90 percent of individuals who lose weight gain it back. By ignoring the fundamental rules of weight reduction, they are doing little more than slenderizing their pocketbooks.

It is simply foolish for anyone who has spent years building up a storage of fat to believe that he or she can safely get rid of those stores overnight. The best way for the public to avoid being taken in by inaccurate or fraudulent claims is to have accurate information concerning the nature and causes of obesity; know the role of diet, drugs, exercise, and psychological factors in weight control management; know the difference between "fad" programs and sound diet management; and know how to recognize legitimate sources of information concerning weight loss.

THE WORTH OF POPULAR COMMERCIAL DIETS

There is a constant parade of "miracle diets" and "reducing formulas" worded to appeal to fat people from every walk of life. Testimonials such as "I thank you for my new body" or "my husband asked me for a date" play upon emotions rather than appeal to intelligence.

Many fad diets operate on the assumption that certain foods, or combinations of foods, are more fattening than others. Actually there are no fattening or slimming foods—just too much or too little. The idea that you can eat all you want of certain foods without regard to calories and lose weight is false. Most popular fad diets that claim calories don't count actually aim at caloric decrease even if they don't state it out loud. One diet claims, "Don't worry about calories—eat all the steak and cottage cheese you want." What it doesn't mention is that too much of any one food naturally reduces the appetite. On the third or fourth day when you can't stand to look at another bowl of cottage cheese, you naturally stop eating as much, your caloric intake is reduced, and you lose weight. It only takes a few days or weeks to find that you can't continue eating that way forever. Back to your regular eating you go, and back comes the fat.

Some diets temporarily help you lose weight—but not fat. Weight loss in crash diets can be due to initial water loss in body tissues rather than actual burning of excess fatty tissue. The consumers' bathroom scales measure only total body weight. They don't distinguish between water loss and actual loss of fat stores.

For long-term weight control, commercial diets and fad reducing plans are ineffective and may be physically harmful. Nearly all diets, balanced or unbalanced, will produce initial weight loss if the total number calories consumed in twenty-four hours is less than the individual's caloric requirement for maintaining weight. But there is more to proper dieting than just losing weight. A sensible diet should use common foods and provide for proper nutrition to maintain health. It must involve permanent changes in eating habits to be safe and effective.

Independent of caloric requirements, every person needs certain daily amounts of carbohydrates, fats, proteins, vitamins, minerals, and water to maintain proper nutritional balance and health. Adjusted nutrient diets are unlikely to provide sufficient amounts of all daily nutrients; they can be a hazard to your health, even if you are losing weight. The balance of daily nutrients should include 50 percent carbohydrates, 30 percent fats, and 20 percent proteins. A nutritionally sound diet lowers the amount of calories ingested, not the proportion of nutrients.

Obesity is not cured, it is only controlled. Just like the diabetic and hypertensive patient, the obese person should remain on a supervised diet throughout his or her life.

Experts suggest that a constant moderate degree of overweight may be healthier than constantly losing and gaining back weight in what Jean Mayer calls the "rhythm method of girth control." Mayer contends that during periods of weight gain, the level of cholesterol in the blood is likely to rise, and fatty deposits are laid down in the walls of blood vessels. These deposits don't shrink proportionately during the losing periods, so the vessels continue to narrow with each gaining bout, increasing the risk of a heart attack or stroke.[1]

Weight gain also tends to follow an upward curve. A crash diet takes one's weight down five pounds. A period of compensatory eating follows, which often adds seven or ten pounds back on, carrying the weight above what it was before. All people fluctuate up and down one or two pounds, but large gains are dangerous.

When choosing a diet, consider the safety factors involved. Adherence to a faulty diet can upset a person's nutritional equilibrium and produce malnutrition. Concentration on one or two nutrients to the exclusion of others can upset body metabolism. Inadequate levels of carbohydrates and essential amino acids, for example, can result in fatigue and depression which in turn helps the dieter return to old habits of overeating. A crash diet program may cause high blood pressure, psychiatric disorders, and depression, especially in persons with previous mental illness.[2]

Medical experts stress that many weight-reducing regimes are especially dangerous for that large percentage of obese people who unknowingly suffer from other ailments. One study of 6,000 overweight persons showed that, of those who were overweight by 10 percent or more, 72 percent suffered from anemia, 18 percent from diabetes, 22 percent from heart disease, 37 percent from nervous or psychogenic disturbances, and 7 percent from gall bladder disease.[3] Each required special diet and special treatment. It could be most risky for an obese person suffering from one or more of these disorders to go on a diet not designed for his or her particular needs.

The following nutrient diets have been called by many different names (the names are changed regularly to benefit the manufacturer, but the contents remain the same). Regardless of what they're called, they are potentially dangerous to health. A summary of these diets is found in Table 17-1.

Low-Fat Diet

Because fats are the most concentrated source of calories, low-fat diet proponents assume lowering fat intake will result in weight loss. However, the body is unable to manufacture certain essential fats which must be part of the daily diet. A low-fat diet will result in dry skin and scalp and decreased joint mobility due to decreased lubrication. Fats are a concentrated form of energy and combine with phosphorus as part of every cell. A layer of fat under the skin cushions the nerves and muscles and insulates the body against sudden temperature changes. Studies demonstrate that rats fed fat-free diets become emaciated and develop skin rashes and kidney disorders.[4]

High-Carbohydrate Diet

A high carbohydrate–low-fat diet may cause hypercholesterolemia, hypertriglyceridemia (associated with increased risk of developing coronary heart disease), and high blood pressure. For a dieter with hypoglycemia, a high-carbohydrate diet can trigger increased insulin production and dangerous lowering of blood sugar.

Low-Carbohydrate Diet

Also known as "Drinking Man's Diet," "Dr. Atkins's Diet Revolution," "Mayo Clinic Diet," "Air Force Diet," "Eat Fat and Grow Slim," "Calories Don't Count," "Doctor's Quick Weight Loss Diet," and "Ketorganic Diet," a low-carbohydrate diet operates on the assumption that when few carbohydrates are ingested, large amounts of ketone bodies (incompletely burned fat particles) are produced and eliminated in the urine. This supposedly results in weight loss. Research shows that ketone losses rarely, if ever, exceed 100 kilo calories per day, an insufficient amount to account for remarkable weight loss. Ketogenic diets can cause a significant increase in blood uric acid concentration. By competing with uric acid for renal tubular excretion, elevated blood ketones can promote hyperurecemia. This is dangerous, especially in persons with gouty diathesis (predisposition to gout). If it is necessary to administer a drug to counteract hyperuricemia, then the side effects of the drug will be added to the already present nausea, anorexia, and fatigue.

Other possible conditions initiated by the diet include weakness, apathy, dehydration, calcium depletion, lack of stamina for prolonged exertion, nausea, hyperlipidemia, kidney failure, tendency to fainting, cardiac irregularity, and potential danger to an unborn child.

Table 17-1.

Popular Names of Diet	Composition	What It Purports to Do	Adequacy	Comments
Dr. Atkins's Diet Revolution The Drinking Man's Diet Calories Don't Count "Air Force" Diet Stillman Diet	Low carbohydrate	Cause weight loss without restricting caloric intake. Carbohydrate intake severely limited.	Does not meet RDA for vitamin C, calcium, and possibly vitamin A. Meets or exceeds RDA for B vitamins. Lacks bulk.	High in saturated fats and probably high in cholesterol. Because of incomplete oxidation, ketone bodies are formed, leading to development of ketosis. Places burden on kidneys to eliminate. Risk of development of dehydration, faintness, shaking, and blackouts.
800-Calorie Liquid Diet (under many trade names)	Moderate carbohydrate Moderate protein Low fat	Cause weight loss on totally liquid diet.	Meets RDA for nutrients. Lacks bulk.	Not normal pattern of eating for adults. Lack of bulk and chewing ingredients may lead to intestinal problems and periodontal problems.
Grapefruit and Steak Diet	Low carbohydrate High protein Moderate to high fat	Cause weight loss by grapefruit's ability to "burn fat."	Meets RDA for vitamin C, protein.	In reality food intake limited by limited selection of foods. Grapefruit and grapefruit juice have no known special metabolic function of "burning fat."
Zen Macrobiotic Diets	High carbohydrate Low protein Low fat	Create "spiritual awakening." Cure disease by "proper" therapy which consists of natural food, no medicine, no surgery.	Most levels are inadequate. Highest level (#7) consisting of only brown rice, is grossly inadequate.	May cause weight loss through general emaciation. Has caused recorded deaths. May interfere with individual's obtaining needed medical or surgical treatment for serious disease.
Carbo-Calorie Diet	60 grams of carbohydrates Moderate protein Moderate fat	Use "carbo-calorie" values to limit food intake.	Depends on individual selection of foods.	Originator's list of carbo-calories of food must be available. Substitutes one method of counting calories for another. Nutritional adequacy of diet not assured in any way.

Diet				
Vegetarian Diets	Moderate to high carbohydrate Moderate to low protein Moderate to high fat	Limit or eliminate sources of animal protein. May cause weight loss if insufficient caloric levels are maintained.	May be inadequate in high quality protein, iron, and B vitamins. Adequate in other vitamins depending on food selections.	Consistent with health if sufficient knowledge of nutrients and body's needs is applied. Requires careful selection of adequate amounts and combinations of foods. Anemia, B vitamin deficiencies, menstrual irregularities, and hypervitaminosis A (overdose) are potential hazards.
Weight Watchers Diet	Moderate Carbohydrates Moderate to high protein Moderate fat	Cause weight loss through use of normal foods restricted in amounts. Saturated fat sources limited. Polyunsaturated fat sources emphasized.	Meets RDA for all nutrients.	Based on cholesterol-lowering diet principles. Diet pattern not individualized. Might be too rigid.
Liquid Protein Diet Protein-Sparing Fast	No food (except for non-caloric beverages such as coffee, tea, and water) Protein supplement to prevent lean mass loss	Provides minimum amount of protein needed to preserve lean body mass in fasting patients.	Nutritionally incomplete. Requires nutrient supplements prescribed by physician.	Designed only for massively obese (50 pounds or more over-weight). Hospital supervision necessary. Numerous side effects including heart irregularities (from potassium imbalance), rapid drops in blood pressure, muscle weakness, cramps, dry skin, hair loss. Numerous contraindications.
Fasting	No food except supervised non-caloric liquid intake and vitamin supplements	Totally stop caloric intake.	Nutritionally incomplete. Liquid and nutrient supplements prescribed by physician.	Any fast lasting longer than 24 hours can be hazardous if done without medical supervision. Not normal eating pattern.

Modified after "Fad Type Diets," prepared by Mary J. Pfeffer, R.D., M.P.H. Director of Public Health Nutrition, Nassau County, Department of Health, Mineola, New York.

A normal diet needs at least one hundred grams of carbohydrates daily to prevent **ketosis,** excessive protein breakdown, and other undesirable metabolic responses. A small amount of carbohydrate is also necessary to protect the cells in the liver, kidney, spleen, heart, and skeletal muscles, as well as all the other vital structures of the body.

Muscles work most efficiently burning carbohydrates, and the brain burns nothing but a carbohydrate glucose. Carbohydrates also help to oxidize fat. Most of the low-carbohydrate diets do not emphasize lower caloric intake as well. There is no evidence to prove that sedentary subjects who consume a low-carbohydrate diet providing 5,000 calories a day will lose weight, as Dr. Atkins's diet claims.

Although low-carbohydrate diets seem to cause greater initial water loss than other diets, diuretics can be administered by a physician to control abnormal water and salt retention that masks or counterbalances weight loss in a low-calorie, balanced-nutrient diet. There is no need to eliminate carbohydrates from the normal diet.

A low-carbohydrate diet has no advantage over other diets. There is no inherent reason to associate a diet rich in carbohydrates with obesity. A lifetime diet must be palatable and have appeal; much variety and taste in foods is provided by carbohydrates.

Dr. Atkins stresses in his book that hypoglycemia is an underdiagnosed disease. A low-carbohydrate diet supposedly helps this condition. Because of the possible misunderstanding about the matter, the American Diabetes Association, the Endocrine Society, and the American Medical Association have issued the following statement for the public concerning the diagnosis and treatment of hypoglycemia:

> Hypoglycemia means a low level of blood sugar. When it occurs, it is often attended by symptoms of sweating, shakiness, trembling, anxiety, fast heart action, headache, hunger sensations, brief feelings of weakness, and occasionally, seizures and coma. However, the majority of people with these kinds of symptoms do not have hypoglycemia; a great many patients with anxiety reactions present similar symptoms. Furthermore, there is no good evidence that hypoglycemia causes depression, chronic fatigue, allergies, nervous breakdowns, alcoholism, juvenile delinquency, childhood behavior problems, drug addiction or inadequate sexual performance . . .[5]

According to Dr. Atkins, most overweight people are hypoglycemic. A majority of physicians probably would not agree with this statement, since it is well known that obese patients tend to be resistant to their own insulin. Moreover, there is no sound evidence to suggest that Dr. Atkins's recommendations of megadoses of B-complex, C, and especially E vitamins will help keep blood sugar at an even level. Blood sugar remains remarkably stable without the help of super doses of vitamins.[6]

It is curious that hypoglycemia does not appear to be a problem in parts of the world where carbohydrates provide up to 80 percent of dietary calories. Indeed, in those same high-carbohydrate areas **diabetes mellitus** is less common than in the United States. Also, it has been shown that diabetic patients consuming a diet low in cholesterol (100 milligrams per 24 hours), high in carbohydrate (64 percent of total calories) maintain good to excellent regulation without an increase in insulin requirements and with a decrease in plasma cholesterol levels. Plasma triglycerides did not increase, which means a decrease in heart disease risk.

Alias "Quick Weight Loss Diet," "Calories Don't Count," "Eat All You Want," "All the Meat You Want," "Doctors' Quick Weight Loss Diet," and the "Super C Grapefruit Diet," the high-protein diet contains a high proportion of protein to a low (or no) proportion of carbohydrates and fats. Meat, cheese, eggs, and fish are the main foods, allowed in unlimited amounts. This diet increases urine excretion, which puts an extra load on the kidneys. Kidney infection or malfunction may result in urea retention, coma, and sometimes death.

High-Protein Diet

Protein provides essential amino acids for maintenance of body structure. If sufficient protein is not supplied (about a gram of proteins per kilo of desirable body weight), as in a low-protein diet, the body will break down its own lean mass tissue in organs and muscles. The body will lose weight—but not from fatty stores. This is a very dangerous way to lose weight. Muscle tissue uses many more calories at rest than does fat tissue. By reducing muscle tissue, you are lowering your caloric expenditure and encouraging obesity. Further tissue depletion is hazardous to anyone who already has organ damage due to liver, kidney, heart disease, anemia, etc.

Low-Protein Diet

HCG (Human Chorionic Gonadotropin) is a growth hormone secreted in the urine of pregnant women. It is used to treat menstrual dysfunction, threatened abortion, dwarfism associated with hypogonadism, and mental retardation in males. The HCG Diet, devised by a Dr. Simeon, consists of hormone injections along with a 500-calorie, near-starvation diet. He claims it can cause weight reduction without hunger and can be used in spot reducing.

HCG Diet

There is no scientific evidence supporting the use of HCG in obesity. Weight loss is most likely due to the strict diet, and the HCG has only a placebo effect. According to Charles Cargille, M.D., of the National Institute of Child Health and Human Development:

> In my opinion, a five hundred calorie diet without chorionic gonadotropin, if combined with daily interviews and encouragement, would be an equally effective, short-term management for obesity, while less costly and painful than if chorionic gonadotropin were used additionally. However, it is indeed possible that deep intragluteal daily needle-sticks per se are an indispensible component of the Simeons' regimen. This painful experience may enhance patient acceptance of the stringent dietary restrictions imposed.[7]

Weight loss should occur on a 500-calorie diet, but there are few persons who are likely able to spend the rest of their lives on such a potentially dangerous diet. The HCG diet does not help form new and stable eating habits. After completing such a diet, most persons will revert back to their old eating habits and will regain all the weight they lost.

While the controversy wages over the effect of the hormone, HCG weight clinics are mushrooming across the country. Clinics charge from $450 and $700 for a diet program—a pretty expensive way to lose weight. Many not only advertise for patients, but offer to pay physicians $50,000 to $100,000 a year for weekly lectures or the use of their name as an endorsement. According to Dr. Asher of the American Society of Bariactric Physicians,

> We are violently opposed to this exploitative type of thing. There is a confusion between what these clinics are doing and what the ASBP is doing. I think most of these are run by lay people, and I think they are mostly concerned about the money.[8]

Fasting   A fasting diet prescribes the ingestion of noncaloric liquids and no protein. It is based on the faulty logic that since eating too much food causes overweight, eating no food at all should reduce weight quickly. Fasting is psychologically frustrating because 65 percent of the weight loss which does occur is due to breakdown of lean body tissue. Only 35 percent of the loss is from adipose tissue stores. When normal diet is resumed, replacement of body weight quickly occurs as the body replaces the lost protein. (It takes four pounds of added body weight to replace one pound of protein). Consequences of fasting include:

1. Initial rapid weight loss due to decreased body water.
2. Electrolyte shift, with increased urinary loss of sodium, potassium, magnesium, and calcium.
3. Decreased volume of plasma and extracellular fluid, with postural hypotension.
4. Loss of lean body mass due to increased urinary nitrogen loss.
5. Ketonemia, ketonuria, milk metabolic acidosis.
6. Hyperuricemia, secondary gout, renal urate stones.
7. Decreased blood glucose levels (not symptomatic).
8. Transient decreased serum cholesterol.
9. Vitamin depletion, unless supplements are taken.
10. Depletion of body stores of fat.[9]

Total fasting for extended periods can lead to heart failure, renal failure, lactic acidosis (disturbance in acid-base balance) in diabetics, and acute volvulus of the small bowel.

**Liquid Protein
Diet**   Liquid protein diets are designed for massively obese persons (50 pounds or more overweight) who for health reasons must take off and keep off weight but have been unable to do so by ordinary, low-calorie diets. The individual completely abstains from food (except for noncaloric beverages such as coffee, tea, and water) and takes a special protein supplement four or five times a day to prevent great losses of lean muscle and organ tissue.

Liquid protein diets are made from hydrolized (predigested) collagen or gelatin obtained from animal hides, tendons, and bones (predigested meaning the protein has already been broken down into essential amino acids). Some are fortified with a limited number of other essential amino acids, vitamins, and minerals. None is nutritionally complete. Liquid protein drinks contain about 60 calories per one-ounce serving. Women on the diets consume three to five ounces a day and men four to seven ounces.

Because the diet is nutritionally incomplete, the use of the diet alone can, and often does, lead to serious nutritional deficiencies, including potassium imbalance, which can cause fatal heart irregularities, rapid drops in blood pressure upon standing up, muscle weakness and cramps, dry skin, nausea, hypoglycemia, menstrual irregularity, or hair loss. Long-term effects of the diet have not yet been assessed. Nutrient supplements, especially potassium supplements, must be carefully prescribed to prevent overdosage. People coming off the diet and re-introducing their bodies to solid food should be especially careful.

The Food and Drug Administration has received reports of more than 40 deaths associated with very low-calorie protein diets. The Center for Disease Control (CDC) found that in at least 15 deaths, diet was highly suspect as a contributing factor. In these 15 cases, the victims were obese women between the ages of twenty-five and fifty-one who lost an average of 83 pounds after being on low-calorie protein diets for two to eight months. None had a history of heart disease. All died suddenly, without previous symptoms of heart irregularities—either while on the diet or shortly after going off it.[10]

In addition to reports of these deaths, the FDA has received reports of more than 100 people who said they became ill due to use of protein products that are promoted for weight control. The FDA convened a panel of medical experts to review the use of protein products in very low-calorie diets. The panel concluded that these products should be used only under the careful supervision of medical personnel trained in their use. These diets are still experimental and are being developed for use by extremely obese people under the strict monitoring of a physician, the panel pointed out, but promotional material aimed at the public plays down the strain on the body caused by the restrictive nature of the diet.

In addition to discouraging general use of protein products in the very low-calorie diets, the panel said that the diets could be especially dangerous to certain groups of people. It recommended against use by individuals taking prescription medications (especially diuretics, oral hypoglycemic agents, insulin, or thyroid drugs); by individuals with kidney, liver, or heart disease or high blood pressure; by the elderly; by preschoolers and adolescents; or by pregnant women or nursing mothers.

Because of the evidence that very low-calorie protein diets are no more effective than other diets and may actually be hazardous when used improperly, the FDA has proposed a mandatory warning label for all protein supplements intended for use in weight reduction or maintenance programs. The label would say:

> WARNING: Very low-calorie protein diets may cause serious illness or death. Do not use for weight reduction or maintenance without medical supervision. Do not use for any purpose without medical advice if you are taking medication. Not for use by infants, children, or pregnant or nursing women.

FDA also proposed a warning label for protein supplements not intended for use in weight reduction or maintenance but nonetheless often used for this purpose by consumers. The label would say:

> WARNING: Very low-calorie protein diets may cause serious illness or death. Do not use for weight reduction or maintenance.

FDA has asked the manufacturers of protein products to put these warnings on the labels of their products immediately, even while FDA is initiating the necessary legal steps to make these or similar warnings mandatory. At the same time, FDA is considering possible ways to remove some or all of these products from the market if the label warnings do not prove adequate to protect the public health.

Zen Macrobiotic Diet   Considered a means of creating a spiritual awakening or rebirth, the Zen Macrobiotic diet recommends an extreme regimen of natural and organic foods. Aside from the fact that so-called natural foods are twice as expensive but only as or less nutritious as regular food, the macrobiotic diet can be nutritionally dangerous. Not all unusual or religious dietary philosophies are hazardous to health, but the Zen macrobiotic diet is obviously so. The diet, consisting of cereals and a few liquids, has resulted in at least one death, and cases of scurvy, anemia, hypoproteinemia, hypocalcemia, emaciation, and loss of kidney function. One young woman followed the diet faithfully for nine months. She ate nothing but natural cereals, as little water as possible, sesame seeds, and "sea salt." She was eventually hospitalized, but medicine was unable to save her life. An autopsy revealed she had died of emaciation due to starvation. Claims that the macrobiotic diet can cure cancer, apoplexy, arthritis, anemia, and other ailments are false.

Vegetarianism   The vegetarian diet dates back at least to the Egyptians. Today, a few follow a pure vegetarian diet, others are lacto-vegetarians who include dairy products in their diet, and some are ovo-lacto-vegetarians who also eat eggs.

All vegetarians, but especially the strict ones, must be careful that their diet is nutritionally sound. The body does not manufacture certain amino acids (isoleucine, tryptophan, valine, and histidine) which must be supplied in food. Meat, fowl, fish, milk, and eggs supply all of them. A diet composed only of commonly used vegetables with no supplementary fruit will lack these essential amino acids. Vitamin B_{12} is another nutrient commonly lacking in a strict vegetarian diet. To avoid nutritional deficiencies, anyone contemplating going on a vegetarian diet should consult a physician first.

It is possible but difficult to construct a vegetarian diet which supplies all necessary nutrients. A common tendency in vegetarianism is to concentrate on one or two foods. Further information on vegetarianism is supplied in Chapter 11.

PRESCRIPTION REDUCING DRUGS

In a medication-oriented society, drug abuse is common in all health areas. Obesity therapy is no exception. Everyone seems to be searching for a magic pill that will make up for lack of self-control to lose weight. Anorectics used to suppress appetite and aid in weight loss are not as effective as advertised and are potentially dangerous to health. Anorectics should be used only under the direction of a physician on a short-term basis as adjunctive aids in obesity treatments where diet control is the prime factor. Most such drugs contain amphetamines, a psychoactive, habit-forming drug which can cause psychotic behavior, drug dependence, and withdrawal if sufficiently abused.

The amphetamines are the most important group of appetite suppressant drugs from a commercial standpoint. Because of the potent effects of such stimulants, the majority are classified under the Drug Abuse Prevention and Control Act. A panel of medical consultants advised the FDA that the value of amphetamine-related diet drugs was "clinically trivial" and that, in view of their potential for misuse, such drugs should be brought under tighter controls.[11]

When given in large doses, amphetamine drugs can temporarily suppress appetite, but the dose varies with the individual. Side effects include dry mouth, irritability, restlessness, insomnia, rapid heartbeat, and lightheadedness. Effectiveness of the drugs wears off with usage, but dependence continues to build. A five-year study showed excellent results in weight reduction usually were obtained in the first month or two of treatment under a physician's guidance, whether or not drugs were employed, and regardless of type. The patients treated by diet alone did as well as those treated with a combination of diet and drugs.[12] The danger was always present, however, that a patient could end up a fat drug addict instead of just a fat person. Most overweight persons should diet without drugs of any kind.

NON-PRESCRIPTION DIET PRODUCTS

Beginning with the Metrecal 900-calorie formula, diet foods have become standard items in supermarkets. They include ready-to-use liquids in cans, powder envelopes to be mixed with milk, cookies, wafers, and soups.

Formula Diets

Slender, a popular diet product, is composed of sucrose, sodium, caseinate, vegetable oil, and various stabilizing chemicals, vitamins, and minerals. Four cans of ready-to-drink Slender yield 900 calories (65 grams of protein; 20 grams of fat; 115 grams of carbohydrates) and are recommended by the manufacturers as a daily substitute for all other foods for stringent dieters.[13]

Diet formulas are convenient and easy to prepare, and nearly everyone who restricts caloric intake to 900 calories daily can expect to lose weight, even without exercise. For many, it is easier to use a formula diet than to juggle regular foods to prepare a balanced diet low in calories. However, few persons can stay on such a drastic and monotonous diet for more than a few weeks, and thus these diets fail to provide long-term maintenance of reduced weight.

Diet formulas may induce gastrointestinal side effects (gas, diarrhea, or constipation) and, rarely, emotional disturbances. Synthetic diets also run the risk, especially when used as sole nourishment for long periods, of inadvertently omitting essential nutrients usually supplied in regular meals.

Some mislabeling is found in formula diet products, but for the most part, the products are what they purport to be. The biggest problem is that many dieters do not understand the correct use of such products and so do not use them safely. The FDA now requires diet food labels to contain this statement: "Weight control by diet requires limiting total intake of calories." The purpose of this statement is to remind consumers that the product is useful for weight control only when considered with the total diet.

Individuals wishing to begin a weight reduction program with a formula diet should consult a physician first. High costs of such a diet can be eliminated by substituting a homemade formula for the commercial product. This can be done by blending about 7 ounces of nonfat powdered skim milk (a little more than the amount recommended for making 2 quarts of milk), 2/3 ounce of corn oil, and a quart or somewhat less of water. The drink can be flavored to taste with a flavoring agent and sweetened with saccharin. The formula should be supplemented with a vitamin/mineral capsule recommended by a physician.[14]

Before-Meal Candies

Other supposed dietary products are caramels and other candies to be taken prior to a meal. The idea is that eating these candies just before a meal causes blood sugar level to rise and appetite to diminish, and the dieter will no longer want to eat rich sauces, gravies, and desserts. There is no evidence that before-meal candies suppress appetite or that they significantly raise blood sugar level in recommended amounts. Some contain even more calories than regular candies.

Many candies are accompanied by low-calorie diets which actually cause the weight loss if followed, while the candies have only a **placebo** effect. Many reducing candies also claim to contain vitamin and mineral supplements. Two popular candies are Ayds and RDX.

Ayds.   Ayds are caramels made with a synthetic sweetener and cream, possibly for taste. This makes Ayds higher in calories than ordinary caramels. Ayds are not harmful physically, but they do not produce weight loss. Inside the package is a low-calorie diet sheet which would help the consumer lose weight with or without the use of the candy. Cost at the time of this writing was three dollars per pound.

RDX.   RDX is a reducing wafer advertised on television. It is made of powdered milk with small amounts of lemon juice and vitamins. It does not produce weight loss.

Phenyl-propanolamine

Phenylopropanolamine, a drug related to ephedrine and amphetamine, is found in over-the-counter (nonprescription) preparations such as Diet-Trim, Hungrex, and Slender-Z. It is also used in nasal decongestants. The *AMA Drug Evaluation* states "this agent is probably ineffective in the dose provided (25 mg)." Overuse of this drug is dangerous, especially to anyone suffering from thyroid trouble, heart disease, diabetes, hypertension, or any other serious disorder.

Benzocaine

Benzocaine, a popular ingredient in over-the-counter (**OTC**) reducing drugs, is a local anaesthetic. The theory behind its use in capsules or chewing gum is to coat the lining of the mouth or the mucous membranes of the stomach and thereby inhibit a person's desire for food. No evidence exists to support the theory. Currently marketed preparations containing benzocaine are Rexule, Pondosan, Reducets, Slim-Mint, Way-Dex, and Diet-Trim. The dosage of benzocaine in products such as Anapex Diet plan tablets is small enough that it cannot affect the stomach. Severe illness can result from overuse of this drug.

Bulk Producers

Bulk producers, which swell up when they absorb water, supposedly suppress appetite by filling up the gastrointestinal tract, thereby giving a false sense of fullness. Bulk producers usually pass quickly into the small intestine, particularly when taken on an empty stomach. Appetite is governed by complicated psychological as well as physical factors. It has not been shown that bulk producers have any effect on hunger contractions or that they prevent one from eating more food. People who overeat frequently do so even when their hunger pains are satisfied. Studies show that ethyl cellulose and sodium methyl cellulose, two common bulk producers, have no weight-reducing effect when given in recommended amounts. If taken in larger than recommended doses, these products can have a laxative effect.

Diuretics, more commonly called water pills, help the body reduce water retention by increasing urine flow. Abuse of diuretics can result in severe dehydration, vital mineral loss, and possible death. While they may help reduce body weight, they do not reduce fatty stores. They should be used only under a physician's direction.

Diuretic Compounds

QUICK-REDUCING GADGETS

Most quick-reducing gadgets are worthless and may even be dangerous. There are no federal laws requiring manufacturers to prove the worth and effectiveness of any device before they market it. Ads are frequently worded to imply weight loss without specifically saying so. The consumer should be wary of any of the following (or similar) items whether advertised in the newspaper, on television, or by mail.[15]

One company sells shorts and belts that can be inflated like an inner tube. When worn during simple exercises, it is claimed, they create a sauna effect which causes the area under the clothing to shrink several inches in only three days. No dieting is necessary, and inches will disappear without weight loss.

Inflatable Clothing

Actually, it is not possible to permanently reduce waistline measurements without reducing weight, nor is it possible to spot reduce an area such as the thighs by "melting the fat away."

Several companies claim that wearing a belt weighted with ten to fifteen pounds of lead or steel shot will cause you to use more calories, thus causing you to lose weight. Investigation by the Federal Trade Commission reveals that such claims are false.[16] Weighted belts will not reduce the waistline or weight. To lose even 1 pound, a six-foot, 200-pound man would have to wear a 10-pound belt eight hours every day for forty-five days. Weighted belts can also be physically damaging.

Weighted Waist Belts

Constricting bands, of semiporous material wrapped around the waist, thighs, upper arms, or chin, supposedly cause weight loss through sweating. A slight volume of water may temporarily be lost through perspiration, but the weight returns as soon as fluids are taken back into the body.

Constricting Bands

Suits of nylon mesh to be worn during exercise and sleep are also claimed to cause weight loss through sweating and a massage action caused by friction between the

Body Suits

body and the suit. It is also claimed to firm, tone, and smooth muscles without any effort on the part of the wearer. The fact remains that weight reduction during sweating is due to temporary water loss. Muscles can only be strengthened and toned with active exercise. These suits and bands can be dangerous to anyone suffering from diabetes or diseases of the arteries and veins of the legs.

Muscle Stimulators According to FDA studies, Americans have spent millions of dollars on electrical body and facial muscle stimulators. These devices bombard the skin with electrical charges, causing muscle contractions that supposedly reduce girth, tone muscles, and destroy wrinkles. The best selling machine, the Relaxacizor (marketed for as much as four hundred fifty dollars), was removed from the market by federal injunction since it could induce miscarriage and damage the heart and other vital organs. Despite this decision, and evidence that such devices are grossly ineffective, similar muscle stimulators are reportedly still being sold.[17]

Creams, Oils, There is no medical evidence that any topical applicant, such as a cream or
Lotions emolient, can have the effect of reducing weight. The manufacturer of XR-6 entices buyers with the possibility of a weight loss of 61 pounds if two XR-6 capsules are put into a bath for five successive baths. This is, of course, impossible.

Exercise Machines Unicycle wheels, hand-grippers, spring platforms for jogging, push-pull gadgets, stationary bicycles and treadmills, and a hundred other devices on the market fall into the category of exercise machines. Treadmills and stationary bicycles, for instance—when used long and hard enough at a stretch—can provide exercise that will benefit the heart and lungs in the same way as long-distance swimming, running, or cycling. It is really difficult to use these machines in a manner that will induce any cardiovascular-pulmonary benefits, however, and people are being deluded about the kind of exercise they are getting in the use of such equipment.

Various health clubs and spas throughout the country advertise programs for fast, guaranteed weight loss (at a price, of course). The problem with many of these programs is that one receives benefits from exercise only in proportion to the amount of effort one puts into the movements. If you let a machine push, pull, vibrate, or massage you, you may find it relaxing, but it will not tone your muscles or use up fat stores. Exercise is an important component of obesity control, but it must be the proper kind of exercise in connection with a proper diet.

RECOGNIZING GOOD AND FAD DIETS

Despite the abundance of fad reducing regimens, you can locate a sound diet and exercise program if you are willing to spend a little time and effort. Consider the following characteristics of reduction programs when evaluating a new diet or exercise gadget:

EARMARKS OF A SOUND DIET

1. Based on a negative caloric balance.
2. Is a long-term program. Once ideal weight is achieved, the diet can be adjusted slightly to maintain the weight for life.
3. Limits calories but maintains balance of daily nutrient requirements.
4. Based on slow, regular weight loss.
5. Emphasizes self-control. There is no guaranteed success.
6. Includes an exercise program.
7. Is an exaggeration of proper eating habits with food you normally eat.
8. Provides for social, cultural, and psychological needs relating to over-eating.
9. Is adjusted to individual's percent of body fat and metabolism.

EARMARKS OF A FAD OR FRAUDULENT DIET

1. Claims that calories don't count.
2. Promises quick, easy weight loss but does not provide a permanent program for maintenance of ideal weight.
3. Alters proportions or omits certain nutrients. Claims some foods are naturally more fattening than others.
4. Guarantees sudden weight loss or spot reduction.
5. Promises weight control without effort.
6. Recommends diet or exercise but not both.
7. Recommends drastic change in the types of foods you are used to eating.
8. Ignores emotional and psychological factors involved in overeating.
9. Promises cures for disease through diet.
10. Carries spectacular advertising appealing to the emotions.
11. Guarantees success for everyone.

RECOGNIZING ACCURATE DIET LITERATURE

As there are no government standards requiring information to be scientifically sound before it is published, it is left to the consumer to distinguish between valid diet advice and quack literature. Judging by the number of fad diet books which reach the best-selling list, the current trend seems to be in favor of the quack. Consumers tend to assume authorship of a physician assures effectiveness.

The book *Calories Don't Count* by Dr. Herman Taller sold some 300,000 copies at $3.95 each in four months. Attacks from the FDA and physicians in the nutrition field that information contained in the book was false had little effect on sales. Faller's success doesn't compare with the success of Dr. Atkins's *Diet Revolution*. Within a year after he published a revised version of an old diet, he had sold more than a million hardcover copies at $6.95 apiece.

The following is a list of characteristics of misleading or fraudulent weight-reduction literature.

EARMARKS OF QUACK BOOKS

1. Jacket design for popular, not scholarly appeal.
2. Collaboration of a popular-style writer.
3. Involvement of a product or idea that is as yet unrecognized by the medical profession as an effective therapeutic agent.
4. Appeal to a mass market; clear and simple enough to be grasped by the layperson and basic enough for anyone "interested in his own health and his children's."
5. Provision made for self-diagnosis and self-treatment, and a cureall promise is made.
6. Undocumented claims of success by testimonial-type evidence offered.
7. A semblance of authority by promotional methods (world's leading authority), by bogus degree, or by recognized degree in a professional discipline but without relevance to the field in which the book is written.
8. The citation of research and wide practice from institutions which may or may not enjoy renown in the field.
9. Respectability conjured up by association with respected institutions and individuals.
10. Complaint of lack of recognition, persecution.
11. Fosters controversy with unqualified theses.
12. The development of seemingly plausible scientific mechanisms.
13. Assurances spreading false hope following outright misinformation.
14. The exorcism of devils (big government, taxes, overworked soil, processed foods, white sugar, and white flour are favorite topics).
15. Prominent missionary zeal.
16. Claims for enhancement of sexual potency.
17. Recommendations of dosage and products.[18]

A list of recommended books is located in Appendix D. If you have a question about the validity or pertinence of a new or popular nutrition book, check with your physician before purchasing the book and following its advice. If you have questions or doubts about any commercial diet, exercise program, or diet book, you can contact any of the following resources for reliable information.

Federal Trade Commission
Bureau of Investigation
Washington, D.C. 20580

The United States Postal Service
1200 Pennsylvania Avenue NW
Washington, D.C. 20260
(for mail-order products)

Council of Better Business Bureaus, Inc.
845 Third Avenue
New York, New York 10022

American Medical Association
Department of Investigation
535 North Dearborn Street
Chicago, Illinois 60610

U.S. Food and Drug Administration's
District Offices
Washington, D.C. 20201
(district offices are listed in local telephone books)

State or Local Health Department

Local Medical Society

Local Food and Drug Enforcement
    Agency

Local Consumer Affairs or Consumer
    Frauds Agency

Local University Nutrition Department

Local College or University Health
    Department

COMMON FALLACIES ABOUT FOOD AND WEIGHT LOSS

A Fat Baby Is a Healthy Baby.   No medical evidence supports this. A high correlation has been shown between obese children and obese parents, and if one or both parents are obese or tend toward obesity, special attention should be directed to the diet and activity pattern of an infant from birth.

The earlier a child becomes obese, the less likely the child is to lose weight later. Research shows that gross overfeeding of infants and children is producing adults who have a larger than normal number of fat storage cells. Once these cells are formed, they do not seem to break down. Throughout life, these persons are much more likely to be overweight.

In general, parents should have a physician determine if a child is overweight and prescribe the proper food program for the child. Parents should not put children on a weight control diet without consulting a physician. Improper nutrition can interfere with a child's growth and development.

It's Natural to Get Fatter as You Get Older.   One may get the impression that it is natural because so many people grow fatter as they get older. During childhood and youth, a certain amount of extra weight is desirable to meet the demands of our growing years. However, as a person grows older, metabolism and physical activity often decrease faster than the appetite. Fat begins to accumulate as a person takes in more food day after day than the body uses. Any weight which is accumulated after age twenty-five (when growth has ceased) is likely to be essentially fat and therefore undesirable.

For Older People Trying to Lose Weight, a Balanced Diet Doesn't Matter So Much.   Balance is important whatever your age. The weakness and ill health of many old people comes from malnourishment. Oldsters who live alone often do not take the trouble to eat properly. For them, the following food tips are worth bearing in mind:

> Use nutritious, non-fattening dry milk. For flavor's sake, mix only one or two glasses at a time. For a good animal protein which needs no cooking, buy small cans of sardines, tuna or salmon. Eat yogurt or cottage cheese for protein. Use enriched or whole-grain breakfast foods as an easy-to-serve source of protein and the B vitamins. Also add dry gelatin to milk and drink it; there is as much protein in one envelope of gelatin as in an egg—and no

cholesterol. But it should be consumed with milk, not water. For snacks and sandwiches, buy enriched or whole-grain crackers (graham, rye, rusks). They keep better than bread, are more nourishing than the usual boxed nibbling foods. Eat as many fruits and vegetables as you like—fresh, frozen or canned.[19]

Overweight People Are Generally Happy, Healthy People.   In actual fact, most overweight people are much more content after they have lost their excess weight. They become unhappy if they regain the weight they lost.

As Long As a Fat Person Feels Well, It Is Not Necessary to Lose Weight.   Excess weight creates an extra hazard for otherwise healthy persons and can affect normal body functions. A fat person may experience respiratory difficulties or less tolerance for exercise. Obesity can aggravate conditions such as gall bladder disease, gout, diabetes, hypertension, cardiovascular diseases, and arthritis. An overweight patient faces more risks in surgery, and mortality rates are higher among overweight persons compared with normal-weight individuals.

Fat People Eat the Wrong Kinds of Food.   Naturally, some of the foods people love to eat, such as rich desserts and carbohydrate foods, are converted to fat more readily than are protein and fat. Overemphasizing carbohydrates in the diet may be a factor in obesity, but the main problem of the obese is that day after day they are sedentary and eat too much of all kinds of foods, not just the wrong ones.

Thin People Naturally Eat Less.   Many lean people are hearty eaters, but their bodies may utilize food less efficiently than an overweight person, whose body stores unused calories as fat. However, being underweight, like being overweight, depends on many factors—genetic, environmental, cultural, economic, and familial influences and the amount of physical activity the person undertakes.

It Is Easier to Gain Than to Lose Weight.   For the underweight person, gaining pounds can be as difficult as reducing is for the overweight. To gain a pound a week, a person must eat an additional 500 calories worth of food a day, and often a constitutionally lean person has a difficult time eating this additional food.

Dieting Is the Best Way to Lose Weight.   If "dieting" refers to a long-term change in eating and living habits, then this statement is true. Dieting should provide for maintenance of weight loss in addition to the initial loss of fat. Too often, however, we think of dieting as a crash eating program at a near-starvation level. Crash diets are doomed to failure because of their short-term nature and inadequate nutrition. They are physically and emotionally wearing.

Certain Pills Make Weight Loss Easy.   Pills actually make weight loss much more difficult. The first thing you should remember is that any diet pills you buy in a drug store or supermarket without a prescription contain little medicine and have very limited effectiveness. The potent pills a physician can prescribe are almost always only chemical crutches for desperate dieters to lean on. Here's why:

A person on a strict diet usually loses weight very quickly at first, and then levels off to a slow weight loss over a period of weeks or months. Along the way, the dieter often gets discouraged and is ready to give up. What's happened is that the body is retaining water. During this discouraging period, the dieter's doctor may prescribe a diuretic to trigger water weight loss. It gives the patient inspiration to stay on the diet, and there's no great harm in that. Less justified is the use of amphetamine drugs, which stimulate a person physically while curbing appetite. These pep pills can be habit forming, and once hooked on them, an individual may have to resort to still other pills to relax. This is the road to drug dependency—and there's a greater danger in that than in being overweight.

Equally hazardous are the "miracle drugs" pushed by some diet doctors. These can be, for example, pep pills with thyroid extract to boost metabolic rate and some digitalis thrown in to spur your heart. You seriously risk weakening your heart if you try to lose weight this way.

It Is Better to Lose Weight as Rapidly as Possible Whatever Reducing Diet One Follows.   The real trouble that can result when weight is lost too rapidly is not caused by the weight reducing itself, but by the kind of weight that is lost. A too-rapid drop in weight almost always means that large amounts of protein (particular, muscle and liver tissue) are being lost instead of fat (adipose tissue). Many popular reducing fads are based on diets that are very low in protein foods. They often produce a rapid loss of body weight, but at the risk of exposing the dieter to serious illness. The loss of weight to be looked for each month by a moderately overweight person is between five and eight pounds. Too-rapid loss of weight in some persons, even on a good reducing diet, may result in weakness, dizziness, and the tendency to anginal attacks. Rapid weight reduction should not be attempted except under the close supervision of a physician who can prescribe a proper diet that will ensure the weight loss is in fat tissue.

You Should Eat Only Three Meals a Day.   Many experts feel we'd all be better off if we ate five or six small meals a day instead of three big ones. Such a nibbling diet can reduce fat and even lower weight. The idea is to feed the body machinery with an even stream of calories during the day, rather than with two fair-sized portions at breakfast and lunch and a huge input at dinner. When we consume small amounts throughout the day, the body uses calories as they come. This doesn't mean, however, that you can forget about total daily calories. Even with the nibbling diet, you still have to watch the crucial balance of calories eaten and calories burned.

Weight management authorities agree, however, that some people do better eating only one meal a day, if it supplies adequate nutrition but cuts down on daily caloric intake.

Meal Skipping Helps Reducing.   Skipping meals is not a good way to reduce. It usually results in overeating. It is desirable to plan the diet around three or more meals a day, each meal containing adequate protein. When the daily food intake is divided into small portions and eaten at intervals, continued weight loss is more likely to occur.

Snacking Makes You Gain Weight. You can eat snacks so long as the total number of calories you eat in a day does not go over the amount of calories allowed.

Food Eaten Before You Go to Bed Is More Likely to Cause Weight Gain Than If the Same Food Were Eaten for Breakfast. The energy requirements of the body must be met whether you are awake or asleep. Food eaten at bedtime will not put on weight if the calories supplied do not exceed the daily caloric requirements for the given body weight.

Adding a Multiple-Vitamin Capsule to Your Meals Every Day Will Balance Your Nutritional Needs While Dieting. A vitamin supplement is no substitute for food. If you eat a balanced diet, you'll get all the vitamins you need. Without the right food, you could take pounds of vitamin capsules and still die of malnutrition.

A dieter eating a nutritionally well-balanced diet does not generally need to take vitamin preparations. An iron supplement may be needed by women to meet their full iron needs while on a low-calorie diet. A physician or nutritionist should analyze the nutritional adequacy of a diet and decide if supplements are needed.

Vitamin preparations will not make up for inadequate nutrition in fad or crash diets. And while buying unnecessary vitamins will generally hurt only your pocketbook, there are dangers in overconsumption of some vitamins which the body can't excrete.

It Makes a Difference Whether a Person Eats Fast or Slowly. Most overweight people eat too fast. They consume large amounts of food without even realizing it. One should always eat slowly and chew food well. This gives the blood sugar regulatory mechanisms of the body a chance to act on appetite-regulating centers. This reduces appetite and hunger during the meal and allows us to be satisfied with less food.

After One Is on a Diet for Several Weeks, the Stomach Shrinks. The stomach does not shrink, although studies have shown that a person who permanently reduces the total quantity of food eaten will not require as much food to feel full. These studies also show that if a dieter stays away from sweet, rich foods, the body becomes accustomed to not having them. Some dieters actually feel ill when they eat these rich foods once again.

One Should Expect to Feel Weak and Fatigued During Weight Reducing. If one loses weight too rapidly, weakness will generally follow. However, a moderate rate of weight loss adapted by your physician to your individual constitution and activity should not lead to excessive fatigue and weakness.

To Lose Weight, You Must Not Eat Bread, Potatoes, or Any Fat. It is total calories you need to cut down on, and neither a medium-sized potato nor a slice of bread is high in calories. Moreover, whole-grain or enriched breads and cereals provide carbohydrates needed for energy, some protein, and some of the B vitamins and minerals important to nerves and digestion; potatoes supply carbohydrates, minerals, vitamin C, and also some protein.

Though an ounce of fat is twice as fattening as an ounce of protein or carbohydrate, you do need some fat to make food taste good and to keep you from feeling edgy. Unsaturated fats, from vegetable sources, are usually better for your heart than saturated, or animal, fats.

To Get Enough Protein When Dieting, You Must Eat Meat at Least Twice a Day. People can be well nourished with much less meat than most eat. You do need a little animal protein, but you can get that from eggs, fresh or dried milk, cheese, fish, or poultry. The rest of your protein can safely—and economically—come from lentils, dried peas or beans, cereals, or nuts.

When Dieting, Everybody Needs at Least Two Cups of Whole Milk a Day. You do need milk or milk products, and two cups of milk a day—or the equivalent—is about the minimum for anyone. Children, teenagers, pregnant women, and nursing mothers should have three to four cups or more a day. But the intake need not be whole milk; the equivalent may be taken in the form of low-fat milk, buttermilk, ice milk, cottage cheese, or cheese, or by adding powdered milk to cooked cereals, puddings, or other foods.

Crunchy Granola-Type Cereals Are More Nutritious and Contain Less Calories Than Other Cereals. More than 30 brands of granola cereals are now on the market. Many, however, have little nutritional advantage over more conventional cereals, although they are superior to some of the high-sugar cereals. A typical granola cereal has among its ingredients nuts, dried fruits, soy oil, brown sugar, sweeteners, and oils. The result is a rather high-calorie product containing perhaps 300 calories per serving, compared to about 100 in a serving of some of the unsweetened conventional cereals. Most of the granola types are 10 to 13 percent protein; some of the unsweetened conventional cereals are about 10 percent protein. Thus, many people bent on avoiding "empty calories" have been led into eating bowls of calories no less empty for being crunchy.

Toast Has Fewer Calories Than Bread. The toasting process does not change caloric content. Burning bread does not burn away the calories.

Margarine Has Fewer Calories Than Butter. Margarine and butter have the same number of calories (100) per tablespoon. Diet margarine has approximately half the amount of calories of regular margarine and butter.

A Person Who Eats Large Amounts of Fish Will Lose Weight. No single food will cause a weight loss. It is the total number of calories you eat in a single day that is important in a weight control program. Most forms of fish contain less fat and therefore are lower in calories than meat.

Washing Rice and Spaghetti After Cooking Reduces Their Calorie Content.   Washing does not reduce the amount of calories to any important degree, but it does rinse away some vitamins.

It's Okay to Drink Alcohol While Dieting.   Alcohol has no nutritive value. Therefore, alcohol is used by the body only as a source of calories (energy). An equivalent number of food calories become surplus, however, and are stored as fat. Few people realize that a large whiskey or gin, or a pint of beer, is the caloric equivalent of two eggs, or one glass of milk, or a slice of bread and butter, or an average portion of potatoes.

Drinking Vinegar Has a Slimming Effect.   There is no truth to the belief that body fat is melted by drinking vinegar.

Different Salad Oils Have Different Calorie Values.   All oils, including safflower, corn, peanut, and olive, have the same number of calories—approximately 125 per tablespoon. No type of oil can flush out body fat, as some claim.

Grapefruit Burns Up Fat in the Body.   No food dissolves body fat tissue.

One Should Drink Less Water While Dieting.   Water intake does not interfere with the loss of fat during weight reducing. Sufficient water—an average of six glasses between meals—should be included in the daily diet.

You Can Actually Exercise Fat Away.   This is a half-truth. Exercise contributes to expenditure of part of the daily caloric budget. An individual who eats the same number of calories and starts exercising will lose weight. Moderate exercise should not increate appetite. However, there is a negative side to this idea. Too many people forget the diet part of their calorie account. They feel that if they exercise regularly, they don't have to worry about what they eat.

Certain Diets Are Good for Spot Reducing.   A person on a diet tends to lose weight uniformly over the body. There are exercises that will strengthen muscle tone in problem areas and make you appear firmer once weight is lost through dieting.

Steam Baths and Massages Help a Person Lose Weight.   No scientific evidence shows that steam baths and massages are of value in a reducing program. A steam bath does cause a quick loss of water through sweating, but when the person drinks water, the loss is replaced.

SUMMARY

The obese are victims of many individuals and groups who prey on their desire for miraculous solutions to weight control problems. Sound and accurate knowledge about the nature and causes of obesity, weight control management, and sources of legitimate information are necessary to combat misinformation and fraudulent schemes sold to the consumer.

For long-term weight control, commercial fad reducing diets are ineffective and often nutritionally incomplete. Fad diets stress quick or instant weight reduction. However, stores of fat that have been built up over years must be removed gradually to maintain the weight loss. A sensible diet should not only help the body lose fat stores, but it should do so safely and with the least variance from a diet of commonly used foods. Actually, despite the drawbacks in fad and crash diets, they are of some value—they are of great financial value to those who promote them.

A sound diet is based on negative caloric and nutritional balance. It is individually adjusted for percent of body fat and metabolism. A sound diet is just an exaggeration of regular eating patterns and provides for slow, regular, and maintained weight loss. No one can guarantee any diet, because success is based upon self-control—not on the diet.

Countless quick reducing gadgets flood the market each year with claims to cause effortless weight reduction, but most are ineffective. Exercise machines and health spa programs claim they can cause weight reduction. Although exercise is an important component of obesity control, it must be the proper kind of exercise in connection with a proper diet. Exercise is beneficial only in proportion to the amount of effort an individual puts into it. Machines or programs that provide movement without effort will not bring about weight loss.

NOTES

1. Jean Mayer, "Exercise and Weight Control," *Family Health,* June 1973, pp. 33–35.
2. Richard B. Stuart, "Exercise Prescription in Weight Management: Advantages, Techniques, and Obstacles," *Obesity and Bariatric Medicine,* Vol. 4, No. 1, 1975.
3. "Weight Loss: Diets, Drugs, and Devices," *Medicine Show* (Mount Vernon, N.Y.: Consumers Union, 1974), pp. 208–227.
4. Ibid.
5. "A Critique of Low-Carbohydrate Ketogenic Weight Reduction Regimes," *Journal of the American Medical Association,* Vol. 224, No. 10, June 4, 1973, p. 682.
6. Ibid.
7. Robert Sherrill, "Before You Believe Those Exercise and Diet Ads, Read the Following Report," *Today's Health,* August 1971.
8. Leland Cooley and Lee Morrison Cooley, "The Great Diet Dupery," *Pre-Medicated Murder* (Radnor, Pa.: Chilton Book Co., 1974), Chap. 13.
9. "The Endless Fight Against Fat," *Current Prescribing,* March 1976, pp. 49–60.
10. "CDC Uncovers High Death Rate from Liquid Protein Diets," *Medical World News,* August 7, 1978.

11. Philip L. White, "The Dangers in Diet Advice," *Medical Insight,* July/August 1973.
12. Ibid.
13. Ibid.
14. Ibid.
15. Handouts: "A Common Sense Diet That Works," "Activity Calorie Costs," "Those So-Called Weight Reducers," "Let's Have No More Nonsense About Weight."
16. Sherrill, "Before You Believe Those Ads."
17. Handouts.
18. Frederick J. Stare, "Diet Books: Facts, Fads, and Frauds," *Medical Opinion,* December 1972.
19. Frederick J. Stare, "Common Sense on Calories," *Alive and Well,* December 1974.

18

Psychological and Sociological Aspects of Overweight and Obesity

There is no question that reduction of food intake and increased exercise bring about predictable weight loss; and millions control their weight, consciously or unconsciously, by regulating these factors. However, a glance at the creeping waistlines of our population reveals that the obvious does not work for everyone. Obesity is not merely a state of body weight; it is also a state of mind. Psychological problems may precipitate development of obesity or may be created within the obese by negative cultural attitudes and even by weight reduction effort itself.

Doctors and psychologists agree that the lack of understanding of the multi-faceted psychological problems facing the obese has hindered successful weight reduction programs.

PSYCHOLOGICAL ASPECTS OF OBESITY

Americans have attached a very real stigma to obesity. Ridicule and disdain are directed toward even the slightly overweight person. Beatrice Kalish feels that stigmatizing stems from self-concept.[1] Upon seeing a threatening distortion which reminds us of our own unearned good luck and our vulnerability, we stigmatize the object to increase our feelings of well-being, safety, and superiority. The ability to stigmatize allows us to dissociate or deny our common condition of vulnerability with the afflicted. Those with strong egos or strong self-concepts have less need to reject than those with weak ones.

The Stigma of Obesity

When children were shown pictures of children with various handicaps and obese children, the pictures of the obese children were considered the least desirable and likeable. Studies show that obese college applicants are less likely to be accepted than the nonobese, despite lack of difference in academic achievement, social class, and motivation. Physicians often display negative attitudes toward obese patients, whom they feel are more uncooperative and awkward than other patients.[2]

Nearly always, obesity is associated with gluttony and self-indulgence, regardless of whether the condition is caused by overeating or lack of activity. Regardless of whether the individual is totally responsible for the "excess baggage," the obese are held accountable and are not allowed to forget for a moment they are overweight and undesirable.

Obese children are often exposed to damaging pressures and difficult situations which intensify the underlying psychological factors which caused the obesity. Studies comparing obese youngsters to normal-weight youngsters have shown that obese children often exhibit personality characteristics similar to traits typical of youngsters in oppressed minority groups who are victims of intense prejudice. These traits include heightened sensitivity to status, passivity, withdrawal, and feelings of isolation and rejection. Many obese youngsters expect to be rejected. When shown a picture of a group of children with one child standing outside, walking toward the group, the normal-weight children assume he or she is joining the group; two-thirds of the obese children will see the child as being excluded from the group.[3]

Cultural circumstances can be ego destructive, and permanent emotional damage can result if the obese accept the negative attitude. Not all obese persons are affected by such attitudes, however. Individuals most susceptible to negative cultural stigma are those who have pre-obese personalities—those suffering from self-doubt, poor body image, inadequate self-concept, and constant, extreme dependence on others' opinions in all areas of living, not just in regard to weight and appearance.[4]

Fifty percent of those obese from childhood have a history of distorted body image. Fat as well as anorexic patients suffer from the misconception of being the misshapen product of somebody else's actions. They do not feel and act as if they had an identity of their own, and they suffer from a conviction of not even owning their own bodies.

Adult-onset obesity less frequently results in body distortion, but body distortion can be seen in some middle-aged people who let their appearance dwindle as they lose pride in their body image.

However, an impaired body image cannot be looked upon as solely a cultural phenomenon. It has been found that obese children who are accepted and encouraged by their families tend to develop good self-concepts and positive body images despite negative cultural attitudes. They are able to control their weight, though perhaps at a higher-than-average level. On the other hand, fat children showing early emotional disturbances associated with severe intrafamilial problems adjust poorly. These children interpret negative cultural attitude as a personal rejection. Those with severe psychological problems come from this second group.[5]

Habituation and Compulsion

Many persons do not recognize the close link between eating and emotional factors. From the beginning of life, food plays a basic part in human existence. Early nutrition is dependent upon the care of others. Food may convey affection, interest, caring, tenderness, and love; it is a source of comfort for most people. If the normal need for food and its accompanying symbolic meaning is distorted, however, addiction to eating for emotional support may result. In super-obese persons, the overuse of food is often an early formed pattern of overeating for pleasure or to reduce psychological or physical disequilibrium. Physical causes include overactive appetite center, impaired satiety center, disordered glucostatic mechanisms, and alteration of fat enzymes. Psychological causes include conditioned behavior, symbolic satisfaction of unfulfilled wants, anxiety, depression, desire for isolation, and socioeconomic frustration. In these cases, the obese individual may be using food as a drug and the condition can be regarded as an habituation syndrome.

A psychological dependence is created when food is used to such an extent that it produces sedation and a compulsion to use it to excess and to continually increase the amount. When the customary intake of food is restricted, behavioral changes occur which may have detrimental effects on the person and the person's family.

Dr. Albert Stunkard cites three compulsive eating patterns. The "night-eating syndrome" in which evening **hyperphagia** (increase in appetite) and insomnia are precipitated by stressful life situations (usually occurring until stress is eliminated); the "binge-eating syndrome" in which there is a self-condemnation, drastic dieting, and recurrent eating binges as a reaction to stress and frustration; and "eating-without-satisfaction," a situation unrelated to stress where the subject cannot stop eating despite the absence of hunger.[6]

Compulsive eating ranges from mild to severe addiction. Slight overweight is not necessarily connected with a disease state, just as social drinking is not alcoholism. Addicted eaters can be identified and separated from social eaters who enjoy abundant food and good company. The addict often eats in secret and gorges himself or herself to the point of sickness. Such an individual may even suffer withdrawal symptoms if dietary restriction is imposed. Leon Salzman indicates:

> The loneliness and emptiness of the compulsive eater are suggested by his symbolic attempt to swallow everything in order to fill his own emptiness. Nothing can be left in the refrigerator or on the table, since it might not be there tomorrow. Like a squirrel storing nuts for the winter, he cannot leave anything behind.[7]

Lack of Hunger Awarness

Some obese persons have lost or not developed a hunger awareness. The old charge that obese people have no willpower describes an important functional deficit, their inability to be discriminantly aware of their bodily sensations. Instead of responding to nutritional needs, they respond to a variety of internal states of tension. Adolescents in one study indicated that they ate when they felt bad, nervous, tense, depressed, bored, and worried.[8] It is not known exactly why this occurs; perhaps learned patterning in reaction to stress is involved. Parents can condition a child to identify outward stimuli rather than inward hunger pains as reason to eat. The children then lose awareness of their own body signals.

The sight of food alone can cause some people to eat. They do not receive any internal signals to stop eating; they stop because they are told or because they have learned polite, socially approved behavior. During eating binges, they feel compulsively driven to eat, in spite of the urgent wish not to gain weight, and they experience neither hunger while eating nor pleasure or satiation afterwards.

Hunger awareness must be conceived of as a function that requires organizing learning experiences early in life for accurate conceptualization. If these learning experiences are inappropriate or confusing, hunger awareness will develop in a distorted and falsified way.[9] For instance, if children learn to eat to pacify anxiety or as a reward, they will not know just to eat when hungry.

In a situation where they were unaware that their eating responses were being studied, the obese continued eating whether their stomachs were full or empty. They ate when they thought it was time to do so, regardless of the interval since their last meal, and responded to fear by increasing feeding activities. The response of nonobese persons was just the opposite. The obese are unable to resist the stimuli of external factors such as smell, sight, taste, and other people's actions. However, when placed in situations where food is bland and uninteresting and the taking of food is completely devoid of any ritualistic or social implications, obese people almost give up eating altogether. Thus when learned signals, such as sociability or exciting food, are removed, obese people are less likely to eat. Persons who are highly sensitive to environmental, food-related cues have extreme difficulty sustaining long-term obesity management.

Psychological Disturbance During Dieting

Obesity is an integrated condition within the mind and the body and can be considered a state of equilibrium. When it is altered for any length of time, as during weight reduction, a new equilibrium must be established.

Experiments with overfeeding in humans showed that body weight resists permanent change. Once overfeeding was discontinued, the subjects returned to old eating patterns and normal weight. Similarly, obesity is not easily changed, especially if it is juvenile-onset.[10] Dieting, which threatens the current equilibrium, is likely to be consciously or unconsciously resisted. This leads to minor emotional upsets and occasional major psychological disorders. Eating, along with many other activities, may be used as a defense against psychological pathology. If this is taken away from the patient, something constructive must replace the activity.

At present, there is no evidence to show that dieting causes significant depression in the average individual, but there is no doubt that starvation or enforced diets produce serious consequences in unstable persons. It is important to assess the pre-diet personality, because dieting can cause neurotic symptoms, depression, suicide, or psychosis.

Some persons can reduce successfully while under strictly controlled conditions, such as in a hospital or reducing institution, where they can adhere to a drastic regimen, even total starvation, without much discomfort. Once back in their old environment, however, they quickly gain the weight back. Perhaps the hospital has provided psychological support or removed the patient from negative interpersonal family influences where obesity began or is perpetuated. A sterile hospital atmosphere where food is out of sight makes it easier to not eat, while at home, food is constantly and easily available. Many are not even aware of their attraction to food.

Family interaction may also affect the success of attempted weight reduction. For example, a slim marriage partner may rebel against the necessity for a diet for the plumper partner. A husband or wife may fear that the partner will slim down, develop self-esteem, and no longer be dependent. Such emotional fears can thwart dieting attempts just as constant ridicule or nagging that "you can't do it" may undermine the husband, wife, or child. Some husbands have been known to change the entire personality and turn their dieting over to the wife. They then blame the wife if the diet does not work or is not strictly followed.

Once weight is lost, it may still represent only a pseudocure if other functional and emotional problems have not yet been shed. Layers of fat sometimes represent layers of insulation against threatening situations. When the fat is gone, no longer preventing one from testing unrealistic desires, emotional problems occur. The dieting girl who insists she is not attractive to men because of her obesity suddenly faces the same social situations and pressures but without an excuse. She may actually be happier at a socially safe level of overweight. Weight reduction is positive only after other coping mechanisms are also conquered.

People with juvenile-onset obesity often use fat as a convenient shelter and have more difficulty reducing than do others who become obese later and do not expect to solve all their problems by losing weight. Hilde Bruch describes three types of outcomes for people who reduce with the unrealistic goal of expecting a changed life before they have experienced the inner emotional changes which make these new adjustments possible.[11] Most will try and try, will lose some weight, and then, suddenly, will give up, regain, and often overshoot their former weight. For others, the stress of starving themselves, or the loss of their expectations, may prove too much, and serious disturbances, even frank psychotic behavior, may break through. A third group of people succeed in becoming and staying thin, but their conflicts are far from solved by having lost weight. Because the ugliness of being fat no longer prevents them from putting their unrealistic dreams to the test, their difficulties have a chance to flourish. They resemble fat people with all their unsolved problems, conflicts, and exaggerated expectations, only they no longer show their fat. Bruch refers to this group as "thin fat people."

Anorexia Nervosa

Most normal dieters plan to reduce to a selected normal weight and maintain the weight loss. As the dieter loses weight, the usual battles with willpower and perhaps lethargy or apathy are experienced if a large amount of weight is lost. However, weight loss is usually accompanied by increased sociability and happiness as the dieter nears his or her goal. There is a rare and severe psychological illness, **anorexia nervosa,** which closely resembles a normal diet in the initial stages but contines even to the point of starvation. Anorexics try to lose weight to a level way below normal. In addition to starving themselves, they take enormous amounts of laxatives or diuretics or go on eating binges and then vomit. Some individuals exist on a 200-calorie per day regimen and claim they are not hungry. In the advanced stages of the disease, severe emaciation, isolation, annoyance, and resentment within the family often develop. When signs of starvation appear, anorexics still look at their skeleton-like bodies in the mirror and believe they are grossly overweight. They feel as though they are reaching an aesthetic ideal by losing more and more weight. These distorted thoughts and compulsions are purely delusional. About 10 percent of anorexics are successful in starving themselves to death.[12]

Many anorexics are young females attempting to assert their autonomy and to gain identity apart from their parents. Starving themselves is their declaration of independence.

The origin of the disease appears to be cultural. The need to be accepted, upwardly mobile, and fashionable can bring on anorexia nervosa. There is no organic cause for the disease; however, whenever severe malnutrition exists for any length of time, an enormous range of functional disturbances appear and secondary physiological damage may maintain the disorder.

Anorexia nervosa is seldom recognized during the early stages because it so closely resembles regular dieting. Parents should become concerned if a youngster has lost about 10 pounds in a month, or if a smaller weight loss occurs and the child has

- begun a bizarre diet (too often looked on as good by parents anxious for the child to lose weight, or considered typical behavior for a teenager)
- stopped menstruating
- become hyperactive
- allowed social relationships to deteriorate (become withdrawn, begun to complain about silly or immature friends, become uninterested in going out with boys)
- become depressed
- begun to have trouble sleeping
- developed physical symptoms: dryness of skin, subnormal temperature, slower than normal basal metabolism rate[13]

Initial treatment of anorexia nervosa is to halt the starvation and then treat the psychological and emotional aspects of the disease. The family must also be treated because of the established familial pattern that leads to the illness. The worst thing that can be done is to force the weight up without changing the underlying psychological problems.

SOCIAL ASPECTS OF OBESITY

Sociological factors involved reveal some interesting insights into obesity development and management. For example, people tend to become obese when their environment offers abundant food and leisure. Adults become fatter with age, as they become more affluent and able to provide large stores of food for themselves. Obesity is much more extensive in developed and mechanized societies than in underdeveloped areas where life is hard and food is scarce. Obesity is also prevalent among the lower classes, perhaps because the use of fattening, starchy food is more prevalent among these classes.

Other factors such as religion and social mobility also affect obesity. Ideal weight varies with role, function, age, sex, and so on. In our own society, young women are slim, but matronly figures are plumper. The image for men has been somewhat different. The image of the successful businessman in the upper classes is a man with a large stomach. This is gradually changing due to increased knowledge of the relationship of obesity to heart malfunctioning and other diseases.

Race is also a factor in the sociology of obesity. A national health survey showed that the mean weight of American black women (of equal height) was eleven pounds greater than that of white women. Black men, however, are four pounds lighter than their white counterparts.[14]

In our contemporary society, consumption is a prized social virtue and physical activity is declining in most occupations. Even leisure-time activities have become passive—traveling by car, watching TV, and watching movies. Exercise is designed to wear us out as little as possible, with tastefully decorated health spas where workout equipment is impressive looking but often of little value to actual physical fitness. Thus preoccupation with dieting has become especially prevalent.

Living Patterns

The giving and taking of food symbolizes love and affection, friendliness and pleasure, and may become a conscious or unconscious compensation for frustration or neurotic problems. It can become an important part of a cultural predisposition to obesity.

Eating Patterns

An example of such a phenomenon may be found among data concerning Americans of Eastern European extraction. Joffe notes that the Czechs love food and are less Americanized than the Poles as far as cooking habits are concerned. Among the Czechs, there is a great deal of visiting on Sundays during which time large quantities of food are consumed. Refusing a second or even a third helping of food is considered impolite. Research data reflects the results of these customs. In one study, of the lower-class Czechs, 41% were obese as compared with only 18% of the lower-class Polish-Russian-Lithuanians that were obese.[15]

Dieting patterns reveal other interesting facts about obesity within our culture. Wyden notes that although only about 11 percent of the total United States population is in the upper- or upper-middle classes, these classes contain 24 percent of all dieters.[16] Furthermore, obesity seems to be a greater disadvantage for a woman, as noted by the greater number of women dieters than men dieters. While physical desirability seems more important for women, financial status, education, and occupation outweigh slimness for men on the social ladder.

Social Goals

Within any given culture, definitions of beauty and ugliness may vary widely. We cannot always view obesity as an abnormal response of the individual. It can also be found to be a normal response of individuals in certain subgroups to the perceived expectations of their sociological environment.

Cultural Standards of "Normal" Obesity

Given the scarcity of food and the ever-present fear of famine in many tribal societies, the significant social role of food, and the lasting impact of the infant's first sensory satisfactions, it is not surprising to find that stoutness or some degree of obesity is often regarded with favor. This is particularly true for the concept of female attractiveness. Among the Banyankole, a pastoral people in East Africa, when a girl began to prepare for marriage at the age of eight, she was not permitted to play and run about but kept in the house and made to drink large quantities of milk daily so that she would grow fat. By the end of a year she could only waddle. "The fatter she grew the more beautiful she was considered and her condition was a marked contrast to that of the men, who were athletic and well-developed." The royal women, the king's mother and his wives, vied with each other as to who should be the stoutest. They took no exercise, but were carried in litters when going from place to place.

Summarizing briefly for tribal pre-literate societies, we note that hunger was common and that a high proportion of men's and women's energy was spent in producing enough food to stay alive; that food was not only a biological necessity, but that its social and psychological functions were also very significant. The giving of food was a prominent part of all relationships: between kindred, between clans, with dead ancestors, and with gods. Food played a role in ritual, magic, and witchcraft, and in hospitality. The accumulation of food was a mark of great prestige. Fatness was a mark of beauty and desirability in women.[17]

Most theories about obesity are formulated by doctors and psychiatrists working with the middle- and upper-class women, in whom obesity is a social liability. In other classes, while obesity may be unhealthy, it is not always abnormal. Obesity is certainly not abnormal in certain lower socioeconomic groups.

Many middle- and upper-class dieters are actually carrying the cultural standard to an extreme:

> Many women make a fetish of being thin and follow reducing diets without awareness of or regard for the fact that they can do so only at the price of continuous strain and tension and some degree of ill health. There are millions of young girls and women who starve themselves in order to look like these envied models for whom slimness is a well-paid professional pose. Ordinary young women do not get paid for being slim. When they become young mothers, they will continuously complain about fatigue, about their children's problems, and about their own irritability. Little attention has been paid to the fact that their attempt to fulfill fashion's demands to be skinny is directly related to these problems. Having grown up with the concept that thinness is identical with beauty and attractiveness and is desirable for its own sake, they have become used to living on a semi-starvation diet, never eating more than their bony figures show. Never having permitted themselves to eat adequately, they are unaware of how much of their tension, bad disposition, irritability, and inability to pursue an educational or professional goal is the direct result of chronic undernutrition.[18]

In actuality, some people function better at a higher-than-average weight.

Kelly West cites an interesting cultural note:

> From a recent informal and unscientific poll, I learned that most Americans still believe that Santa Claus ought to be fat. A majority told me they would make him at least a little fat even if they had an opportunity to reinvent him. None of my interviewees had given much thought to the possibility that Santa might be sustaining an increased risk of diabetes, arthritis, and hypertension. Apparently, it was the popular view that, if he could fly a well-stocked and very heavy sled without the assistance of wings or jets, he could be expected to attend successfully to the trivial problems of operating his metabolism. It is, however, noteworthy that the degree of corpulence of Santa Claus, Kriss Kringle, Saint Nicholas, and Father Christmas has varied among cultures, and over time in the same culture.
>
> I did not gather enough data to determine definitely why America expects Santa to be fat. But it would appear to be mainly attributable to the still prevalent feeling that the various degrees of adiposity have associations with certain characteristics of personality, mood, and behavior. Santa is fat; villains are usually lean; the devil is usually very lean; and witches are always skinny to extreme. Even those who believe it is unhealthy to be fat usually "feel" a certain association between generosity of adiposity and generosity of spirit, while leanness and meanness are still linked to some degree by most cultures.[19]

SUMMARY

Obesity is not simply a physical characteristic of an individual. Emotional, psychological, and social factors play an important role in obesity onset and complicate its understanding and treatment.

The need and enjoyment of food is a normal part of human existence. However, if the normal need for food and its accompanying symbolic meaning is distorted, addiction to eating for emotional support may result. Compulsive eating patterns range from mild to severe addiction with lack of hunger awareness. In the severely obese, the overuse of food is often an early formed pattern of overeating for pleasure or to reduce psychological or physical disequilibrium.

While obesity may always be unhealthy, it is not always abnormal. Obesity can be found to be a normal response of individuals in certain subgroups to the perceived expectations of their sociological environment. In general, however, a real stigma is attached to obesity and ridicule and disdain are directed toward even the slightly overweight person. Exposure to damaging pressures and difficulties can intensify the underlying psychological factors which caused or contributed to the obesity.

Individuals who develop obesity early in life are especially vulnerable to development of distorted self-concept and loss of identity. Obese children often exhibit personality characteristics similar to traits typical of youngsters in oppressed minority groups who are victims of intense prejudice. Impaired body image is not solely a cultural phenomenon. Obese children who are accepted and encouraged by their families tend to develop good self-concepts and positive body image despite negative influences. It is children showing early emotional disturbance associated with severe intrafamilial problems who develop severe psychological problems and interpret negative cultural attitude as personal rejection.

Psychological disturbance in an obese person can also be produced by attempts to alter his or her obese state. When a person's equilibrium is altered for any length of time, as during weight reduction, a new equilibrium must be established. The body's tendency to resist permanent change, especially in a short period of time, may explain some of the difficulty the obese have in adhering to weight loss programs for a significant length of time.

Sociological factors also affect development of obesity. People tend to become obese when their environment offers abundant food combined with increasing lack of activity. Obesity is more extensive in developed and mechanized societies than in underdeveloped areas where life is hard and food scarce.

NOTES

1. Beatrice J. Kalish, "The Stigma of Obesity," *American Journal of Nursing,* Vol. 72, pp. 1124–27.
2. Ibid.

3. Donald D. Gold, "Psychological Factors Associated with Obesity," *AFP,* Vol. 13, No. 6, June 1976, p. 6.
4. Hilde Bruch, "Psychological Aspects of Obesity," *Medical Insight,* July/August 1973, pp. 23–28.
5. Ibid.
6. Swanson and Dinello, "Severe Obesity as a Habituation Syndrome." Reprinted from Archives of General Psychiatry, 22(2): 120–27, 1970, Copyright 1970, American Medical Association.
7. Leon Salzman, "Obesity—Understanding the Compulsion," *Medical Insight,* July 1970, pp. 52-62.
8. Ibid.
9. Hilde Bruch, "The Psychological Handicaps of the Obese," in George A. Bray (ed.), *Obesity in Perspective,* National Institute of Health, DHEW Publication No. (NIH) 75-708, 1975, p. 111.
10. Joel Grinker, "Behavioral and Metabolic Consequences of Weight Reduction," *Journal of the American Dietetic Association,* January 1973.
11. Bruch, "Handicaps of the Obese," p. 111.
12. "Dieting to Death," *Emergency Medicine,* October 1976, p. 127.
13. Ibid.
14. Kelly M. West, "Culture, History and Adiposity, or Should Santa Claus Reduce?" *Obesity/Bariatric Medicine,* No. 3, 1974, pp. 48-52.
15. P. B. Goldblatt et al., "Social Factors in Obesity," *Journal of the American Medical Association,* Vol. 192, 1965, pp. 97-100.
16. Kalish, "Stigma of Obesity," pp. 1124-1127.
17. H. Powdermaker, "An Anthropological Approach to the Problem of Obesity," *Bulletin of the New York Academy of Medicine,* Vol. 36, 1960, pp. 75-83.
18. Hilde Bruch, "Thin Fat People," in *Eating Disorders: Obesity, Anorexia Nervosa, and the Person Within* (New York: Basic Books, 1974), Chap. 11.
19. West, "Should Santa Claus Reduce?," pp. 48-52.

19

Development of Obesity in Childhood and Adolescence

The rosy, rotund cheeks of a pleasantly plump infant used to signify to physicians and mothers alike a healthy, happy baby. Unfortunately, baby fat is not much different from adult fat, and most of it does not wear off before adulthood. Approximately 10 to 40 percent of school-age children are overweight, and this proportion is steadily rising. Since 50 to 85 percent of overweight children remain obese as adults, there is an urgent need to understand and to prevent childhood obesity and its consequences.[1] Persons who develop obesity in childhood have more difficulty in losing fat and maintaining fat loss than people who become fat as adults. Aside from the emotional and psychological trauma, the greatest risk factor in childhood obesity seems to be that of becoming an obese adult.

Early-onset or childhood obesity is primarily hyperplastic, meaning that the child has too many fat cells. Adipose (fat) cells of infants are still dividing. An excess caloric intake during this maturational period can cause the cells to increase in number as well as in size. Knittle cites two critical periods in the development of fat cells: the years from birth to age two and the years from age eight to age twelve. The increase in fat cell number will remain a lifelong hazard.[2] Table 19-1 summarizes factors that seem to contribute to juvenile-onset obesity.

The number of fat cells in an individual's body is mostly determined by age sixteen. Obesity which develops after adulthood is usually hypertrophic; in other words, weight gain is due to the filling up of existing adipose cells, not the increase in number of cells. Subsequently, when weight is decreased, the size of the fat cells decreases, but not the number.

PHYSICAL AND PSYCHOLOGICAL IMPLICATIONS OF OBESITY

Fat infants do not appear to have a higher mortality rate than normal weight children, but they are more susceptible to respiratory infections and other illnesses.[3] Obese boys and girls are taller than their lean peers. In addition, skeletal development is advanced in obese youngsters, giving them a body with greater skeletal mass than their peers. Whether this development results from the need to support greater mass weight or whether it is a concomitant result is not known. Obese children also show higher than normal levels of hemoglobin and certain vitamins in their blood. Surprisingly, they have an increase not only in fat tissue, but also in fat-free weight.[4] Puberty comes earlier in the obese.

Table 19-1. Factors That Seem to Contribute to Exogenous Obesity (Obesity Originating Outside the Person)

I.   Genetic influence
    A. If neither parent is obese, 7 percent of offspring will be obese.
    B. If one parent is obese, 40 percent of offspring will be obese.
    C. If both parents are obese, 80 percent of offspring will be obese.

II.   Dietary influence
    A. Hypertrophic obesity: normal numbers of adipocytes are present but each cell is enlarged and excessively fat-laden. This is common in adult-onset obesity and is possibly more responsive to therapy than hyperplastic-hypertrophic obesity.
    B. Hyperplastic-hypertrophic obesity: there is an excess number and size of fat cells. This is thought to be related to overfeeding during critical phases of adipocyte proliferation. It is common in persons obese since infancy and is harder to treat.

III. Restricted physical activity
    A. Primary physical restrictions → second-degree obesity.
    B. Physical inactivity in overweight subjects, especially adolescents, that *may be* a secondary effect of obesity.

IV.   Emotional factors
    A. Many children are given food to "cheer them up" and, by the same measure, many adults respond to stress by overeating. Depression should be strongly suspected in patients with no genetic background of obesity.

From L. Howard, "Obesity: A Feasible Approach to a Formidable Problem," *American Family Physician*, Vol. 12, No. 3, September 1975, p. 154.

Psychological factors may play a large role in juvenile obesity. Atypical physical characteristics are particularly difficult to accept during adolescence. Of all the variations in appearance during adolescence, obesity and lesser degrees of fatness are unique in that they are often linked by the obese person, as well as others (including physicians), not only with unattractiveness in terms of current cultural ideals, but also with guilt and lack of willpower. Although all obese persons suffer somewhat from these negative societal attitudes toward obesity, adolescents are particularly vulnerable. Poor adjustment to home, school, or other emotional problems can lead to further excessive, compensating interest in food.

Tragically, obesity is a serious handicap in the social life of a child, and even more so of a teenager. Obesity interferes with the child's interrelationships with others. Obese teenagers suffer from peer ridicule and exclusion from activities.

Weight problems often bar obese people from successful adult adjustment in their social lives and career choices. The obese adolescent may not stand as good a chance of entering the college of his or her choice as nonobese peers. H. Canning and Jean Mayer found that obesity was not associated with high school performance, academic qualifications, or application rates to colleges, but that acceptance rates into high-ranking colleges were lower for obese students, especially for girls.[5] D. Pargman has also noted the low incidence of obesity (2.4 percent) among college freshmen in a northeastern private college. Perhaps unconscious prejudices, of high school teachers in writing recommendations or among college interviewers when meeting obese adolescents, are responsible.[6]

Family arguments often focus upon obese children. Parents tend to worry more about obesity in girls than they do in boys, and mothers are more likely to worry than fathers. Siblings may also get into the act. Often children are nagged when they fail to follow their diet, and tempted (often deliberately) when they do. It takes mature and understanding parents to deal with adolescent obesity effectively. The topic is often a highly sensitive one for either or both parents who are (or were) obese themselves. Obesity isn't always taken seriously, even by adults, and does not have the "dignity" of other diseases.

Children of obese parents are more likely to become obese than are children of normal-weight parents. If neither parent is obese, the child has a 7 percent chance of being obese. If one parent is obese, the child has a 40 percent chance of being obese, and if both parents are obese, the chance is 80 percent. Certain body types which are inherited can also be associated with obesity.

Genetic Considerations

The greatest difference between most overweight children and normal-weight children is not that the overweight eat more, but that they exercise far less than normal-weight children.[7] Physical inactivity is common among babies and children who are confined to playpens, cribs, or strollers to keep them out of mischief. Young children are camped in front of television sets for hours at a time. Children are driven to and from school. Instead of being allowed to explore their environment and discover and develop their physical capabilities, children are encouraged to remain inactive. Not every child needs to participate in competitive sports, but all children (and adults) should exercise vigorously regularly.

Activity and Obesity Development

One study by M. L. Johnson, B. S. Burke, and Jean Mayer compared diet, maturation, and physical activity of 28 obese and 28 nonobese school girls of similar height, age, and grade. The average daily calorie intake of the obese girls was lower in most cases than that of the nonobese girls. The obese group tended to eat less frequently and tended to omit breakfast and lunch more often. Conversely, the obese group also spent fewer hours per week in active pursuits.[8]

It also appears likely that the psychological results of obesity, including passivity, withdrawal, and oversensitivity to appearance, tend to accentuate physical inactivity of obese youngsters. Obesity becomes even more self-accelerating or at least self-perpetuating.

Obese adolescents may be less fit than their more active peers because they are disinclined to physical activity and thus have less opportunity to practice. Given training, this deficit can be reversed, and the obese child can withstand sports as well as anyone else. More difficult to alter are habits of inactivity, which may be firmly established by adolescence. Obese adolescents (and often their parents) beg school physicians to excuse them from gym classes because of fears of embarrassment or injury. Children and mothers sometimes mistake the effects of overheating (huffing, puffing, and flushing) for an imminent heart attack. Some children apparently have so seldom engaged in vigorous physical activity that the signs of exertion are an unrecognizable and frightening phenomenon. Such stories can easily be put to rest by adequate anticipatory guidance and understanding teachers.

In spite of the fact that the obese can, with proper instruction, become fit and learn to enjoy sports and the more active life, in many school systems obese children never receive the attention they deserve because of undue emphasis on competitive athletics for the fit.

EATING HABITS AND HYPERPLASTIC DEVELOPMENT

It is true that body type and certain other genetic factors influence the development of early obesity. But many infants develop an obese condition because the food patterns established in early infancy and childhood predispose them to hyperplasia. Pediatricians and nutritionists warn that overfeeding and the early introduction of solids to babies can trigger an hyperplastic response resulting in chronic obesity. Overfeeding may lead to excessive secretion of insulin and growth hormone, which will increase fat cell size and number.

The Mechanism of Appetite

The hypothalamus controls the satiety center of the body in humans and signals the brain to terminate the desire to eat more when the body has consumed a quota of calories. The volume of food is not usually the triggering factor. Rather, the body adjusts instantly to changes in calorie content. For example, we find ourselves able to eat only small portions of high-calorie foods such as rich pastries or sweets, yet we can consume large volumes of low-calorie vegetables such as lettuce. We stop when we reach a certain calorie point. The fullness of the stomach is rarely the reason why we stop eating. Even removal of portions of the stomach does not seem to have a bearing on the amount of food eaten. This usually results only in the consumption of a larger number of smaller meals.

The appetite mechanism in newborn infants is different from that in older children and adults. The hypothalamic system is not in full operation, and babies probably stop eating because they are literally full. A baby will turn its head away, close its mouth, refuse to suck, or will regurgitate excess food after the stomach is full. Because of these spontaneous reactions to excess food, it is very difficult to overfeed a baby with extra amounts of food. Most overfeeding is due not to volume, however, but to unnaturally high concentration of calories in a small amount of food. Infant feeding habits have changed rapidly with the introduction of commercially prepared foods. Strict breastfeeding up until at least six months post partum has given way to early introduction of high-calorie formulas and solids into the baby's diet.

In an overconcentrated diet, the baby has little defense against being overfed. It is difficult to overfeed a baby on breast milk, which contains 65 calories per 100 milliliters; but solid and semisolid foods contain up to 200 calories per 100 milliliters. Many baby foods contain as much as two to three times as many calories per unit as breast milk. Prepared baby foods such as egg yolk, cereals, meat, fruit, and desserts may have considerable added sugar. The younger an infant is, the less able he or she is to adjust to highly concentrated foods. Premature infants have the most difficulty adjusting to great variations in calorie content.[9]

Parents who regard early use of solid foods and early weight gain in their infant's life as some sort of status symbol, ranking with early walking and early development of teeth, should take the time to measure the length of their babies. If they did, they would discover that many of the babies are overweight. A study in England showed that 16 percent of 300 infants were obese and over 27 percent were overweight. It was found that the diets of these infants were higher in calories than the recommended allowance and that almost 40 percent had received solids before the fourth week of life. There was a correspondingly low incidence of breastfeeding and an early weaning pattern.[10]

Breastfeeding may be considered as one answer to preventing obesity within the first year of life. Breast milk is biologically related to the infant, is low in calories, and comes in a vehicle which makes it impossible to visually measure milk volume. The mother is more likely to go by the infant's appetite than to force feed. There is a tendency in bottle feeding to encourage the child to finish the bottle so as not to waste milk or because the doctor has prescribed a specific amount of formula. A bottle should not be used as a pacifier either, since it encourages the child to overeat. Parents should allow a baby's normal appetite, stimulated by natural growth, to set the pace of food ingestion. Any dietary change contemplated by parents should be supervised by a physician to prevent overfeeding. *Breastfeeding*

If a mother cannot breastfeed her child, she should find a formula that resembles breast milk as closely as possible. Formulas contain all needed nutrient requirements for babies up to three months of age. Solids are simply not needed until after that time. It should be noted that children grow equally well whether they are fed on breast milk, formula, or evaporated milk as long as the weight factor is not a problem.

As a guideline for feeding an infant, a child is getting enough nourishment if his or her weight increases by ½ pound a week for the first six months.[11]

Caloric content should be carefully controlled when solid foods are added to a baby's diet. Table 19-2 shows a schedule of addition of solids to an infant's diet. *Solid Foods*

Early introduction of a variety of foreign proteins in solid foods may also sensitize an infant to a greater number of allergies.

Once an infant begins eating commercially prepared baby food, some wise shopping may prevent economic and nutritional problems. Too often parents buy baby food according to what would taste good to them rather than what is best for the baby. Home preparation of baby food is preferable to use of commercial brands which have a high content of carbohydrates and often contain starch and sugar additives. If commercial products are used, plain vegetables and meats should be emphasized instead of mixed dinners which are lower in protein and higher in carbohydrates. High sugar and water content of commercial foods is an indication of poor economic value.

A most important aspect in obesity prevention and management in infancy is educating the parents, particularly the one who regularly feeds the baby, about nutritional values of foods, amounts needed by the infant, and age-related feeding behavior. The following suggestions are important nutritional concepts for prevention of infant obesity:

- Encourage breastfeeding for infants for at least three months when possible.
- Do not force a bottle-fed infant to empty the bottle each time.
- Mix all formulas correctly. Check the formula every few weeks to be sure it is not too rich. Your physician can dilute the formula if the baby is gaining too much weight.
- Give water and unsweetened juices as substitutes for milk, especially during hot weather when children are thirstier.
- Discourage introduction of solids until the infant is three to six months old, particularly if iron supplementation is provided.
- Do not force a child to eat more than he or she wants. By the age of one year, a child's appetite and nutritional requirements fluctuate and diminish significantly.
- Learn to decipher an infant's cries, and do not offer food in response to every crying episode.
- Encourage an infant's free movement of extremities and whole body, whether the baby is fat or thin.[12]

The habit of overeating will persist into adolescence and adulthood unless parents teach their children how to eat properly. Parents should recognize just what a good eater is. A good eater is not necessarily the one who cleans a plate quickly and pleasantly and then asks for more food. A truly good eater is the one who knows that his or her body needs have been met and quits eating at that point.[13]

Table 19-2. Schedule for Addition of Solid Foods to Infant Diet

3 months	4 months	5 months	6 months	7 & 8 months
CEREAL—1 srvg. 3 T. Rice Cereal	CEREAL—1 srvg. (3 T. Rice Cereal)	CEREAL—1 srvg. (3 T. Rice Cereal)	CEREAL—1 srvg. 3 T. Rice Cereal	CEREAL—1 srvg. 3 T. Rice Cereal
	FRUIT—1 srvg. (4½ T.)	FRUIT—1 srvg. (4½ T.)	FRUIT—2 srvg. (9 T.)	FRUIT—2 srvg. (9 T.)
	VEGETABLE— ½ srvg. (2 T.)	VEGETABLE— 1 srvg. (4½ T.)	VEGETABLE— 2 srvg. (9 T.)	VEGETABLE— 2 srvg. (9 T.)
		MEAT—½ srvg. (2 T.)	MEAT—1 srvg. (3½ T.)	MEAT—2 srvg. (7 T.)
ALL MEASUREMENTS ARE LEVEL T. = tablespoon 1 jar fruits & veg. = 9 T. (134 gm) srvg. = serving 1 jar meat = 7 T. (100 gm)				

Copyright 1974, *Continuing Education for the Family Physician.* Reprinted with permission.

Infant-onset obesity holds different implications in health and prevention of over-weight than does adult-onset obesity. It is a major concern to those wishing to prevent potential obesity, since the success rate of treatment of hyperplastic (increase in number of fat cells) obesity is extremely low. Jean Mayer cites three warning signs of infant obesity: a) parents or relatives are overweight, b) the baby looks fat or is at least broad rather than long, and c) the baby is unusually in-active.[14] Generally speaking, a baby is considered obese if he or she is 20 percent over expected weight, or if the ratio of weight to height is over the 97th percentile. Infantile obesity is usually diagnosed by a physician with the aid of standard height/weight charts.

Obesity management in an infant is not aimed at weight reduction as it is in the adult. The goal is a slowing of the rate of weight gain commensurate with linear growth. A regular diet is advised to satisfy normal growth requirements, about 110 calories per day for infants under six months and about 90 calories per kilogram of child's weight per day for infants six to twelve months. If the baby consumes over thirty ounces of milk a day, this volume should be reduced and water feedings substituted as needed. It is not recommended that skim milk be used to cut down on calories because of its high solute (substance dissolved in a solution) load due to relatively high protein and carbohydrate content. Two-percent-fat (low-fat) milk is occasionally given to older, obese infants. Infant diets should be carefully super-vised by a physician to prevent severe caloric restriction which can reduce fat-free body tissue, inhibit growth, and deplete energy reserves that handle stress.

MANAGING CHILDHOOD AND ADOLESCENT OBESITY

Teenagers experience rapid linear growth, with almost a doubling of body weight in boys and a somewhat lesser weight gain in girls. Thus, it becomes harder to dif-ferentiate between normal weight gain and excessive gain in adipose tissue. Early recognition by parents of a teenager's tendency toward weight gain is an important factor in preventing what could become an irreversible situation. For the adolescent motivated to lose weight, a reducing program should be outlined under the direction of a knowledgeable physician, and with the full cooperation and under-standing of parents, school nurse, and teachers.

Because teenagers vary greatly in their eating practices, treatment of every patient should begin with an assessment of his or her unique problems. Unlike with adult diet management, the main goal should be weight control, not reduction, which allows the child to grow into his or her correct weight. Severe diet restriction should be avoided. The components of an adolescent obesity management program are outlined in Table 19–3.

Whichever treatment is used, adolescent weight loss must be accomplished slowly in order to preserve normal growth. Because of poor body image and other behavioral difficulties, many adolescents have emotional problems which complicate therapy. Prevention seems to be a key in view of the present success rate in treating obesity in any age group.

Table 19–3.

Evaluation of Patient

Complete medical and social history should be taken.

Establish Diet and Exercise Program

Calories and protein should be adjusted to permit growth and development of lean body mass while decreasing fat deposits. (Children under age twelve should receive approximately sixty kilocalories per kilogram of ideal body weight in the following proportions: 20 percent from protein; 40 percent from carbohydrates, and 40 percent from fat.)

Behavior Modification (Environmental Control)

The environment must be modified and controlled by parents, but the child must take responsibility for his or her own management appropriate to the level of maturity.

Give the child appropriate-size portions of low-calorie food. Do not deny the child the basic family diet.

Avoid the "clean plate syndrome."

Engage the child in conversation while eating. Avoid having the child eat alone.

Allow the child to eat only in a fixed, designated place.

Carefully plan eating strategies for parties, picnics, treats, etc.

Teach the child to distinguish between high- and low-calorie foods. Teach him or her to make knowledgeable and independent food decisions so he or she can take responsibility for his or her own eating.

Provide low-calorie nutritious snacks (such as raw vegetables) for the whole family instead of sweets.

Discourage the child from taking food-handling jobs in the school cafeteria.

Offer food only in response to signals indicating nutritional need so the child will develop a definite concept of hunger, as something to be appeased by food and as a sensation distinct from other tensions or needs which require other activities for their relief. (If the parent's reaction is continuously inappropriate, neglectful, oversolicitous, inhibiting, or indiscriminately permissive, the child will become confused and will not learn to differentiate between being hungry or sated or suffering from some other discomfort.)

Do not allow the child to spend countless inactive hours in front of the television.

Encourage but do not nag the child to follow the diet.

Family Support

Do not snack in front of the child.

Don't use food for bribery, punishment, reward, or as substitute for meaningful interpersonal relationships.

Participate with the child in home or community recreational activities. Encourage the child to exercise.

Teach siblings how to respect and relate positively to an extremely sensitive child.

Work at the problem gradually and utilize community resources (dieticians, hospitals, health departments, nurse practitioners, or other paramedical persons interested in working with obese youngsters). Don't allow the child's problem to seem bigger than it is or eclipse regular family interaction and activity.

From "Obesity: A Weighty Problem at Any Age," *Modern Medicine,* Vol. 45, 1977, p. 90.

SUMMARY

Obesity that develops in childhood and adolescence is primarily hyperplastic. Fat infants do not appear to have a higher mortality rate than normal-weight children, but they are more susceptible to respiratory infections and other illnesses. Psychological factors play an important role in juvenile obesity. Atypical physical characteristics are particularly difficult to accept during adolescence.

The primary factors that contribute to early development of obesity are genetic predisposition, diet and eating patterns, restricted physical activity, and emotional conditioning to respond to stress by overeating.

Children of obese parents are more likely to become obese than are children of normal-weight parents. Obesity occurs more frequently in endomorphic body types than other types. Endomorphy predisposes deposition of additional quantities of fat unless excessive activity, disease or voluntary weight control intervene.

The greatest difference between most overweight children and normal-weight children is not that the overweight eat more, but that they exercise far less than normal-weight children. Oversensitivity to appearance, withdrawal, and passivity tend to accentuate physical inactivity of many obese children.

It is easier to prevent obesity than to treat it. Many develop an obese condition because of food patterns established in early infancy. Overfeeding of infants can lead to excessive secretion of insulin and growth hormone, which increases fat cell size and number. To prevent early development of obesity, wise eating patterns should be developed in infancy. Breastfeeding is recommended if possible. Less calorically dense foods should be emphasized, and food should be offered only in response to hunger. A baby should not be forced to eat beyond his or her natural appetite. Solid foods should not be introduced into the diet before the third to sixth month. Physical activity should be encouraged.

Once obesity has developed in a child or adolescent, management is aimed at slowing the rate of weight gain to make it commensurate with linear growth, rather than reducing weight. Severe caloric restriction in children can reduce fat-free body tissue, inhibit growth, and deplete energy reserves that handle stress.

NOTES

1. *Facts About Obesity,* Department of Health, Education, and Welfare, Public Health Service, DHEW Publication No. (NIH) 76-974.

2. Jerome L. Knittle, "Obesity in Childhood: A Problem in Adipose Tissue Cellular Development," *Journal of Pediatrics,* Vol. 81, 1972, pp. 1048-1059.

3. Myron Winick, "Childhood Obesity," *Nutrition Today,* March/June 1974, pp. 6-12.

4. Ibid.

5. J. Dwyer and J. Mayer, "The Dismal Condition: Problems Faced by Obese Adolescent Girls in American Society," *Obesity in Perspective,* pp. 12, 103.

6. Dwyer and Mayer, "The Dismal Condition," pp. 12, 103.

7. Jean Mayer, "Fat Babies Grow into Fat People," *Family Health,* May 1973, pp. 24-28.

8. Ruth L. Huenemann, "Food Habits of Obese and Nonobese Adolescents," *Postgraduate Medicine,* May 1972, Vol. 51, pp. 99-105.

9. Mayer, "Fat Babies Grow into Fat People," pp. 24-28.

10. Terence Collins, "Infantile Obesity," *American Family Physician,* Vol. 11, No. 3, March 1975, pp. 162-163.

11. "When to Start Dieting? At Birth," *Medical World News,* September 1973, pp. 31-33.

12. Leonard S. Taitx, "Obesity in Pediatric Practice: Infantile Obesity," *Pediatric Clinics of North America,* Vol. 24, No. 1, February 1977, p. 107.

13. Margaret A. Flynn, "The Portly, Corpulent or Obese American," *Continuing Education for the Family Physician,* July 1974, pp. 28-33.

14. Mayer, "Fat Babies Grow into Fat People," pp. 24-28.

20

The Dynamics of Weight Control

The problem with losing weight is that, although many individuals repeatedly succeed in doing it, they invariably put it on again. Their experience resembles that of Mark Twain in giving up smoking, which he found very easy, having done it hundreds of times.

To many people, the idea behind weight loss has nothing to do with permanent, ideal weight control. They plan diets for special occasions, and as soon as they lose the desired poundage, they return to their old eating habits with little thought to the consequences. To some, the inconvenience in spot dieting and seesawing up and down on the weight scales is preferable to maintaining a sound lifetime diet, or perhaps they haven't the self-control to maintain sound eating habits.

The goal of an effective weight loss regimen is not merely to prescribe a diet. Weight control requires a lifelong commitment, an understanding of one's eating habits, and a willingness to change them. Moderate but frequent exercise is necessary, and accomplishment must be reinforced to sustain motivation. Crash dieting, chemical crutches, and magical formulas are ineffective.

At present, a nutrition-wise physician, nutritionist, health educator, or physical educator is probably best equipped to counsel and encourage patients in weight loss. Some doctors are unwilling or unable to spend the amount of time needed by obese patients and may utilize the services of paraprofessionals or some other resource to help them. Regardless of who takes the responsibility for counseling, a sound obesity management program should incorporate five major components:

1. Screening of patients;
2. Establishing support and encouragement;
3. Methods of inducing weight loss;
4. Behavior therapy;
5. Daily exercise program.

SCREENING OF PATIENTS

Not everyone can or should lose weight. Common obesity is not one homogenous entity. Different types of obesity may be characterized by varied eating patterns, tissue morphology (structure and form), and etiology (study of cause of disease). Table 20-1 shows different classifications of obesity. It is a disservice to any person to fail to assess whether his or her physical environment, financial circumstances, level of intelligence, and motivation are adequate to deal with weight loss.

Table 20-1. Classification of Obesity

Anatomic

Hypercellular (hyperplasia)
  With increase in number of adipocytes and variable degrees of enlargement; onset
    usually early or late childhood
Normocellular (hypertrophy)
  With increase in size but not in number of adipocytes; onset usually in adult years
    or during pregnancy

Etiologic

Endocrine
  Excess of insulin or of adrenocortical hormones
  Associated with other endocrine disorder
    diabetes mellitus, non-insulin-dependent
    ovarian dysfunction
    thyroid dysfunction
    Cushing disease
Hypothalamic
Genetic
  Unusual syndromes associated with obesity
  Familial obesity (reserve for obesity with strong familial incidence)
Obesity of undetermined origin

Information Relevant to Obesity

Family history
  obesity
  diabetes mellitus
  hyperlipemia
  accelerated arteriosclerosis
Profile of patient's obesity
  rate of progression at various stages of life
  current rate of weight gain or loss

Contributing Factors

Factors influencing eating behavior, such as circumstances of eating, social factors,
    psychiatric disorders such as depression
Frequency and pattern of eating; nibbling or gorging pattern, night feeding,
    compulsive eating
Factors affecting amount eaten, such as occupation and activity level of cook,
    composition of diet, perceived satiety
Physical activity; previous experience with exercise programs, current physical
    fitness, daily routine, living conditions, opportunities for extra exertion and
    exercise
Pharmacologic and endocrine (relating to endocrine glands which in turn relate to
    metabolism) factors
  use of oral contraceptives
  insulin excess from ill-advised use of insulin or substitutes
  glucocorticoid (steroids that affect carbohydrate metabolism) administration
  phenothiazine drugs or other tranquilizers

Addiction
alcohol (type and amount drunk)
tobacco smoking or recent cessation of smoking
marijuana smoking

Screening devices are often used by physicians in evaluating patients for obesity management problems. A screening device helps the physician identify physical condition, relevant aspects of weight history, level of dietary and nutrition knowledge, problem eating patterns, activity level, influences on eating behavior, and areas of stress related to problem eating. It also becomes a means of education to correct misconceptions and help the patient develop realistic expectations for weight control.

Medical Contraindications

Most obesity is the result of human behavior and not of some special feature of human metabolism. However, a complete physical exam is necessary to identify metabolic disorders, problems which would prevent or alter exercise capabilities, special nutritional needs, and age-related factors.

Pregnant women, for example, should be cautioned about trying to lose weight. The mother who breastfeeds her baby needs nutrients to produce about a quart of milk per day and should be cautioned to get adequate protein. Children and adolescents need added nutrients to build new tissue and should be warned about harmful diets.

Convalescent patients who have lost ten or fifteen pounds during illness need plenty of proteins, vitamins, and minerals in order to regenerate body tissue. Patients who are on medication that can cause malabsorption should never try fad weight loss programs. The elderly require careful supervision because this age group is susceptible to malnutrition.

Onset of Obesity

Persons who have been obese since childhood and are grossly obese as adults generally suffer from hyperplastic obesity and may have more difficulty controlling weight than those individuals who develop obesity in adult life and whose obesity is mild to moderate. Techniques for diagnosing the hyperplastic type of obesity are not yet generally available. These involve measurement of lipid content of adipocytes combined with estimates of total body fat. A presumptive diagnosis is usually made on clinical grounds when the onset is in childhood and the distribution of the fat is universal.

Failure rate in treating severe hyperplastic obesity is high enough to discourage many busy primary-care physicians from spending the time and effort required with these persons. It is unrealistic for these patients to expect dramatic results from a weight control program. They need short-term goals to achieve modest decreases in body weight and then maintain that weight loss rather than unrealistic goals of bringing body weight down to a normal level.[1] In adult onset obesity, nutritional counseling may be sufficient to initiate an effective program.

SUPPORT AND ENCOURAGEMENT

Assessment of obese patients extends beyond diagnosing specific metabolic disorders or disease states. There are many contributory factors that must be taken into consideration in caring for the patients and aiding them in changing their eating behavior. It is essential that an obese patient's emotional resources be adequate to support and maintain morale and self-respect throughout the program.

If, for example, a thorough examination of eating reveals that oral gratification is the only comfort and solace in a life otherwise devoid of satisfaction, eating habits should be left alone until new interests and solutions have been found to unacceptable situations. Otherwise, profound depression and anxiety may result.

Every program must be suited to the individual metabolic rate, which will influence the determination of daily input and output of energy. The 2,000-calorie diet that takes weight off Harry may cause Alice to gain. The three-mile-a-day run that keeps May fit and happy may give Jack sore ankles and shin splints. The physician must be prepared to effectively evaluate each aspect of an individual's case and to educate the patient to expect predictable patterns of weight loss.

Quick water and protein loss accounts for a good part of initial weight loss when a diet begins. As the body adapts to lower energy intake, it takes a higher energy deficit to lose a pound of weight, so the rate of weight loss will slow down. In addition, the decrease in body fat may be larger than the average decrease in body weight. Anyone on a diet can reach a plateau where he or she will temporarily stop losing weight because of changes such as in the natural water balance of the body. Eventually a dieter will lose more pounds if he or she continues to follow the diet. It is during these plateau phases that the patient needs support and assurance to allay discouragement.

Not only does the individual need treatment, but it is important that other key members of the family are worked with as well. An individual changes as he or she loses weight, and power relationships within a family can change because of this. Family members who do not want the relationship to change can sabotage a successful weight reduction plan. Spouses who try to lose weight together should be warned that men appear to lose weight more quickly than women. This can be quite disturbing when a woman and her husband are on the same program and are competing with each other.

Steady and maintained weight reduction is no fun for anyone. Patients are generally happier when they lose weight rapidly but they tend to regain it more readily than those who lose slowly. Unless education and change in lifestyle occur, weight loss is rarely maintained.[2]

After a trial period, a physician may need to redesign the regimen or advise a patient that this is not the time or place to continue this endeavor.

METHODS OF PRODUCING WEIGHT LOSS

Obesity management programs vary with the degree of obesity. The risks associated with mild degrees of overweight are minimal, and the potential therapies to be used involve lower risk. Table 20–2 outlines management strategies sometimes used by physicians according to a general obesity index.

Table 20–2. Management Plan for Weight Reduction

Mild exogenous obesity (not more than 20 percent overweight):
  A. Outline reasonable diet therapy (not less than 1,200 calories per day) and exercise program.
  B. Refer the patient to community diet organization.
  C. Recommend a reliable diet manual.

Moderate exogenous obesity (20 to 50 percent overweight):
  A. Outline the components of a balanced deficit diet and exercise program.
  B. Stress behavior modification, using techniques such as asking patient to keep a diary, or a reward system.
  C. Consider a modified fast.

Severe (morbid) exogenous obesity (50 percent or more overweight):
  A. Start with balanced deficit, exercise, and behavior modification.
  B. Use a modified or protein-sparing fast.
  C. Consider wiring the patient's jaws.
  D. Consider a jejunileal bypass procedure.

From L. Howard, "Obesity: A Feasible Approach to a Formidable Problem," *American Family Physician,* Vol. 12, No. 3, September 1975, p. 153.

Weight Control Through Diet

The basic concept behind any dietary attempt at weight control is to produce a negative caloric balance by eliminating a certain number of calories not needed by the overweight person.

In developing an eating program, it is not enough to simply follow a standard form diet. Every patient has a unique management problem and needs a program adjusted to individual needs. A sound diet is personal, nutritionally adequate, appealing, and liveable. An improper diet can cause headaches, dizziness, diarrhea, fatigue, indigestion, skin disorders, and constipation, as well as psychological disturbance such as irritability and depression. You should not try to lose more than ten pounds in a year without medical supervision.

Important steps in planning a reducing diet are as follows:

1. Determine desirable body weight.
2. Calculate caloric deficit to achieve slow, steady weight loss.
3. Ensure intake of essential nutrients.
4. Adjust for eating patterns.
5. Set up maintenance diet when desired weight is reached.[3]

Determining Desirable Body Weight

There is no such thing as a one-size-fits-all ideal weight. That's why you can't rely just on height-weight charts to tell you your right weight. But you can get some idea of where you stand from a chart such as Table 20–3. Small frame means a slight, delicate build with narrow feet, thin chest, small ankles and wrists. Medium frame indicates a muscular, athletic build with V-shaped chest, sturdy ankles and wrists. A person with a large frame is built stockily, with heavy muscles, big hands, husky looking ankles and wrists.

A look in the mirror may be enough to tell you you're carrying excess weight, but other factors besides frame enter into the determination of desirable weight, so check with your doctor before drastically altering your patterns of eating or exercising.

Table 20-3. Desirable Body Weights

Height (in shoes)	Small Frame		Medium Frame		Large Frame	
	Men	Women	Men	Women	Men	Women
4'10"		95		101		111
5'0"		100		107		117
5'2"	116	106	123	113	133	123
5'4"	122	112	129	119	140	129
5'6"	128	119	136	127	147	137
5'8"	136	127	145	135	156	146
5'10"	145	135	153	143	165	154
6'0"	153	143	162	151	174	163
6'2"	161		171		183	

Department of Health, Education, and Welfare, U.S. Department of Health.

Caloric Cutbacks   Dietary therapy requires various degrees of cutbacks depending largely upon desired results and the present condition of obesity. On all caloric-cutback diets, the quality of the food should not be changed. It is important that the dieter receive adequate amounts of protein, carbohydrates, and fats. A good vitamin supplement is frequently added. To prevent possible nutrient deficiencies in their diets, women should not reduce their caloric intake below 1,200 calories nor men below 1,500 calories without consulting a physician.

There are four general diets for caloric reduction.

Common Sense Reduction in Calories. For mild weight reduction, caloric intake can be reduced without specifically counting calories by cutting down on high-calorie foods (remembering, however, that nutrient values should not be lowered).

WHERE THE CALORIES ARE

Preparing good food that is not fattening depends on knowing which foods contain the most calories. Food is made up of water, undigestible bulk, calories, and minerals. Water content and undigestible bulk are major factors in determining how many calories there are in any food. A good example here is raw round steak with all the visible fat removed. The remaining meat is over 70 percent water and that is why a whole pound of separable lean round steak will contain only about 600 calories. Fish is about 80 percent water and is a low calorie food. Fresh fruits and vegetables contain lots of water. Many vegetables, particularly those used for salads, contain lots of water and undigestible bulk. That is why raw lettuce is such a low calorie food. Whole milk is 87 percent water. Most of the foods you use are calories diluted with water and undigestible bulk, whether they are solid such as meat or liquids such as milk or fruit juice.

The high calorie foods are those which contain little water or undigestible bulk. Sugar is a good example. Less than one percent of its weight is water. So, 100 grams (3½ ounces) of sugar contains 385 calories. The same weight of raw separable lean round steak contains only 135 calories. Sugar contains almost three times as many calories. The same amount of all-purpose flour (12 percent of its weight is water) contains 364 calories. It is mostly carbohydrate with some protein and fat.

Fat is the highest calorie food. Lard is the supreme example as it contains no water. One hundred grams (3½ ounces) of lard contains 902 calories. A gram of fat contains nine calories while a gram of protein or carbohydrate contains about four calories per gram. That's important—but how much water and undigestible bulk is in a food item is equally important. The various cooking oils contain no water either and 100 grams (3½ ounces) contains 884 calories—just slightly less than lard.[4]

Although many people are painstakingly conscious of the calories in the food they eat, they forget that what they drink also contributes to caloric intake. When the body oxidizes alcohol, seven kilocalories (those used to measure weight) are produced per gram of pure alcohol. (One fluid ounce of pure alcohol [200 proof] has 160 k calories.) Additional k calories are contributed from such items as orange juice, tonic water or sugar.

It is not necessary to stop eating the types of foods you normally eat and like in order to lose weight. An easy way to eliminate excess calories without unbalancing or cutting out nutritional needs is to substitute foods with lower caloric content that are just as nourishing and filling for foods currently eaten. Table 20-4 shows how a typical meal and snack can be trimmed of many calories that add excess body weight. More detailed low-calorie food selections and substitutions are found in Table 20-5.

1,000-Calorie Deficit.   In the 1000-calorie deficit diet, the number of calories needed by the body and those required for normal activity are added, and 1,000 calories are subtracted from that total. This creates an elimination of 7,000 calories a week or about two pounds, which is an ideal rate of reduction as it does not cause the weakness that rapid weight loss often does and generally the weight is not as rapidly regained.

1,000-to-1,200-Calorie Diet.   The 1,000-to-1,200-calorie diet is similar to the preceding one, only on a stricter scale. It is quite effective for the middle-aged or elderly, but is probably too extreme for the younger, more active patient who would find it rather weakening.

Table 20-4. Sample of How Calorie Intake Can Be Reduced through Sensible Substitution

BREAKFAST

From:		To:	
½ glass (4 oz.) orange juice	50	½ glass (4 oz.) orange juice	50
1 scrambled egg	120	1 boiled egg	78
2 slices bacon	100	1 slice bacon	50
2 slices white bread	126	2 slices Gluten bread (white) 35 Calories per slice	70
2 pats butter	100	Low Calorie margarine 17 Calories per pat	34
2 cups coffee, each with sugar (2 lumps) and cream (2 tbsp.)	220	2 cups coffee with no Calorie sweetener and non dairy cream, 11 Calories per tbsp.	22
Total Calories	**716**	**Total Calories**	**304**

MID-MORNING SNACK

From:		To:	
1 cup coffee with sugar (2 lumps) and cream (2 tbsp.)	110	1 cup coffee with no Calorie sweetener and non dairy cream	11
1 small Danish pastry	140	2 low Calorie cookies 25 Calories per cookie	50
Total Calories	**250**	**Total Calories**	**61**

LUNCH

From:		To:	
Hamburger	350	Hamburger	350
1 slice apple pie	338	Low Calorie pudding	123
1 glass (8 oz.) whole milk	165	1 glass (8 oz.) skim milk	80
Total Calories	**853**	**Total Calories**	**553**

MID-AFTERNOON SNACK

From:		To:	
1 bottle cola beverage	105	Low Calorie cola	2
1 custard (4 oz. cup)	205	2 low Calorie cookies	50
Total Calories	**310**	**Total Calories**	**52**

DINNER

From:		To:	
½ glass (4 oz.) tomato juice	25	Consomme, 1 cup	10
6 oz. meat loaf	680	6 oz. club steak, broiled, lean	320
with 4 tbsp. gravy (41 Calories per tbsp.)	164		
½ cup mashed potatoes	123	1 medium potato, baked	100
½ cup green peas	72	12 spears asparagus	40
2 slices French bread	160	2 pats low Calorie margarine	34
with 2 pats butter	100		
Tossed Salad	20	Hearts of lettuce	20
w/1½ tbsp. Roquefort Cheese dressing (100 Calories per tbsp.)	150	with low Calorie salad dressing	15
Iced plain layer cake	290	1 cup low Calorie whipped dessert	123
1 cup coffee with sugar (2 lumps) and cream (2 tbsp.)	110	1 cup coffee with no Calorie sweetener and non dairy cream	11
Total Calories	**1894**	**Total Calories**	**673**
Total Calories for day	**4023**	**Total Calories for day**	**1643**
		A saving of 2380 Calories	

From *Are You Really Serious About Losing Weight?* (Rochester, N.Y.: PennWalt Corporation, Pharmaceutical Division, 1975), pp. 37–39.

Table 20-5.   **279**

For This   Substitute This

Beverages	Calories		Calories	Calories saved
☐ Milk (whole), 8 oz.	165	Milk (buttermilk, skim) 8 oz.	80	85
☐ Prune juice, 8 oz.	170	Tomato juice, 8 oz.	50	120
☐ Soft drinks, 8 oz.	105	Diet soft drinks, 8 oz.	1	104
☐ Coffee (with cream and 2 tsp. sugar)	110	Coffee (black with artificial sweetener)	0	110
☐ Cocoa (all milk), 8 oz.	235	Cocoa (milk and water), 8 oz.	140	95
☐ Chocolate malted milk shake, 8 oz.	500	Lemonade (sweetened), 8 oz.	100	400
☐ Beer (1 bottle), 12 oz.	175	Liquor (1½ oz.), with soda or water, 8 oz.	120	55
Breakfast foods				
☐ Rice flakes, 1 cup	110	Puffed rice, 1 cup	50	60
☐ Eggs (scrambled), 2	220	Eggs (boiled, poached), 2	160	60
Butter and Cheese				
☐ Butter on toast	170	Apple butter on toast	90	80
☐ Cheese (Blue, Cheddar, Cream, Swiss), 1 oz.	105	Cheese (cottage, uncreamed), 1 oz.	25	80
Desserts				
☐ Angel food cake, 2″ piece	110	Cantaloupe melon, ½	40	70
☐ Cheese cake, 2″ piece	200	Watermelon, ½″ slice (10″ diam.)	60	140
☐ Chocolate cake with icing, 2″ piece	425	Sponge cake, 2″ piece	120	305
☐ Fruit cake, 2″ piece	115	Grapes, 1 cup	65	50
☐ Pound cake, 1 oz. piece	140	Plums, 2	50	90
☐ Cupcake, white icing, 1	230	Plain cupcake, 1	115	115
☐ Cookies, assorted (3″ diam.), 1	120	Vanilla wafer (dietetic), 1	25	95
☐ Ice cream, 4 oz.	150	Yoghurt (flavored), 4 oz.	60	90
Pie				
☐ Apple, 1 piece (1/7 of a 9″ pie)	345	Tangerine (fresh), 1	40	305
☐ Blueberry, 1 piece	290	Blueberries (frozen, unsweetened), ½ cup	45	245
☐ Cherry, 1 piece	355	Cherries (whole), ½ cup	40	315
☐ Custard, 1 piece	280	Banana, small, 1	85	195
☐ Lemon meringue, 1 piece	305	Lemon flavored gelatin, ½ cup	70	235
☐ Peach, 1 piece	280	Peach (whole), 1	35	245
☐ Rhubarb, 1 piece	265	Grapefruit, ½	55	210
☐ Pudding (flavored), ½ cup	140	Pudding (dietetic, non-fat milk), ½ cup	60	80
Fish and Fowl				
☐ Tuna (canned), 3 oz.	165	Crabmeat (canned), 3 oz.	80	85
☐ Oysters (fried), 6	400	Oysters (shell w/sauce), 6	100	300

From *Are You Really Serious About Losing Weight?* (Rochester, N.Y.: PennWalt Corporation, Pharmaceutical Division, 1975), pp. 37–39.

For This   Substitute This

For This	Calories	Substitute This	Calories	Calories saved
☐ Ocean perch (fried), 4 oz.	260	Bass, 4 oz.	105	155
☐ Fish sticks, 5 sticks or 4 oz.	200	Swordfish, (broiled), 3 oz.	140	60
☐ Lobster meat, 4 oz. with 2 tbsp. butter	300	Lobster meat, 4 oz., with lemon	95	205
☐ Duck (roasted), 3 oz.	310	Chicken (roasted), 3 oz.	160	150

Meats

For This	Calories	Substitute This	Calories	Calories saved
☐ Loin roast, 3 oz.	290	Pot roast (round), 3 oz.	160	130
☐ Rump roast, 3 oz.	290	Rib roast, 3 oz.	200	90
☐ Swiss steak, 3½ oz.	300	Liver (fried), 2½ oz.	210	90
☐ Hamburger (av. fat, broiled), 3 oz.	240	Hamburger (lean, broiled), 3 oz.	145	95
☐ Porterhouse steak, 3 oz.	250	Club steak, 3 oz.	160	90
☐ Rib lamb chop (med.), 3 oz.	300	Lamb leg roast, (lean only), 3 oz.	160	140
☐ Pork chop (med.), 3 oz.	340	Veal chop (med.), 3 oz.	185	155
☐ Pork roast, 3 oz.	310	Veal roast, 3 oz.	230	80
☐ Pork sausage, 3 oz.	405	Ham (boiled, lean), 3 oz.	200	205

Potatoes

For This	Calories	Substitute This	Calories	Calories saved
☐ Fried, 1 cup	480	Baked (2½" diam.)	100	380
☐ Mashed, 1 cup	245	Boiled (2½" diam.)	100	140

Salads

For This	Calories	Substitute This	Calories	Calories saved
☐ Chef salad with oil dressing, 1 tbsp.	180	Chef salad with dietetic dressing, 1 tbsp.	40	120
☐ Chef salad with mayonnaise, 1 tbsp.	125	Chef salad with dietetic dressing, 1 tbsp.	40	85
☐ Chef salad with Roquefort, Blue, Russian, French dressing, 1 tbsp.	105	Chef salad with dietetic dressing, 1 tbsp.	40	65

Sandwiches

For This	Calories	Substitute This	Calories	Calories saved
☐ Club	375	Bacon and tomato (open)	200	175
☐ Peanut butter and jelly	275	Egg salad (open)	165	110
☐ Turkey with gravy, 3 tbsp.	520	Hamburger, lean, (open), 3 oz.	200	320

Snacks

For This	Calories	Substitute This	Calories	Calories saved
☐ Fudge, 1 oz.	115	Vanilla wafers, (dietetic) 2	50	65
☐ Peanuts (salted), 1 oz.	170	Apple, 1	100	70
☐ Peanuts (roasted), 1 cup, shelled	1375	Grapes, 1 cup	65	1305
☐ Potato chips, 10 med.	115	Pretzels, 10 small sticks	35	80
☐ Chocolate, 1 oz. bar	145	Toasted marshmallows, 3	75	70

Soups

For This	Calories	Substitute This	Calories	Calories saved
☐ Creamed, 1 cup	210	Chicken noodle, 1 cup	110	100
☐ Bean, 1 cup	190	Beef noodle, 1 cup	110	80
☐ Minestrone, 1 cup	105	Beef bouillon, 1 cup	10	95

Vegetables

For This	Calories	Substitute This	Calories	Calories saved
☐ Baked beans, 1 cup	320	Green beans, 1 cup	30	290
☐ Lima beans, 1 cup	160	Asparagus, 1 cup	30	130
☐ Corn (canned), 1 cup	185	Cauliflower, 1 cup	30	155
☐ Peas (canned), 1 cup	145	Peas (fresh), 1 cup	115	30
☐ Winter squash, 1 cup	75	Summer squash, 1 cup	30	45
☐ Succotash, 1 cup	260	Spinach, 1 cup	40	220

Total Caloric Restriction. When totally restricting calories, the patient fasts from one to two days under the supervision of a physician in a hospital setting. The fasting patient is generally satisfied with the fast, as it causes a feeling of anorexia and euphoria. It also has the psychological advantage of rapid weight loss.

However, in one recent study on weight loss by fasting it was found that all those who lost weight eventually returned to their prefasting weight. Those who were obese since infancy tended to ultimately exceed their prefast weight.[5]

Many experts feel that due to an error in metabolism, severely obese persons have a daily caloric requirement for maintenance of ideal weight which is far below the Recommended Dietary Allowance set by the Food and Nutrition Board of the National Research Council (2,800 calories for men, 2,000 for women). Severe obesity is caused by this lower caloric requirement combined with ingestion of excess calories. Without the error in metabolism, these people would still become fat but probably not severely obese. A severely obese dieter, therefore, may have to lower daily caloric intake to between 800 and 1,400 calories in order to experience weight loss.

Weight reduction is difficult and is made more so by the nagging hunger pains a caloric cutback can bring. Numerous drugs are prescribed by physicians to promote weight loss. These include:

Drugs in the Treatment of Obesity

- anorectics to reduce appetite
- drugs to cause nausea
- drugs to prevent gastrointestinal absorption
- hormones to increase metabolism and lypolysis
- tranquilizers
- diuretics to eliminate water (which is the cause of a good percentage of the weight and fatness in obese persons)

Drugs cannot miraculously cause fat to melt away without effort or discipline. When diet is unrestricted, most drugs are little more effective than placebo therapy. In sound weight loss regimens, drugs are prescribed conservatively only as short-term initial boosts to diet and exercise programs. After a month or so, anorectics lose their appetite-suppressant effects and often have unwanted side effects, including abuse potential and severe psychological dependence.

Even in cases where drug treatment may be indicated, it is clear that no one drug approach is best.

For many extreme cases of obesity (100 pounds or more over normal), when no other method of weight control has had a positive effect, jejunileal or intestinal bypass surgery can be performed to reduce the digesting and absorbing surface of the jejunum and ilium.

Jejunileal Surgery

This surgical procedure is effective but drastic—with significant complications and side effects. Expected weight loss is about 30 percent the first year and 10 percent the second year. Much of the loss is attributed to patients' not eating as much.[6] Thereafter, loss levels off and remains fairly stable indefinitely, with minor fluctuations. Complications of jejunileal bypass surgery include diarrhea, liver failure, infection, malabsorption of vitamins, blood clots, and death.

Because the side effects and potential complications of this procedure are dangerous enough to be fatal if unrecognized or inappropriately treated, selected patients must be psychologically stable, reliable, and capable of understanding the risks of surgery and the necessity for frequent postoperative evaluations after such a procedure.

Behavior Therapy   Most obesity is a function of food ingestion and activity behaviors that have developed over a lifetime. Behavior therapy, or modification, is a new concept in weight control that focuses on helping change habits and lifestyle on a long-term basis. Behavior control tries to guide people away from the all-or-nothing approach to losing weight. Modifying eating habits is not necessarily a drastic procedure. The focus is not solely on eating, but also on the patient's knowledge, misconceptions, activity, time management, and life stresses. The program stresses control of the hows, whys, and whens of eating.

The theoretical underpinnings of behavior therapy come from the findings of Dr. Albert Stunkard, who claims that overweight and obese people are very susceptible to food cues. "Put a cue—say, a bowl of potato chips—in front of a normal-weight person who's just eaten, and he will ignore them. But put the bowl in front of an obese individual and he will devour them, even if he's just gotten up from a large meal." A decrease in weight alone doesn't lead to a decrease in susceptibility to cues. "In all our studies, we observed that formerly obese people reacted to cues the same way currently obese individuals did."[7]

Cues which can stimulate desire include pizza shops, baker's windows, everybody else's leftovers, a last piece of cheesecake, watching television or reading.

Many physicians utilize a behavior assessment evaluation to identify specific behavior patterns and what influences these patterns, and to help the patient recognize and control cues or make them less tempting. Here is an outline of one program:

1. *Keep a Food Intake Sheet.* Keep track of what you eat for two weeks. Your record should be very detailed, including a remark on where you ate, when, your emotional state while eating, etc.
2. *Try to Pinpoint Your Eating Problems.* Check your eating speed. This may prove vital. Also check places where you ate, how you felt when you ate, and when.
3. *Make Eating a Pure Experience.* Learn to eat just for the joy of eating. Sit in the same place each time you eat and just eat. No television, no newspaper, nothing else. Eat more slowly by beginning after others or cutting your food into smaller pieces or putting down your fork after every third bite; for snacking problems, create an alternative set of activities at the time you usually snack, i.e., walking, hobbies.
4. *Reduce Temptations.* Make a shopping list and purchase only those things that are on your list. Snacking is much less likely if you have to spend fifteen to twenty minutes preparing the snack.

5. *Enlist Your Family's Support.* Explain your plans to them and ask for their moral support. Requesting that they have fewer snack foods around would also help.
6. *Cope with Emotions.* Don't eat when you get upset or angry; try jogging instead.
7. *Take It Slowly.* Aim at a gradual weight loss; keep a record, but don't starve yourself.
8. *Get More Exercise.* You are more likely to do this (jogging, calisthenics, etc.) if you have a partner to do it with.
9. *Special Situations.* If you are going to a wedding, party, or church social, eat something substantial before you leave the house, so that you won't arrive at the function hungry. To avoid temptation while you are there, dance a lot, engage in conversation. In short, keep yourself busy.[8]

These general rules apply to everyone, but authorities emphasize that habit changes should be individually worked out and applied. For example, some persons can easily eliminate all between-meal snacking, while others cannot.

The constant eater should be advised to satisfy his or her need with a handy, plentiful supply of high-bulk, low-calorie foods (celery, carrots, cucumber sticks, lettuce, raw cauliflower, radishes, green peppers, apples, fruit sticks, etc.). This person will not be very hungry at meal times and can round out meals with leafy salads to get a filled feeling without eating lots of high-calorie foods.

Research indicates that some persons, including children, are better off eating one large meal a day and skipping all others than taking small quantities of food at shorter intervals. These are people who need to feel gorged, and with careful planning they can satisfy this need and achieve and maintain normal weight and adequate nutrition.[9] A more comprehensive set of suggestions for altering habits to aid in weight loss can be found in Table 20-6.

Table 20-6. Changing Habits to Change Weight

Changing Eating Habits

Many of us overeat because we eat too fast. Satiety—the feeling of fullness—comes on slowly. Eating more slowly will give satiety a chance to catch up, and you will feel satisfied after eating less.

1. Eat in slow motion.
2. Sip your beverages—don't gulp.
3. After each mouthful, place your utensils on the plate until you have swallowed that mouthful.
4. Before your main meal, drink a low-calorie drink or a cup of boullion to help to take the edge off your appetite.
5. If invited out, eat a few low-calorie snacks before going.
6. Eat the salad before the rest of the meal.
7. Get in the habit of leaving at least two forkfuls of food on the plate at the end of the meal.
8. Eat foods that take time to eat—such as an orange that has to be peeled instead of an apple.
9. Put scraps of food directly in the garbage.

Other tricks to help:

1. If sweets must be kept around the house, put them in a seldom-used cupboard or in an unlikely place, e.g., broom closet, and let others get their own sweets.
2. When the meal is over, do not linger at the table unless all food has been cleared.
3. Make small portions of food appear larger on the plate by a) using smaller plates, and b) spreading your food on the plate.
4. Put your own portions on your plate—preferably in the kitchen.
5. Resist the temptation to eat what others have left when you are cleaning up after a meal.
6. If you envy something someone else is eating, take one small bit of it to satisfy yourself.
7. Reduce or eliminate use of salt at the table.

Changing Shopping Habits

There are other habits you can modify that will help you lose weight, such as your shopping habits.

1. Shop only from a prepared list, and stick to it.
2. Don't buy foods that later may be a problem to resist.
3. Shop after eating, or at least when you are not hungry.
4. Resist the free snacks offered at supermarkets.
5. Buy tuna fish that has been packed in water instead of oil.
6. Buy fruit that is fresh or canned without sugar.
7. Choose canned or frozen vegetables that are plain instead of those containing rich sauces; avoid using the frozen-in-butter vegetables that come in plastic pouches.
8. Don't trust a product's claim of being low-calorie. Compare the ingredients to those in the regular product—often there is only a minor difference!

Changing Cooking Habits

The way you prepare and serve food can also be modified to make your dieting easier.

1. Trim all fat from meat before cooking.
2. Broil meat that you normally would fry, even as a first step to stews and other dishes.
3. Broil, boil, or roast meat without added sauces, flour, or fat.
4. Marinate or baste poultry or meats, using a bottled low-calorie dressing. This also eliminates the need to use fat.
5. When broiling or baking fish, use lemon juice or boullion instead of butter.
6. Use lean meat in all recipes. When you buy ground beef, specify lean round or sirloin; these cuts are usually just as economical because they have no excess fat and so don't "shrink" when cooked.
7. Before cooking chicken, remove the skin and any loose fat.
8. Cook vegetables in a small amount of water with herbs or in boullion instead of with butter.
9. Use whipped butter or whipped margarine for spreads. The air or water they contain reduces the fat content and cuts their calories almost in half.

10. Learn which are the low- or no-calorie foods and serve them often in meals and for snacks. Some are green beans, green peppers, leeks, celery, cauliflower, carrots, water cress, zucchini, lettuce, and cucumbers.
11. Experiment with seasonings. Here are a few ideas: mint on carrots, basil on tomatoes, parsley or chives on boiled potatoes, Italian seasoning on green beans. Juicy lemon wedges, herb vinegar, pickle relish, soy and Worcestershire sauces and seasoned salt all add zip while adding few, if any, calories.
12. Go all out on garnishes, for they brighten any plate, taste good, and cost little in calories.

From *Slim Ideas,* a pamphlet by Riker Laboratories.

The Group Way to Lose Weight. Across the country, groups such as TOPS (Take Off Pounds Sensibly) and Weight Watchers have received great attention and are meeting with much success as weight reduction programs. TOPS, since its birth in 1948, has signed up a total of 350,000 members in the United States, and equally astounding numbers in other countries in the world. In one of the most successful TOPS groups, 62 percent of the members lost twenty pounds or more, compared with 10 percent in one of the least effective groups.[10]

Perhaps the reason behind so much success is that the members are working with other people who have the same problems. They look at each other as intelligent individuals striving to reach similar goals. Some groups are set up along the same lines as AA (Alcoholics Anonymous) and provide great moral support for members. In Table 20-7 is the creed used by one such group—Overeaters Anonymous.

Limitations of Behavior Therapy. Behavior modification techniques are useful for the majority of weight reduction patients but are not designed to treat or relieve underlying emotional causes of obesity. Approximately 10 percent of the obese population, frequently women, are classified as having the night-eating syndrome, which is characterized by morning anorexia, evening hyperphagia (increase in appetite), and insomnia. The heavy eating which occurs almost every night is seen as a response to stressful life situations. Although there is generally no self-condemnation, weight reduction is not successful without alleviation of the stress.[11]

Fewer than 5 percent of the obese population have the so-called binge-eating syndrome, which is characterized by sudden compulsive ingestion of large amounts of food in a very short period. This seems to be closely linked to some obviously frustrating experience. Self-condemnation usually follows these bouts. Although binge-eaters may be able to lose large amounts of weight on diets, the effort is usually interrupted by incredible feats of gluttony.[12] In cases such as these, behavior modification and other methods of weight reduction will not be of extended value until the underlying emotional conditions have been altered.

Exercise—The Forgotten Element

The benefits of exercise in weight reduction programs have been minimized in the past. Research shows that exercise is an essential part of appetite and weight control; a good weight reduction program includes regulation of energy output as well as calorie intake.

Table 20-7.

Table 1: The Twelve Steps

1. We admitted we were powerless over food—that our lives had become unmanageable.

2. Came to believe that a Power greater than ourselves could restore us to sanity.

3. Made a decision to turn our will and our lives over to the care of God *as we understood Him.*

4. Made a searching and fearless moral inventory of ourselves.

5. Admitted to God, to ourselves and to another human being the exact nature of our wrongs.

6. Were entirely ready to have God remove all these defects of character.

7. Humbly asked Him to remove our shortcomings.

8. Made a list of all persons we had harmed, and became willing to make amends to them all.

9. Made direct amends to such people wherever possible, except when to do so would injure them or others.

10. Continued to take personal inventory and when we were wrong, promptly admitted it.

11. Sought through prayer and meditation to improve our conscious contact with God *as we understood Him,* praying only for knowledge of His will for us and the power to carry that out.

12. Having had a spiritual awakening as the result of these steps, we tried to carry this message to compulsive overeaters and to practice these principles in all our affairs.

Table 2: The Twelve Traditions

1. Our common welfare should come first; personal recovery depends upon O.A. unity.

2. For our group purpose there is but one ultimate authority—a loving God as He may express Himself in our group conscience. Our leaders are but trusted servants; they do not govern.

3. The only requirement for O.A. membership is a desire to stop eating compulsively.

4. Each group should be autonomous except in matters affecting other groups or O.A. as a whole.

5. Each group has but one primary purpose—to carry its message to the compulsive overeater who still suffers.

6. An O.A. group ought never endorse, finance or lend the O.A. name to any related facility or outside enterprise, lest problems of money, property and prestige divert us from our primary purpose.

7. Every O.A. group ought to be fully self-supporting, declining outside contributions.

8. Overeaters Anonymous should remain forever non-professional, but our service centers may employ special workers.

9. O.A., as such, ought never be organized; but we may create service boards or committees directly responsible to those they serve.

10. Overeaters Anonymous has no opinion on outside issues; hence the O.A. name ought never be drawn into public controversy.

11. Our public relations policy is based on attraction rather than promotion; we need always maintain personal anonymity at the level of press, radio, films, television, and other public media of communication.

12. Anonymity is the spiritual foundation of all these traditions, ever reminding us to place principles before personalities.

From Linder, "Overeaters Anonymous—Report on a Self-Help Group," *Obesity/Bariatric Medicine,* Vol. 3, No. 4, 1974, pp. 135, 136.

Have you ever wondered why farmers keep their hogs, geese, and steers locked up in pens instead of allowing them to move about freely? One reason is to prevent the increase of connective tissue in the muscles of these animals (a result of exercise) which toughens the meat. But the main reason is so they won't walk off the valuable poundage.

By the same token, it is our increasingly inactive way of life that causes most of the extra weight in America today. Studies show that obese persons tend to be much more sedentary than their active skinny neighbors. Although it's difficult to work exercise into busy schedules, it is one of the best ways to remedy problems of obesity.

Physiological Advantages. In the normally active person, appetite is a precise regulatory device. Sedentary people, on the other hand, tend to overeat slightly and ingest more calories than they expend. Even a surplus of only 100 calories a day—an apple or serving of potato chips—will accumulate into ten pounds of fat a year.[13] Those 100 calories could be used up by walking twenty minutes a day. And if you consumed no extra calories but burned up an excess 100 calories a day, you would lose ten pounds in a year. Small, daily amounts of exercise consume an appreciable number of calories.

An active person tends to maintain a more stable weight than an inactive person. The energy expended in physical activity gets spent, whether you do it in five-minute bursts or three hours at a stretch. Since you've been gaining that excess fat bit by bit over a long period of time, it is not reasonable to expect to lose it overnight in one big lump. It is also true that it will take a thin person longer to use up calories than a fat one doing the same thing because the energy cost of moving the body is proportional to body weight.

It has been shown that an increase in energy is not automatically followed by an increase in food intake.[14] An already active person's appetite may increase slightly with activity, but a sedentary person can increase activity with no increase in appetite. On the other hand, when activity decreases, appetite does not automatically decrease. In fact, it often increases, and the result is fat accumulation. A study of more than two hundred overweight adults by G. Greene showed that the beginning of obesity could be traced directly to a sudden decrease in activity.[15]

Studies also show that weight loss in a reduction program involving diet alone is 75 percent from loss of fat tissue and 25 percent from loss of body fluids and lean body mass. Diet combined with an exercise program causes loss of 98 percent fat and only 2 percent lean body mass. Aside from weight loss, exercise contributes to better cardiovascular functioning and better health.

Psychological and Social Advantages. A variety of investigations of diet programs combined with exercise reported the following psychological factors in addition to the physiological changes:

1. Reduction in tension and stress levels.
2. More adequate sleep and rest.

3. Reduced desire to eat excessively.
4. Increased optimism about the future—particularly among post-cardiac patients.
5. Increased ability to concentrate.
6. Increased psychic energy level.
7. Better attitudes and performance at work.
8. Increased stamina and energy.
9. Greater interest in health related activities in general.
10. Improved self-concept and increased self-confidence.[16]

Exercise Caution. Any overused or misdirected exercise program can be harmful to mental and physical health. Sudden strenuous exercise or exercise on an irregular basis is not the prescription. A regular, lifetime exercise program designed to fit your individual capacity and need is important, just as a long-lasting change in nutritional habits is necessary in order to reduce weight permanently. To avoid a physical overload due to misinformation or overenthusiasm at the outset of an exercise program, consult your physician for a complete physical examination, including an electrocardiogram during rest and physical exertion. You should also have a supervised activity stress test to determine starting and target intensities of exercise. An out-of-condition adult can stand to expend from 500 to 600 calories at the start without discomfort. As the heart and muscle become conditioned, strenuous activity can be increased.

Although the advantages of exercise in connection with weight control have been clearly established, individuals suffering from any of the following conditions may have to forgo vigorous activity: severe (80 to 90 percent) **stenosis** (narrowing) of the three main coronary arteries, progressive angina, impending infarction, certain arrhythmias, valvular diseases, uncontrolled hypertension, acute myocarditus, uncontrolled diabetes mellitus, severe pulmonary hypertension, severe electrolyte imbalance, severe varicose veins, anemia, and other serious health problems. A physician should make this determination.

SUMMARY

The goal of an effective weight loss regimen is not merely to prescribe a diet. Weight control requires a lifelong commitment, an understanding of one's eating habits, and a willingness to change them. Moderate, frequent exercise is necessary, and accomplishment must be reinforced to sustain motivation.

Beginning and maintaining a weight control program requires support and encouragement from many sources. The physician who manages the program should not merely lecture the patient or hand out a standard diet but should be willing to give the patient the time and guidance he or she would offer to a diabetic patient or someone with another chronic condition.

Most physicians recommend a weight loss of one to two pounds a week, unless there is a specific reason the physician wants a patient to lose more rapidly. Fast loss usually means a person resorts to a "crash" or fad diet. These can be hazardous to health if they do not provide a proper balance of nutrients.

A good diet provides all of the nutrients needed for good health but restricts calories. The diet should be within the framework of normal eating habits and should teach the dieter good nutritional habits that will permit continuous weight maintenance.

The basic premise behind dieting is to eliminate a certain number of calories that are not really needed to perform daily activites. A diet, to be beneficial, must be practical and suited to the needs of the dieter. In other words, it must be livable by the person who wants to lose weight.

To plan a reducing diet that is best for you, you must take into account your desirable body weight and how much of a calorie deficit will produce a slow but steady weight loss. You must at the same time ensure an adequate intake of essential nutrients and adjust for your particular eating patterns. Finally, you must plan for maintenance of the desired weight when it is reached.

Behavior therapy is commonly used to encourage weight control and weight loss. Many times, obesity has been produced by a lifetime of poor eating habits. Behavior therapy is aimed at changing the habits and lifestyle that produced obesity. Keeping track of those foods eaten, pinpointing eating problems, making eating a pure experience (unenhanced by any other stimuli), curbing bad eating habits, reducing temptations, gaining support from other family members, learning to cope with emotions, losing weight slowly, exercising more, and learning to cope with eating in special situations (such as weddings and church socials) are techniques commonly used in behavior therapy to modify eating habits.

Proper exercise should accompany any weight loss program to increase energy output and to tone tissues and muscles. A sound weight reduction program should carefully evaluate patients for physical and emotional resources, establish a safe and workable weight reduction program incorporating diet and exercise, and modify eating habits so that weight loss can be maintained for a lifetime. A program that fails to do this is inadequate.

NOTES

1. E. R. Monsen, "Helping Patients Use Foods Effectively in Weight Control," *Medical Digest,* May 1976, pp. 11-5.
2. "Doctors' Methods of Reducing Weight," *Medical World News,* September 5, 1977, p. 34.
3. "The Endless Fight Against Fat," *Current Prescribing,* March 1976, pp. 49-60.
4. "Kitchen Power for Weight Control," *The Health Letter,* Vol. 9, No. 12, June 24, 1977.
5. "Morbid Obesity—Long-Term Results of Therapeutic Fasting," *Nutrition Reviews,* Vol. 36, No. 1, January 1978, pp. 6-7.
6. Lyn Howard, "Obesity: A Feasible Approach to a Formidable Problem," *American Family Physician,* Vol. 12, No. 3, September 1975, p. 153.
7. John Kelly, "Who Controls Your Eating Habits," *Family Health,* Vol. 5, April 1973, pp. 36-37.
8. Excerpts from "Who Controls Your Eating Habits," by John Kelly, *Family Health Magazine,* April 1973, pp. 36-37. Reprinted with permission of *Family Health Magazine,* April 1973 ©. All rights reserved.

9. A. David and Doris F. Jonas, "Obesity: Separating the Herbivores from the Carnivores," *Modern Medicine,* May 15, 1976, p. 84.

10. Albert J. Stunkard, "The Success of TOPS, A Self-Help Group," *Postgraduate Medicine,* Vol. 51, May 1972, pp. 143-147.

11. Donald D. Gold, "Psychologic Factors Associated with Obesity," *American Family Physician,* Vol. 13, No. 6, June 1976, p. 6.

12. Ibid.

13. "Fighting Obesity: Developments You May Have Overlooked," *Current Prescribing,* January 1978, pp. 103-104, 106.

14. "Morbid Obesity—Long-Term Results of Therapeutic Fasting," pp. 6-7.

15. Ibid.

16. Harold Hopkins, "Controlling Diet Food Claims," *FDA Consumer,* October 1977, p. 16.

APPENDIXES

APPENDIX A

Nutritive Values of the Edible Parts of Foods

The following tables are from the United States Department of Agriculture, Home and Gardens Bulletin No. 72.

NUTRITIVE VALUES OF THE EDIBLE PART OF FOODS

(Dashes (—) denote lack of reliable data for a constituent believed to be present in measurable amount)

NUTRIENTS IN INDICATED QUANTITY

DAIRY PRODUCTS (CHEESE, CREAM, IMITATION CREAM, MILK; RELATED PRODUCTS)

Butter. See Fats, oils; related products, items 103-108.

Item No. (A)	Foods, approximate measure, units, and weight (edible part unless footnotes indicate otherwise) (B)	Grams	Water (C) Per cent	Food energy (D) Calories	Protein (E) Grams	Fat (F) Grams	Fatty Acids Saturated (total) (G) Grams	Unsaturated Oleic (H) Grams	Unsaturated Linoleic (I) Grams	Carbo-hydrate (J) Grams	Calcium (K) Milligrams	Phos-phorus (L) Milligrams	Iron (M) Milligrams	Potas-sium (N) Milligrams	Vitamin A value (O) International units	Thiamin (P) Milligrams	Ribo-flavin (Q) Milligrams	Niacin (R) Milligrams	Ascorbic acid (S) Milligrams
	Cheese:																		
	Natural:																		
1	Blue — 1 oz	28	42	100	6	8	5.3	1.9	0.2	1	150	110	0.1	73	200	0.01	0.11	0.3	0
2	Camembert (3 wedges per 4-oz container) — 1 wedge	38	52	115	8	9	5.8	2.2	.2	1	147	132	.1	71	350	.01	.19	.2	0
	Cheddar:																		
3	Cut pieces — 1 oz	28	37	115	7	9	6.1	2.1	.2	Trace	204	145	.2	28	300	.01	.11	Trace	0
4	1 cu in	17.2	37	70	4	6	3.7	1.3	.1	Trace	124	88	.1	17	180	Trace	.06	Trace	0
5	Shredded — 1 cup	113	37	455	28	37	24.2	8.5	.7	1	815	579	.8	111	1,200	.03	.42	.1	0
	Cottage (curd not pressed down):																		
	Creamed (cottage cheese, 4% fat):																		
6	Large curd — 1 cup	225	79	235	28	10	6.4	2.4	.2	6	135	297	.3	190	370	.05	.37	.3	Trace
7	Small curd — 1 cup	210	79	220	26	9	6.0	2.2	.2	6	126	277	.3	177	340	.04	.34	.3	Trace
8	Low fat (2%) — 1 cup	226	79	205	31	4	2.8	1.0	.1	8	155	340	.4	217	160	.05	.42	.3	Trace
9	Low fat (1%) — 1 cup	226	82	165	28	2	1.5	.5	.1	6	138	302	.3	193	80	.05	.37	.3	Trace
10	Uncreamed (cottage cheese dry curd, less than 1/2% fat) — 1 cup	145	80	125	25	1	.4	.1	Trace	3	46	151	.3	47	40	.04	.21	.2	0
11	Cream — 1 oz	28	54	100	2	10	6.2	2.4	.2	1	23	30	.3	34	400	Trace	.06	Trace	0
	Mozzarella, made with—																		
12	Whole milk — 1 oz	28	48	90	6	7	4.4	1.7	.2	1	163	117	.1	21	260	Trace	.08	Trace	0
13	Part skim milk — 1 oz	28	49	80	8	5	3.1	1.2	.1	1	207	149	.1	27	180	.01	.10	Trace	0
	Parmesan, grated:																		
14	Cup, not pressed down — 1 cup	100	18	455	42	30	19.1	7.7	.3	4	1,376	807	1.0	107	700	.05	.39	.3	0
15	Tablespoon — 1 tbsp	5	18	25	2	2	1.0	.4	Trace	Trace	69	40	Trace	5	40	Trace	.02	Trace	0
16	Ounce — 1 oz	28	18	130	12	9	5.4	2.2	.1	1	390	229	.3	30	200	.01	.11	.1	0
17	Provolone — 1 oz	28	41	100	7	8	4.8	1.7	.1	1	214	141	.1	39	230	.01	.09	Trace	0
	Ricotta, made with—																		
18	Whole milk — 1 cup	246	72	428	28	32	20.4	7.1	.7	7	509	389	.9	257	1,210	.03	.48	.3	0
19	Part skim milk — 1 cup	246	74	340	28	19	12.1	4.7	.5	13	669	449	1.1	308	1,060	.05	.46	.2	0
20	Romano — 1 oz	28	31	110	9	8	—	—	—	1	302	215	—	—	160	—	.11	—	0
21	Swiss — 1 oz	28	37	105	8	8	5.0	1.7	.2	1	272	171	Trace	31	240	.01	.10	Trace	0
	Pasteurized process cheese:																		
22	American — 1 oz	28	39	105	6	9	5.6	2.1	.2	Trace	174	211	.1	46	340	.01	.10	Trace	0
23	Swiss — 1 oz	28	42	95	7	7	4.5	1.7	.1	1	219	216	.2	61	230	Trace	.08	Trace	0
24	Pasteurized process cheese food, American — 1 oz	28	43	95	6	7	4.4	1.7	.1	2	163	130	.2	79	260	.01	.13	Trace	0
25	Pasteurized process cheese spread, American — 1 oz	28	48	82	5	6	3.8	1.5	.1	2	159	202	.1	69	220	.01	.12	Trace	0
	Cream, sweet:																		
26	Half-and-half (cream and milk) — 1 cup	242	81	315	7	28	17.3	7.0	.6	10	254	230	.2	314	260	.08	.36	.2	2
27	1 tbsp	15	81	20	Trace	2	1.1	.4	Trace	1	16	14	Trace	19	20	.01	.02	Trace	Trace
28	Light, coffee, or table — 1 cup	240	74	470	6	46	28.8	11.7	1.0	9	231	192	.1	292	1,730	.08	.36	.1	2
29	1 tbsp	15	74	30	Trace	3	1.8	.7	.1	1	14	12	Trace	18	110	Trace	.02	Trace	Trace

(A)	(B) Foods, approximate measures, units, and weight	Grams	(C) Water %	(D) Food energy (cal)	(E) Protein (g)	(F) Fat (g)	(G) Saturated fatty acids (g)	(H) Oleic (g)	(I) Linoleic (g)	(J) Carbohydrate (g)	(K) Calcium (mg)	(L) Phosphorus (mg)	(M) Iron (mg)	(N) Potassium (mg)	(O) Vitamin A (IU)	(P) Thiamin (mg)	(Q) Riboflavin (mg)	(R) Niacin (mg)	(S) Ascorbic acid (mg)
	Whipping, unwhipped (volume about double when whipped):																		
30	Light—— 1 cup	239	64	700	5	74	46.2	18.3	1.5	7	166	146	0.1	231	2,690	0.06	0.30	0.1	1
31	1 tbsp	15	64	45	Trace	5	2.9	1.1	.1	Trace	10	9	Trace	15	170	Trace	.02	Trace	Trace
32	Heavy—— 1 cup	238	58	820	5	88	54.8	22.2	2.0	7	154	149	.1	179	3,500	.05	.26	.1	1
33	1 tbsp	15	58	80	Trace	6	3.5	1.4	.1	Trace	10	9	Trace	11	220	Trace	.02	Trace	Trace
34	Whipped topping, (pressurized)—— 1 cup	60	61	155	2	13	8.3	3.4	.3	7	61	54	Trace	88	550	.02	.04	Trace	0
35	1 tbsp	3	61	10	Trace	1	.4	.2	Trace	Trace	3	3	Trace	4	30	Trace	Trace	Trace	0
36	Cream, sour—— 1 cup	230	71	495	7	48	30.0	12.1	1.1	10	268	195	.1	331	1,820	.08	.34	.2	2
37	1 tbsp	12	71	25	Trace	3	1.6	.6	.1	1	14	10	Trace	17	90	Trace	.02	Trace	Trace
	Cream products, imitation (made with vegetable fat):																		
	Sweet:																		
	Creamers:																		
38	Liquid (frozen)—— 1 cup	245	77	335	2	24	22.8	.3	Trace	28	23	157	.1	467	[1]220	0	0	0	0
39	1 tbsp	15	77	20	Trace	1	1.4	Trace	0	2	1	10	Trace	29	[1]10	0	0	0	0
40	Powdered—— 1 cup	94	2	515	5	33	30.6	.9	.4	52	21	397	Trace	763	[1]190	0	.16	0	0
41	1 tsp	2	2	10	Trace	1	.7	Trace	0	1	Trace	8	Trace	16	[1]Trace	0	Trace	0	0
	Whipped topping:																		
42	Frozen—— 1 cup	75	50	240	1	19	16.3	1.0	.2	17	5	6	.1	14	[1]650	0	0	0	0
43	1 tbsp	4	50	15	Trace	1	.9	.1	Trace	1	Trace	Trace	Trace	1	[1]30	0	0	0	0
44	Powdered, made with whole milk.—— 1 cup	80	67	150	3	10	8.5	.6	.1	13	72	69	Trace	121	[1]290	.02	.09	Trace	1
45	1 tbsp	4	67	10	Trace	1	.4	Trace	Trace	1	4	3	Trace	6	[1]110	Trace	Trace	0	0
46	Pressurized—— 1 cup	70	60	185	1	16	13.2	1.4	.2	11	4	13	Trace	13	[1]330	Trace	Trace	0	0
47	1 tbsp	4	60	10	Trace	1	.8	.1	Trace	1	Trace	1	Trace	1	[1]120	Trace	Trace	0	0
48	Sour dressing (imitation sour cream) made with nonfat dry milk.—— 1 cup	235	75	415	8	39	31.2	4.4	1.1	11	266	205	.1	380	[1]120	.09	.38	.2	2
49	1 tbsp	12	75	20	Trace	2	1.6	.2	.1	1	14	10	Trace	19	[1]Trace	.01	.02	Trace	Trace
	Ice cream. See Milk desserts, frozen (items 75-80).																		
	Ice milk. See Milk desserts, frozen (items 81-83).																		
	Milk:																		
	Fluid:																		
50	Whole (3.3% fat)—— 1 cup	244	88	150	8	8	5.1	2.1	.2	11	291	228	.1	370	[2]310	.09	.40	.2	2
	Lowfat (2%):																		
51	No milk solids added—— 1 cup	244	89	120	8	5	2.9	1.2	.1	12	297	232	.1	377	500	.10	.40	.2	2
	Milk solids added:																		
52	Label claim less than 10 g of protein per cup.—— 1 cup	245	89	125	9	5	2.9	1.2	.1	12	313	245	.1	397	500	.10	.42	.2	2
53	Label claim 10 or more grams of protein per cup (protein fortified).—— 1 cup	246	88	135	10	5	3.0	1.2	.1	14	352	276	.1	447	500	.11	.48	.2	3
	Lowfat (1%):																		
54	No milk solids added—— 1 cup	244	90	100	8	3	1.6	.7	.1	12	300	235	.1	381	500	.10	.41	.2	2
	Milk solids added:																		
55	Label claim less than 10 g of protein per cup.—— 1 cup	245	90	105	9	2	1.5	.6	.1	12	313	245	.1	397	500	.10	.42	.2	2
56	Label claim 10 or more grams of protein per cup (protein fortified).—— 1 cup	246	89	120	10	3	1.8	.7	.1	14	349	273	.1	444	500	.11	.47	.2	3
	Nonfat (skim):																		
57	No milk solids added—— 1 cup	245	91	85	8	Trace	.3	.1	Trace	12	302	247	.1	406	500	.09	.37	.2	2

[1] Vitamin A value is largely from beta-carotene used for coloring. Riboflavin value for items 40-41 apply to products with added riboflavin.

[2] Applies to product without added vitamin A. With added vitamin A, value is 500 International Units (I.U.).

(Dashes (—) denote lack of reliable data for a constituent believed to be present in measurable amount)

Item No.	Foods, approximate measures, units, and weight (edible part unless footnotes indicate otherwise)		Water	Food energy	Protein	Fat	Fatty Acids Saturated (total)	Unsaturated Oleic	Unsaturated Linoleic	Carbo-hydrate	Calcium	Phos-phorus	Iron	Potas-sium	Vitamin A value	Thiamin	Ribo-flavin	Niacin	Ascorbic acid
(A)	(B)	Grams	(C) Per cent	(D) Cal-ories	(E) Grams	(F) Grams	(G) Grams	(H) Grams	(I) Grams	(J) Grams	(K) Milli-grams	(L) Milli-grams	(M) Milli-grams	(N) Milli-grams	(O) Inter-national units	(P) Milli-grams	(Q) Milli-grams	(R) Milli-grams	(S) Milli-grams
	DAIRY PRODUCTS (CHEESE, CREAM, IMITATION CREAM, MILK; RELATED PRODUCTS)—Con.																		
	Milk—Continued																		
	Fluid—Continued																		
	Nonfat (skim)—Continued																		
	Milk solids added:																		
58	Label claim less than 10 g of protein per cup. 1 cup	245	90	90	9	1	0.4	0.1	Trace	12	316	255	0.1	416	500	0.10	0.43	0.2	2
59	Label claim 10 or more grams of protein per cup (protein forti-fied). 1 cup	246	89	100	10	1	.4	.1	Trace	14	352	275	.1	446	500	.11	.48	.2	3
60	Buttermilk. 1 cup	245	90	100	8	2	1.3	.5	Trace	12	285	219	.1	371	[3]80	.08	.38	.1	2
	Canned:																		
	Evaporated, unsweetened:																		
61	Whole milk. 1 cup	252	74	340	17	19	11.6	5.3	.4	25	657	510	.5	764	[4]610	.12	.80	.5	5
62	Skim milk. 1 cup	255	79	200	19	1	.3	.3	Trace	29	738	497	.7	845	[4]1,000	.11	.79	.4	3
63	Sweetened, condensed. 1 cup	306	27	980	24	27	16.8	6.7	.7	166	868	775	.6	1,136	[3]1,000	.28	1.27	.6	8
	Dried:																		
64	Buttermilk. 1 cup	120	3	465	41	7	4.3	1.7	.2	59	1,421	1,119	.4	1,910	[3]260	.47	1.90	1.1	7
	Nonfat instant:																		
65	Envelope, net wt., 3.2 oz[5]. 1 envelope	91	4	325	32	1	.4	.1	Trace	47	1,120	896	.3	1,552	[6]2,160	.38	1.59	.8	5
66	Cup[7]. 1 cup	68	4	245	24	Trace	.3	.1	Trace	35	837	670	.2	1,160	[6]1,610	.28	1.19	.6	4
	Milk beverages:																		
	Chocolate milk (commercial):																		
67	Regular. 1 cup	250	82	210	8	8	5.3	2.2	.2	26	280	251	.6	417	[3]300	.09	.41	.3	2
68	Lowfat (2%). 1 cup	250	84	180	8	5	3.1	1.3	.1	26	284	254	.6	422	500	.10	.42	.3	2
69	Lowfat (1%). 1 cup	250	85	160	8	3	1.5	.7	.1	26	287	257	.6	426	500	.10	.40	.2	2
70	Eggnog (commercial). 1 cup	254	74	340	10	19	11.3	5.0	.6	34	330	278	.5	420	890	.09	.48	.3	4
	Malted milk, home-prepared with 1 cup of whole milk and 2 to 3 heaping tsp of malted milk powder (about 3/4 oz):																		
71	Chocolate. 1 cup of milk plus 3/4 oz of powder.	265	81	235	9	9	5.5	—	—	29	304	265	.5	500	330	.14	.43	.7	2
72	Natural. 1 cup of milk plus 3/4 oz of powder.	265	81	235	11	10	6.0	—	—	27	347	307	.3	529	380	.20	.54	1.3	2
	Shakes, thick:[8]																		
73	Chocolate, container, net wt. 10.6 oz. 1 container	300	72	355	9	8	5.0	2.0	.2	63	396	378	.9	672	260	.14	.67	.4	0
74	Vanilla, container, net wt., 11 oz. 1 container	313	74	350	12	9	5.9	2.4	.2	56	457	361	.3	572	360	.09	.61	.5	0
	Milk desserts, frozen:																		
	Ice cream:																		
	Regular (about 11% fat):																		
75	Hardened. 1/2 gal	1,064	61	2,155	38	115	71.3	28.8	2.6	254	1,406	1,075	1.0	2,052	4,340	.42	2.63	1.1	6
76	1 cup	133	61	270	5	14	8.9	3.6	.3	32	176	134	.1	257	540	.05	.33	.1	1
77	3-fl oz container	50	61	100	2	5	3.4	1.4	.1	12	66	51	Trace	96	200	.02	.12	.1	Trace
78	Soft serve (frozen custard). 1 cup	173	60	375	7	23	13.5	5.9	.6	38	236	199	.4	338	790	.08	.45	.2	1
79	Rich (about 16% fat), hardened. 1/2 gal	1,188	59	2,805	33	190	118.3	47.8	4.3	256	1,213	927	.8	1,771	7,200	.36	2.27	.9	5
80	1 cup	148	59	350	4	24	14.7	6.0	.5	32	151	115	.1	221	900	.04	.28	.1	1
	Ice milk:																		
81	Hardened (about 4.3% fat). 1/2 gal	1,048	69	1,470	41	45	28.1	11.3	1.0	232	1,409	1,035	1.5	2,117	1,710	.61	2.78	.9	6
82	1 cup	131	69	185	5	6	3.5	1.4	.1	29	176	129	.1	265	210	.08	.35	.1	1

(A)	(B)	Weight (g)	(C)	(D)	(E)	(F)	(G)	(H)	(I)	(J)	(K)	(L)	(M)	(N)	(O)	(P)	(Q)	(R)	(S)
83	Soft serve (about 2.6% fat)—1 cup	175	70	225	8	5	2.9	1.2	0.1	38	274	202	0.3	412	180	0.12	0.54	0.2	1
84	Sherbet (about 2% fat)—1/2 gal	1,542	66	2,160	17	31	19.0	7.7	.7	469	827	594	2.5	1,585	1,480	.26	.71	1.0	31
85	—1 cup	193	66	270	2	4	2.4	1.0	.1	59	103	74	.3	198	190	.03	.09	.1	4
	Milk desserts, other: From home recipe:																		
86	Custard, baked—1 cup	265	77	305	14	15	6.8	5.4	.7	29	297	310	1.1	387	930	.11	.50	.3	1
	Puddings: From home recipe: Starch base:																			
87	Chocolate—1 cup	260	66	385	8	12	7.6	3.3	.3	67	250	255	1.3	445	390	.05	.36	.3	1
88	Vanilla (blancmange)—1 cup	255	76	285	9	10	6.2	2.5	.2	41	298	232	Trace	352	410	.08	.41	.3	2
89	Tapioca cream—1 cup	165	72	220	8	8	4.1	2.5	.5	28	173	180	.7	223	480	.07	.30	.2	2
	From mix (chocolate) and milk:																			
90	Regular (cooked)—1 cup	260	70	320	9	8	4.3	2.6	.2	59	265	247	.8	354	340	.05	.39	.3	2
91	Instant—1 cup	260	69	325	8	7	3.6	2.2	.3	63	374	237	1.3	335	340	.08	.39	.3	2
	Yogurt: With added milk solids: Made with lowfat milk:																			
92	Fruit-flavored[9]—1 container, net wt., 8 oz	227	75	230	10	3	1.8	.6	.1	42	343	269	.2	439	[10]120	.08	.40	.2	1
93	Plain—1 container, net wt., 8 oz	227	85	145	12	4	2.3	.8	.1	16	415	326	.2	531	[10]150	.10	.49	.3	2
94	Made with nonfat milk—1 container, net wt., 8 oz	227	85	125	13	Trace	.3	.1	Trace	17	452	355	.2	579	[10]20	.11	.53	.3	2
	Without added milk solids:																			
95	Made with whole milk—1 container, net wt., 8 oz	227	88	140	8	7	4.8	1.7	.1	11	274	215	.1	351	280	.07	.32	.2	1
	EGGS																			
	Eggs, large (24 oz per dozen): Raw:																			
96	Whole, without shell—1 egg	50	75	80	6	6	1.7	2.0	.6	1	28	90	1.0	65	260	.04	.15	Trace	0
97	White—1 white	33	88	15	3	Trace	0	0	0	Trace	4	4	Trace	45	0	Trace	.09	Trace	0
98	Yolk—1 yolk	17	49	65	3	6	1.7	2.1	.6	Trace	26	86	.9	15	310	.04	.07	Trace	0
	Cooked:																			
99	Fried in butter—1 egg	46	72	85	5	6	2.4	2.2	.6	1	26	80	.9	58	290	.03	.13	Trace	0
100	Hard-cooked, shell removed—1 egg	50	75	80	6	6	1.7	2.0	.6	1	28	90	1.0	65	260	.04	.14	Trace	0
101	Poached—1 egg	50	74	80	6	6	1.7	2.0	.6	1	28	90	1.0	65	260	.04	.13	Trace	0
102	Scrambled (milk added) in butter. Also omelet.—1 egg	64	76	95	6	7	2.8	2.3	.6	1	47	97	.9	85	310	.04	.16	Trace	0
	FATS, OILS; RELATED PRODUCTS																			
	Butter: Regular (1 brick or 4 sticks per lb):																			
103	Stick (1/2 cup)—1 stick	113	16	815	1	92	57.3	23.1	2.1	Trace	27	26	.2	29	[13]3,470	.01	.04	Trace	0
104	Tablespoon (about 1/8 stick)—1 tbsp	14	16	100	Trace	12	7.2	2.9	.3	Trace	3	3	Trace	4	[14]430	Trace	Trace	Trace	0
105	Pat (1 in square, 1/3 in high; 90 per lb)—1 pat	5	16	35	Trace	4	2.5	1.0	.1	Trace	1	1	Trace	1	[11]150	Trace	Trace	Trace	0
	Whipped (6 sticks or two 8-oz containers per lb):																			
106	Stick (1/2 cup)—1 stick	76	16	540	1	61	38.2	15.4	1.4	Trace	18	17	.1	20	[12]2,310	Trace	.03	Trace	0
107	Tablespoon (about 1/8 stick)—1 tbsp	9	16	65	Trace	8	4.7	1.9	.2	Trace	2	2	Trace	2	[13]290	Trace	Trace	Trace	0
108	Pat (1 1/4 in square, 1/3 in high; 120 per lb)—1 pat	4	16	25	Trace	4	1.9	.8	.1	Trace	1	1	Trace	1	[11]120	0	Trace	Trace	0

[3]Applies to product without vitamin A added.
[4]Applies to product with added vitamin A. Without added vitamin A, value is 20 International Units (I.U.).
[5]Yields 1 qt of fluid milk when reconstituted according to package directions.
[6]Applies to product with added vitamin A.
[7]Weight applies to product with label claim of 1 1/3 cups equal 3.2 oz.
[8]Applies to products made from thick shake mixes and that do not contain added ice cream. Products made from milk shake mixes are higher in fat and usually contain added ice cream.
[9]Content of fat, vitamin A, and carbohydrate varies. Consult the label when precise values are needed for special diets.
[10]Applies to product made with milk containing no added vitamin A.
[11]Applies to product made with whole milk containing no added vitamin A.
[11]Based on year-round average.

NUTRITIVE VALUES OF THE EDIBLE PART OF FOODS - Continued

(Dashes (—) denote lack of reliable data for a constituent believed to be present in measurable amount)

Item No. (A)	Foods, approximate measures, units, and weight (edible part unless footnotes indicate otherwise) (B)	Grams	Water (C) Percent	Food energy (D) Calories	Protein (E) Grams	Fat (F) Grams	Fatty Acids Saturated (total) (G) Grams	Unsaturated Oleic (H) Grams	Unsaturated Linoleic (I) Grams	Carbohydrate (J) Grams	Calcium (K) Milligrams	Phosphorus (L) Milligrams	Iron (M) Milligrams	Potassium (N) Milligrams	Vitamin A value (O) International units	Thiamin (P) Milligrams	Riboflavin (Q) Milligrams	Niacin (R) Milligrams	Ascorbic acid (S) Milligrams
	FATS, OILS; RELATED PRODUCTS—Con.																		
109	Fats, cooking (vegetable shortenings). 1 cup	200	0	1,770	0	200	48.8	88.2	48.4	0	0	0	0	0	—	0	0	0	0
110	1 tbsp	13	0	110	0	13	3.2	5.7	3.1	0	0	0	0	0	—	0	0	0	0
111	Lard 1 cup	205	0	1,850	0	205	81.0	83.8	20.5	0	0	0	0	0	0	0	0	0	0
112	1 tbsp	13	0	115	0	13	5.1	5.3	1.3	0	0	0	0	0	0	0	0	0	0
	Margarine: Regular (1 brick or 4 sticks per lb):																		
113	Stick (1/2 cup) 1 stick	113	16	815	1	92	16.7	42.9	24.9	Trace	27	26	.2	29	[12]3,750	.01	.04	Trace	0
114	Tablespoon (about 1/8 stick) 1 tbsp	14	16	100	Trace	12	2.1	5.3	3.1	Trace	3	3	Trace	4	[12]470	Trace	Trace	Trace	0
115	Pat (1 in square, 1/3 in high; 90 per lb). 1 pat	5	16	35	Trace	4	.7	1.9	1.1	Trace	1	1	Trace	1	[12]170	Trace	Trace	Trace	0
116	Soft, two 8-oz containers per lb. 1 container	227	16	1,635	1	184	32.5	71.5	65.4	Trace	53	52	.4	59	[12]7,500	.01	.08	.1	0
117	1 tbsp	14	16	100	Trace	12	2.0	4.5	4.1	Trace	3	3	Trace	4	[12]470	Trace	Trace	Trace	0
	Whipped (6 sticks per lb):																		
118	Stick (1/2 cup) 1 stick	76	16	545	Trace	61	11.2	28.7	16.7	Trace	18	17	.1	20	[12]2,500	Trace	.03	Trace	0
119	Tablespoon (about 1/8 stick) 1 tbsp	9	16	70	Trace	8	1.4	3.6	2.1	Trace	2	2	Trace	2	[12]310	Trace	Trace	Trace	0
	Oils, salad or cooking:																		
120	Corn 1 cup	218	0	1,925	0	218	27.7	53.6	125.1	0	0	0	0	0	—	0	0	0	0
121	1 tbsp	14	0	120	0	14	1.7	3.3	7.8	0	0	0	0	0	—	0	0	0	0
122	Olive 1 cup	216	0	1,910	0	216	30.7	154.4	17.7	0	0	0	0	0	—	0	0	0	0
123	1 tbsp	14	0	120	0	14	1.9	9.7	1.1	0	0	0	0	0	—	0	0	0	0
124	Peanut 1 cup	216	0	1,910	0	216	37.4	98.5	67.0	0	0	0	0	0	—	0	0	0	0
125	1 tbsp	14	0	120	0	14	2.3	6.2	4.2	0	0	0	0	0	—	0	0	0	0
126	Safflower 1 cup	218	0	1,925	0	218	20.5	25.9	159.8	0	0	0	0	0	—	0	0	0	0
127	1 tbsp	14	0	120	0	14	1.3	1.6	10.0	0	0	0	0	0	—	0	0	0	0
128	Soybean oil, hydrogenated (partially hardened). 1 cup	218	0	1,925	0	218	31.8	93.1	75.6	0	0	0	0	0	—	0	0	0	0
129	1 tbsp	14	0	120	0	14	2.0	5.8	4.7	0	0	0	0	0	—	0	0	0	0
130	Soybean-cottonseed oil blend, hydrogenated. 1 cup	218	0	1,925	0	218	38.2	63.0	99.6	0	0	0	0	0	—	0	0	0	0
131	1 tbsp	14	0	120	0	14	2.4	3.9	6.2	0	0	0	0	0	—	0	0	0	0
	Salad dressings: Commercial: Blue cheese:																		
132	Regular 1 tbsp	15	32	75	1	8	1.6	1.7	3.8	1	12	11	Trace	6	30	Trace	.02	Trace	Trace
133	Low calorie (5 Cal per tsp) 1 tbsp	16	84	10	Trace	1	.5	.3	Trace	1	10	8	Trace	5	30	Trace	.01	Trace	Trace
	French:																		
134	Regular 1 tbsp	16	39	65	Trace	6	1.1	1.3	3.2	3	2	2	.1	13	—	—	—	—	—
135	Low calorie (5 Cal per tsp) 1 tbsp	16	77	15	Trace	1	.1	.1	.4	2	2	2	.1	13	—	—	—	—	—
	Italian:																		
136	Regular 1 tbsp	15	28	85	Trace	9	1.6	1.9	4.7	1	2	1	Trace	2	Trace	Trace	Trace	Trace	—
137	Low calorie (2 Cal per tsp) 1 tbsp	15	90	10	Trace	1	.1	.1	.4	Trace	2	1	Trace	2	Trace	Trace	Trace	Trace	—
138	Mayonnaise 1 tbsp	14	15	100	Trace	11	2.0	2.4	5.6	Trace	3	4	.1	5	40	Trace	.01	Trace	—
	Mayonnaise type:																		
139	Regular 1 tbsp	15	41	65	Trace	6	1.1	1.4	3.2	2	2	4	Trace	1	30	Trace	Trace	Trace	—
140	Low calorie (8 Cal per tsp) 1 tbsp	16	81	20	Trace	2	.4	.4	1.0	2	3	4	Trace	1	40	Trace	Trace	Trace	—
141	Tartar sauce, regular 1 tbsp	14	34	75	Trace	8	1.5	1.8	4.1	1	3	4	.1	11	30	Trace	Trace	Trace	Trace
	Thousand Island:																		
142	Regular 1 tbsp	16	32	80	Trace	8	1.4	1.7	4.0	2	2	3	.1	18	50	Trace	Trace	Trace	Trace
143	Low calorie (10 Cal per tsp) 1 tbsp	15	68	25	Trace	2	.4	.4	1.0	2	2	3	.1	17	50	Trace	Trace	Trace	Trace
	From home recipe:																		
144	Cooked type [13] 1 tbsp	16	68	25	1	2	.5	.6	.3	2	14	15	.1	19	80	.01	.03	Trace	Trace

FISH, SHELLFISH, MEAT, POULTRY; RELATED PRODUCTS

(A)	(B)	(C)	(D)	(E)	(F)	(G)	(H)	(I)	(J)	(K)	(L)	(M)	(N)	(O)	(P)	(Q)	(R)	(S)
	Fish and shellfish:																	
145	Bluefish, baked with butter or margarine. 3 oz — 85	68	135	22	4	—	—	—	0	25	244	0.6	—	40[12]	.09	.08	1.6	—
	Clams:																	
146	Raw, meat only. 3 oz — 85	82	65	11	1	0.2	Trace	Trace	2	59	138	5.2	154	90	.08	.15	1.1	8
147	Canned, solids and liquid. 3 oz — 85	86	45	7	1	—	—	—	2	47	116	3.5	119	—	.01	.09	.9	—
148	Crabmeat (white or king), canned, not pressed down. 1 cup — 135	77	135	24	3	.6	.4	.1	1	61	246	1.1	149	—	.11	.11	2.6	—
149	Fish sticks, breaded, cooked, frozen (stick, 4 by 1 by 1/2 in). 1 fish stick or 1 oz — 28	66	50	5	3	—	—	—	2	3	47	.1	—	0	.01	.02	.5	—
150	Haddock, breaded, fried[14]. 3 oz — 85	66	140	17	5	1.4	2.2	1.2	5	34	210	1.0	296	—	.03	.06	2.7	2
151	Ocean perch, breaded, fried[14]. 1 fillet — 85	59	195	16	11	2.7	4.4	2.3	6	28	192	1.1	242	—	.10	.10	1.6	—
152	Oysters, raw, meat only (13-19 medium Selects). 1 cup — 240	85	160	20	4	1.3	.2	.1	8	226	343	13.2	290	740	.34	.43	6.0	—
153	Salmon, pink, canned, solids and liquid. 3 oz — 85	71	120	17	5	.9	.8	.1	0	[15]167	243	.7	307	60	.03	.16	6.8	—
154	Sardines, Atlantic, canned in oil, drained solids. 3 oz — 85	62	175	20	9	3.0	2.5	.5	0	372	424	2.5	502	190	.02	.17	4.6	—
155	Scallops, frozen, breaded, fried, reheated. 6 scallops — 90	60	175	16	8	—	—	—	9	—	—	—	—	—	—	—	—	—
156	Shad, baked with butter or margarine, bacon. 3 oz — 85	64	170	20	10	—	—	—	0	20	266	.5	320	30[12]	.11	.22	7.3	—
	Shrimp:																	
157	Canned meat. 3 oz — 85	70	100	21	1	.1	.1	Trace	1	98	224	2.6	104	50	.01	.03	1.5	—
158	French fried[16]. 3 oz — 85	57	190	17	9	2.3	3.7	2.0	9	61	162	1.7	195	70	.03	.07	2.3	—
159	Tuna, canned in oil, drained solids. 3 oz — 85	61	170	24	7	1.7	1.7	.7	0	7	199	1.6	—	—	.04	.10	10.1	—
160	Tuna salad[17]. 1 cup — 205	70	350	30	22	4.3	6.3	6.7	7	41	291	2.7	—	590	.08	.23	10.3	2
	Meat and meat products:																	
161	Bacon, (20 slices per lb, raw), broiled or fried, crisp. 2 slices — 15	8	85	4	8	2.5	3.7	.7	Trace	2	34	.5	35	0	.08	.05	.8	—
	Beef,[18] cooked: Cuts braised, simmered or pot roasted:																	
162	Lean and fat (piece, 2 1/2 by 2 1/2 by 3/4 in). 3 oz — 85	53	245	23	16	6.8	6.5	.4	0	10	114	2.9	184	30	.04	.18	3.6	—
163	Lean only from item 162. 2.5 oz — 72	62	140	22	5	2.1	1.8	.2	0	10	108	2.7	176	10	.04	.17	3.3	—
	Ground beef, broiled:																	
164	Lean with 10% fat. 3 oz or patty 3 by 5/8 in — 85	60	185	23	10	4.0	3.9	.3	0	10	196	3.0	261	20	.08	.20	5.1	—
165	Lean with 21% fat. 2.9 oz or patty 3 by 5/8 in — 82	54	235	20	17	7.0	6.7	.4	0	9	159	2.6	221	30	.07	.17	4.4	—
	Roast, oven cooked, no liquid added: Relatively fat, such as rib:																	
166	Lean and fat (2 pieces, 4 1/8 by 2 1/4 by 1/4 in). 3 oz — 85	40	375	17	33	14.0	13.6	.8	0	8	158	2.2	189	70	.05	.13	3.1	—
167	Lean only from item 166. 1.8 oz — 51	57	125	14	7	3.0	2.5	.3	0	6	131	1.8	161	10	.04	.11	2.6	—
	Relatively lean, such as heel of round:																	
168	Lean and fat (2 pieces, 4 1/8 by 2 1/4 by 1/4 in). 3 oz — 85	62	165	25	7	2.8	2.7	.2	0	11	208	3.2	279	10	.06	.19	4.5	—

[12] Based on average vitamin A content of fortified margarine. Federal specifications for fortified margarine require a minimum of 15,000 International Units (I.U.) of vitamin A per pound.

[13] Fatty acid values apply to product made with regular-type margarine.

[14] Dipped in egg, milk or water, and breadcrumbs; fried in vegetable shortening.

[15] If bones are discarded, value for calcium will be greatly reduced.

[16] Dipped in egg, breadcrumbs, and flour or batter.

[17] Prepared with tuna, celery, salad dressing (mayonnaise type), pickle, onion, and egg.

[18] Outer layer of fat on the cut was removed to within approximately 1/2 in of the lean. Deposits of fat within the cut were not removed.

NUTRITIVE VALUES OF THE EDIBLE PART OF FOODS - Continued

(Dashes (—) denote lack of reliable data for a constituent believed to be present in measurable amount)

FISH, SHELLFISH, MEAT, POULTRY: RELATED PRODUCTS—Con.

Item No. (A)	Foods, approximate measure, units, and weight (edible part unless footnotes indicate otherwise) (B)	Grams	Water (C) Per-cent	Food energy (D) Calories	Protein (E) Grams	Fat (F) Grams	Saturated (total) (G) Grams	Oleic (H) Grams	Linoleic (I) Grams	Carbohydrate (J) Grams	Calcium (K) Milligrams	Phosphorus (L) Milligrams	Iron (M) Milligrams	Potassium (N) Milligrams	Vitamin A value (O) International units	Thiamin (P) Milligrams	Riboflavin (Q) Milligrams	Niacin (R) Milligrams	Ascorbic acid (S) Milligrams
	Meat and meat products—Continued																		
	Beef,[18] cooked—Continued																		
	Roast, oven cooked, no liquid added—Continued																		
	Relatively lean such as heel of round—Continued																		
169	Lean only from item 168--- 2.8 oz	78	65	125	24	3	1.2	1.0	0.1	0	10	199	3.0	268	Trace	0.06	0.18	4.3	—
	Steak:																		
	Relatively fat—sirloin, broiled:																		
170	Lean and fat (piece, 2 1/2 by 2 1/2 by 3/4 in.)--- 3 oz	85	44	330	20	27	11.3	11.1	.6	0	9	162	2.5	220	50	.05	.15	4.0	—
171	Lean only from item 170--- 2.0 oz	56	59	115	18	4	1.8	1.6	.2	0	7	146	2.2	202	10	.05	.14	3.6	—
	Relatively lean—round, braised:																		
172	Lean and fat (piece, 4 1/8 by 2 1/4 by 1/2 in.)--- 3 oz	85	55	220	24	13	5.5	5.2	.4	0	10	213	3.0	272	20	.07	.19	4.8	—
173	Lean only from item 172--- 2.4 oz	68	61	130	21	4	1.7	1.5	.2	0	9	182	2.5	238	10	.05	.16	4.1	—
	Beef, canned:																		
174	Corned beef--- 3 oz	85	59	185	22	10	4.9	4.5	.2	0	17	90	3.7			.01	.20	2.9	—
175	Corned beef hash--- 1 cup	220	67	400	19	25	11.9	10.9	.5	24	29	147	4.4	440		.02	.20	4.6	—
176	Beef, dried, chipped--- 2 1/2-oz jar	71	48	145	24	4	2.1	2.0	.1	0	14	287	3.6	142		.05	.23	2.7	0
177	Beef and vegetable stew--- 1 cup	245	82	220	16	11	4.9	4.5	.2	15	29	184	2.9	613	2,400	.15	.17	4.7	17
178	Beef potpie (home recipe), baked[19] (piece, 1/3 of 9-in diam. pie)--- 1 piece	210	55	515	21	30	7.9	12.8	6.7	39	29	149	3.8	334	1,720	.30	.30	5.5	6
179	Chili con carne with beans, canned--- 1 cup	255	72	340	19	16	7.5	6.8	.3	31	82	321	4.3	594	150	.08	.18	3.3	—
180	Chop suey with beef and pork (home recipe)--- 1 cup	250	75	300	26	17	8.5	6.2	.7	13	60	248	4.8	425	600	.28	.38	5.0	33
181	Heart, beef, lean, braised--- 3 oz	85	61	160	27	5	1.5	1.1	.6	1	5	154	5.0	197	20	.21	1.04	6.5	1
	Lamb, cooked:																		
	Chop, rib (cut 3 per lb with bone), broiled:																		
182	Lean and fat--- 3.1 oz	89	43	360	18	32	14.8	12.1	1.2	0	8	139	1.0	200		.11	.19	4.1	—
183	Lean only--- 2 oz	57	60	120	16	6	2.5	2.1	.2	0	6	121	1.1	174		.09	.15	3.4	—
	Leg, roasted:																		
184	Lean and fat (2 pieces, 4 1/8 by 2 1/4 by 1/4 in.)--- 3 oz	85	54	235	22	16	7.3	6.0	.6	0	9	177	1.4	241		.13	.23	4.7	—
185	Lean only from item 184--- 2.5 oz	71	62	130	20	5	2.1	1.8	.2	0	9	169	1.4	227		.12	.21	4.4	—
	Shoulder, roasted:																		
186	Lean and fat (3 pieces, 2 1/2 by 2 1/2 by 1/4 in.)--- 3 oz	85	50	285	18	23	10.8	8.8	.9	0	9	146	1.0	206		.11	.20	4.0	—
187	Lean only from item 186--- 2.3 oz	64	61	130	17	6	3.6	2.3	.2	0	8	140	1.0	193		.10	.18	3.7	—
188	Liver, beef, fried[20] (slice, 6 1/2 by 2 3/8 by 3/8 in.)--- 3 oz	85	56	195	22	9	2.5	3.5	.9	5	9	405	7.5	323	[2]45,390	.22	3.56	14.0	23
	Pork, cured, cooked:																		
189	Ham, light cure, lean and fat, roasted (2 pieces, 4 1/8 by 2 1/4 by 1/4 in.),[22]--- 3 oz	85	54	245	18	19	6.8	7.9	1.7	0	8	146	2.2	199	0	.40	.15	3.1	—
	Luncheon meat:																		
190	Boiled ham, slice (8 per 8-oz pkg.)--- 1 oz	28	59	65	5	5	1.7	2.0	.4	0	3	47	.8		0	.12	.04	.7	—
191	Canned, spiced or unspiced: Slice, approx. 3 by 2 by 1/2 in.--- 1 slice	60	55	175	9	15	5.4	6.7	1.0	1	5	65	1.3	133	0	.19	.13	1.8	—

(A)	(B)	(C)	(D)	(E)	(F)	(G)	(H)	(I)	(J)	(K)	(L)	(M)	(N)	(O)	(P)	(Q)	(R)	(S)
	Pork, fresh,[18] cooked:																	
	Chop, loin (cut 3 per lb with bone), broiled:																	
192	Lean and fat, 2.7 oz	78	42	305	19	25	8.9	10.4	2.2	0	9	209	2.7	216	0	0.75	0.22	4.5	—
193	Lean only from item 192, 2 oz	56	53	150	17	9	3.1	3.6	.8	0	7	181	2.2	192	0	.63	.18	3.8	—
194	Roast, oven cooked, no liquid added: Lean and fat (piece, 2 1/2 by 2 1/2 by 3/4 in), 3 oz	85	46	310	21	24	8.7	10.2	2.2	0	9	218	2.7	233	0	.78	.22	4.8	—
195	Lean only from item 194, 2.4 oz	68	55	175	20	10	3.5	4.1	.8	0	9	211	2.6	224	0	.73	.21	4.4	—
196	Shoulder cut, simmered: Lean and fat (3 pieces, 2 1/2 by 2 1/2 by 1/4 in), 3 oz	85	46	320	20	26	9.3	10.9	2.3	0	9	118	2.6	158	0	.46	.21	4.1	—
197	Lean only from item 196, 2.2 oz	63	60	135	18	6	2.2	2.6	.6	0	8	111	2.3	146	0	.42	.19	3.7	—
	Sausages (see also Luncheon meat (items 190-191)):																	
198	Bologna, slice (8 per 8-oz pkg.), 1 slice	28	56	85	3	8	3.0	3.4	.5	Trace	2	36	.5	65	—	.05	.06	.7	—
199	Braunschweiger, slice (6 per 6-oz pkg.), 1 slice	28	53	90	4	8	2.6	3.4	.8	1	3	69	1.7	—	1,850	.05	.41	2.3	—
200	Brown and serve (10-11 per 8-oz pkg.), browned, 1 link	17	40	70	3	6	2.3	2.8	.7	Trace	—	—	—	—	—	—	—	—	—
201	Deviled ham, canned, 1 tbsp	13	51	45	2	4	1.5	1.8	.4	0	1	12	.3	—	0	.02	.01	.2	—
202	Frankfurter (8 per 1-lb pkg.), cooked (reheated), 1 frankfurter	56	57	170	7	15	5.6	6.5	1.2	1	3	57	.8	—	—	.08	.11	1.4	—
203	Meat, potted (beef, chicken, turkey), canned, 1 tbsp	13	61	30	2	2	—	—	—	0	—	—	—	—	—	Trace	.03	.2	—
204	Pork link (16 per 1-lb pkg.), cooked, 1 link	13	35	60	2	6	2.1	2.4	.5	Trace	1	21	.3	35	0	.10	.04	.5	—
	Salami:																	
205	Dry type, slice (12 per 4-oz pkg.), 1 slice	10	30	45	2	4	1.6	1.6	.1	Trace	1	28	.4	—	—	.04	.03	.5	—
206	Cooked type, slice (8 per 8-oz pkg.), 1 slice	28	51	90	5	7	3.1	3.0	.2	Trace	3	57	.7	—	—	.07	.07	1.2	—
207	Vienna sausage (7 per 4-oz can), 1 sausage	16	63	40	2	3	1.2	1.4	.2	Trace	1	24	.3	—	—	.01	.02	.4	—
	Veal, medium fat, cooked, bone removed:																	
208	Cutlet (4 1/8 by 2 1/4 by 1/2 in), braised or broiled, 3 oz	85	60	185	23	9	4.0	3.4	.4	0	9	196	2.7	258	—	.06	.21	4.6	—
209	Rib (2 pieces, 4 1/8 by 2 1/4 by 1/4 in), roasted, 3 oz	85	55	230	23	14	6.1	5.1	.6	0	10	211	2.9	259	—	.11	.26	6.6	—
	Poultry and poultry products:																	
	Chicken, cooked:																	
210	Breast, fried,[23] bones removed, 2.8 oz (1/2 breast (3.3 oz with bones))	79	58	160	26	5	1.4	1.8	1.1	1	9	218	1.3	—	70	.04	.17	11.6	—
211	Drumstick, fried,[23] bones removed (2 oz with bones), 1.3 oz	38	55	90	12	4	1.1	1.3	.9	Trace	6	89	.9	—	50	.03	.15	2.7	—
212	Half broiler, broiled, bones removed (10.4 oz with bones), 6.2 oz	176	71	240	42	7	2.2	2.5	1.3	0	16	355	3.0	483	160	.09	.34	15.5	—
213	Chicken, canned, boneless, 3 oz	85	65	170	18	10	3.2	3.8	2.0	0	18	210	1.3	117	200	.03	.11	3.7	3
214	Chicken a la king, cooked (home recipe), 1 cup	245	68	470	27	34	12.7	14.3	3.3	12	127	358	2.5	404	1,130	.10	.42	5.4	12
215	Chicken and noodles, cooked (home recipe), 1 cup	240	71	365	22	18	5.9	7.1	3.5	26	26	247	2.2	149	430	.05	.17	4.3	Trace

[18] Outer layer of fat on the cut was removed to within approximately 1/2 in. of the lean. Deposits of fat within the cut were not removed.

[19] Outer layer of fat on the cut was removed within approximately 1/2 in. of the lean. Deposits of fat within the cut were not removed.

[20] Crust made with vegetable shortening and enriched flour.

[21] Regular-type margarine used.

[22] Value varies widely.

[23] About one-fourth of the outer layer of fat on the cut was removed. Deposits of fat within the cut were removed.

Vegetable shortening used.

NUTRITIVE VALUES OF THE EDIBLE PART OF FOODS - Continued

(Dashes (—) denote lack of reliable data for a constituent believed to be present in measurable amount)

Item No. (A)	Foods, approximate measures, units, and weight (edible part unless footnotes indicate otherwise) (B)		Grams	Water (C) Percent	Food energy (D) Calories	Protein (E) Grams	Fat (F) Grams	Fatty Acids Saturated (total) (G) Grams	Unsaturated Oleic (H) Grams	Linoleic (I) Grams	Carbohydrate (J) Grams	Calcium (K) Milligrams	Phosphorus (L) Milligrams	Iron (M) Milligrams	Potassium (N) Milligrams	Vitamin A value (O) International units	Thiamin (P) Milligrams	Riboflavin (Q) Milligrams	Niacin (R) Milligrams	Ascorbic acid (S) Milligrams
	FISH, SHELLFISH, MEAT, POULTRY; RELATED PRODUCTS—Continued																			
	Poultry and poultry products—Continued																			
	Chicken chow mein:																			
216	Canned	1 cup	250	89	95	7	7	—	—	—	18	45	85	1.3	418	150	0.05	0.10	1.0	13
217	From home recipe	1 cup	250	78	255	31	10	2.4	3.4	3.1	10	58	293	2.5	473	280	.08	.23	4.3	10
218	Chicken potpie (home recipe), baked,[19] piece (1/3 or 9-in diam. pie).	1 piece	232	57	545	23	31	11.3	10.9	5.6	42	70	232	3.0	343	3,090	.34	.31	5.5	5
	Turkey, roasted, flesh without skin:																			
219	Dark meat, piece, 2 1/2 by 1 5/8 by 1/4 in.	4 pieces	85	61	175	26	7	2.1	1.5	1.5	0	—	—	2.0	338	—	.03	.20	3.6	—
220	Light meat, piece, 4 by 2 by 1/4 in.	2 pieces	85	62	150	28	3	.9	.6	.7	0	—	—	1.0	349	—	.04	.12	9.4	—
	Light and dark meat:																			
221	Chopped or diced	1 cup	140	61	265	44	9	2.5	1.7	1.8	0	11	351	2.5	514	—	.07	.25	10.8	—
222	Pieces (1 slice white meat, 4 by 2 by 1/4 in with 2 slices dark meat, 2 1/2 by 1 5/8 by 1/4 in).	3 pieces	85	61	160	27	5	1.5	1.0	1.1	0	7	213	1.5	312	—	.04	.15	6.5	—
	FRUITS AND FRUIT PRODUCTS																			
	Apples, raw, unpeeled, without cores:																			
223	2 3/4-in diam. (about 3 per lb with cores).	1 apple	138	84	80	Trace	1	—	—	—	20	10	14	.4	152	120	.04	.03	.1	6
224	3 1/4-in diam. (about 2 per lb with cores).	1 apple	212	84	125	Trace	1	—	—	—	31	15	21	.6	233	190	.06	.04	.2	8
225	Applejuice, bottled or canned.[21]	1 cup	248	88	120	Trace	Trace	—	—	—	30	15	22	1.5	250	—	.02	.05	.2	2[52]
	Applesauce, canned:																			
226	Sweetened	1 cup	255	76	230	1	Trace	—	—	—	61	10	13	1.3	166	100	.05	.03	.1	2[53]
227	Unsweetened	1 cup	244	89	100	Trace	Trace	—	—	—	26	10	12	1.2	190	100	.05	.02	.1	2[52]
	Apricots:																			
228	Raw, without pits (about 12 per lb with pits).	3 apricots	107	85	55	1	Trace	—	—	—	14	18	25	.5	301	2,890	.03	.04	.6	11
229	Canned in heavy sirup (halves and sirup).	1 cup	258	77	220	2	Trace	—	—	—	57	28	39	.8	604	4,490	.05	.05	1.0	10
	Dried:																			
230	Uncooked (28 large or 37 medium halves per cup).	1 cup	130	25	340	7	1	—	—	—	86	87	140	7.2	1,273	14,170	.01	.21	4.3	16
231	Cooked, unsweetened, fruit and liquid.	1 cup	250	76	215	4	1	—	—	—	54	55	88	4.5	795	7,500	.01	.13	2.5	8
232	Apricot nectar, canned	1 cup	251	85	145	1	Trace	—	—	—	37	23	30	.5	379	2,380	.03	.03	.5	2[36]
	Avocados, raw, whole, without skins and seeds:																			
233	California, mid- and late-winter (with skin and seed, 3 1/8-in diam.; wt., 10 oz).	1 avocado	216	74	370	5	37	5.5	22.0	3.7	13	22	91	1.3	1,303	630	.24	.43	3.5	30
234	Florida, late summer and fall (with skin and seed, 3 5/8-in diam.; wt., 1 lb).	1 avocado	304	78	390	4	33	6.7	15.7	5.3	27	30	128	1.8	1,836	880	.33	.61	4.9	43
235	Banana without peel (about 2.6 per lb with peel).	1 banana	119	76	100	1	Trace	—	—	—	26	10	31	.8	440	230	.06	.07	.8	12
236	Banana flakes	1 tbsp	6	3	20	Trace	Trace	—	—	—	5	2	6	.2	92	50	.01	.01	.2	Trace

(A)	(B)		(C)	(D)	(E)	(F)	(G)	(H)	(I)	(J)	(K)	(L)	(M)	(N)	(O)	(P)	(Q)	(R)	(S)
237	Blackberries, raw	1 cup	144	85	85	2	1	—	—	—	19	46	27	1.3	245	290	0.04	0.06	0.6	30
238	Blueberries, raw	1 cup	145	83	90	1	1	—	—	—	22	22	19	1.5	117	150	.04	.09	.7	20
	Cantaloup. See Muskmelons (item 271).																			
	Cherries:																			
239	Sour (tart), red, pitted, canned, water pack.	1 cup	244	88	105	2	Trace	—	—	—	26	37	32	.7	317	1,660	.07	.05	.5	12
240	Sweet, raw, without pits and stems.	10 cherries	68	80	45	1	Trace	—	—	—	12	15	13	.3	129	70	.03	.04	.3	7
241	Cranberry juice cocktail, bottled, sweetened.	1 cup	253	83	165	Trace	Trace	—	—	—	42	13	8	.8	25	60	.03	.03	.1	[27]81
242	Cranberry sauce, sweetened, canned, strained.	1 cup	277	62	405	Trace	1	—	—	—	104	17	11	.6	83	60	.03	.03	.1	6
	Dates:																			
243	Whole, without pits	10 dates	80	23	220	2	Trace	—	—	—	58	47	50	2.4	518	40	.07	.08	1.8	0
244	Chopped	1 cup	178	23	490	4	1	—	—	—	130	105	112	5.3	1,153	90	.16	.18	3.9	0
245	Fruit cocktail, canned, in heavy sirup.	1 cup	255	80	195	1	Trace	—	—	—	50	23	31	1.0	411	360	.05	.03	1.0	5
	Grapefruit:																			
	Raw, medium, 3 3/4-in diam. (about 1 lb 1 oz):																			
246	Pink or red	1/2 grapefruit with peel[28]	241	89	50	1	Trace	—	—	—	13	20	20	.5	166	540	.05	.02	.2	44
247	White	1/2 grapefruit with peel[28]	241	89	45	1	Trace	—	—	—	12	19	19	.5	159	10	.05	.02	.2	44
248	Canned, sections with sirup	1 cup	254	81	180	2	Trace	—	—	—	45	33	36	.8	343	30	.08	.05	.5	76
	Grapefruit juice:																			
249	Raw, pink, red, or white	1 cup	246	90	95	1	Trace	—	—	—	23	22	37	.5	399	([29])	.10	.05	.5	93
	Canned, white:																			
250	Unsweetened	1 cup	247	89	100	1	Trace	—	—	—	24	20	35	1.0	400	20	.07	.05	.5	84
251	Sweetened	1 cup	250	86	135	1	Trace	—	—	—	32	20	35	1.0	405	30	.08	.05	.5	78
	Frozen, concentrate, unsweetened:																			
252	Undiluted, 6-fl oz can	1 can	207	62	300	4	1	—	—	—	72	70	124	.8	1,250	60	.29	.12	1.4	286
253	Diluted with 3 parts water by volume.	1 cup	247	89	100	1	Trace	—	—	—	24	25	42	.2	420	20	.10	.04	.5	96
254	Dehydrated crystals, prepared with water (1 lb yields about 1 gal).	1 cup	247	90	100	1	Trace	—	—	—	24	22	40	.2	412	20	.10	.05	.5	91
	Grapes, European type (adherent skin), raw:																			
255	Thompson Seedless	10 grapes	50	81	35	Trace	Trace	—	—	—	9	6	10	.2	87	50	.03	.02	.2	2
256	Tokay and Emperor, seeded types	10 grapes[30]	60	81	40	Trace	Trace	—	—	—	10	7	11	.2	99	60	.03	.02	.2	2
	Grapejuice:																			
257	Canned or bottled	1 cup	253	83	165	1	Trace	—	—	—	42	28	30	.8	293	—	.10	.05	.5	[25]Trace
	Frozen concentrate, sweetened:																			
258	Undiluted, 6-fl oz can	1 can	216	53	395	1	Trace	—	—	—	100	22	32	.9	255	40	.13	.22	1.5	[31]32
259	Diluted with 3 parts water by volume.	1 cup	250	86	135	1	Trace	—	—	—	33	8	10	.3	85	10	.05	.08	.5	[31]10
260	Grape drink, canned	1 cup	250	86	135	Trace	Trace	—	—	—	35	8	10	.3	88	—	[32].03	[32].03	.3	([32])
261	Lemon, raw, size 165, without peel and seeds (about 4 per lb with peels and seeds).	1 lemon	74	90	20	1	Trace	—	—	—	6	19	12	.4	102	10	.03	.01	.1	39
	Lemon juice:																			
262	Raw	1 cup	244	91	60	1	Trace	—	—	—	20	17	24	.5	344	50	.07	.02	.2	112
263	Canned, or bottled, unsweetened	1 cup	244	92	55	1	Trace	—	—	—	19	17	24	.5	344	50	.07	.02	.2	102
264	Frozen, single strength, unsweetened, 6-fl oz can.	1 can	183	92	40	1	Trace	—	—	—	13	13	16	.5	258	40	.05	.02	.2	81
	Lemonade concentrate, frozen:																			
265	Undiluted, 6-fl oz can	1 can	219	49	425	Trace	Trace	—	—	—	112	9	13	.4	153	40	.05	.06	.7	66
266	Diluted with 4 1/3 parts water by volume.	1 cup	248	89	105	Trace	Trace	—	—	—	28	2	3	.1	40	10	.01	.02	.2	17

[19]Crust made with vegetable shortening and enriched flour.

[24]Also applies to pasteurized apple cider.

[25]Applies to product without added ascorbic acid. For value of product with added ascorbic acid, refer to label.

[26]Based on product with label claim of 45% of U.S. RDA in 6 fl oz.

[27]Based on product with label claim of 100% of U.S. RDA in 6 fl oz.

[28]Weight includes peel and membranes between sections. Without these parts, the weight of the edible portion is 123 g for item 246 and 118 g for item 247.

[29]For white-fleshed varieties, value is about 20 International Units (I.U.) per cup; for red-fleshed varieties, 1,080 I.U.

[30]Weight includes seeds. Without seeds, weight of the edible portion is 57 g.

[31]Applies to product without added ascorbic acid. With added ascorbic acid, based on claim that 6 fl oz of reconstituted juice contain 45% or 50% of the U.S. RDA, value in milligrams is 108 or 120 for a 6-fl oz can (item 258), 36 or 40 for 1 cup of diluted juice (item 259).

[32]For products with added thiamin and riboflavin but without added ascorbic acid, values in milligrams would be 0.60 for thiamin, 0.80 for riboflavin, and trace for ascorbic acid. For products with only ascorbic acid added, value varies with the brand. Consult the label.

NUTRITIVE VALUES OF THE EDIBLE PART OF FOODS - Continued

(Dashes (—) denote lack of reliable data for a constituent believed to be present in measurable amount)

NUTRIENTS IN INDICATED QUANTITY

Item No. (A)	Foods, approximate measure, units, and weight (edible part unless footnotes indicate otherwise) (B)		Water (C) Percent	Food energy (D) Calories	Protein (E) Grams	Fat (F) Grams	Saturated (total) (G) Grams	Oleic (H) Grams	Linoleic (I) Grams	Carbohydrate (J) Grams	Calcium (K) Milligrams	Phosphorus (L) Milligrams	Iron (M) Milligrams	Potassium (N) Milligrams	Vitamin A value (O) International units	Thiamin (P) Milligrams	Riboflavin (Q) Milligrams	Niacin (R) Milligrams	Ascorbic acid (S) Milligrams
		Grams																	
	FRUITS AND FRUIT PRODUCTS—Con.																		
	Limeade concentrate, frozen:																		
267	Undiluted, 6-fl oz can	1 can	50	410	Trace	Trace	—	—	—	108	11	13	0.2	129	Trace	0.02	0.02	0.2	26
268	Diluted with 4 1/3 parts water by volume.	1 cup	89	100	Trace	Trace	—	—	—	27	3	3	Trace	32	Trace	Trace	Trace	Trace	6
	Limejuice:																		
269	Raw	1 cup	90	65	1	Trace	—	—	—	22	22	27	.5	256	20	.05	.02	.2	79
270	Canned, unsweetened	1 cup	90	65	1	Trace	—	—	—	22	22	27	.5	256	20	.05	.02	.2	52
	Muskmelons, raw, with rind, without seed cavity:																		
271	Cantaloup, orange-fleshed (with rind and seed cavity, 5-in diam., 2 1/3 lb).	1/2 melon with rind[33]	91	80	2	Trace	—	—	—	20	38	44	1.1	682	9,240	.11	.08	1.6	90
272	Honeydew (with rind and seed cavity, 6 1/2-in diam., 5 1/4 lb).	1/10 melon with rind[33]	91	50	1	Trace	—	—	—	11	21	24	.6	374	60	.06	.04	.9	34
	Oranges, all commercial varieties, raw:																		
273	Whole, 2 5/8-in diam., without peel and seeds (about 2 1/2 per lb with peel and seeds).	1 orange	86	65	1	Trace	—	—	—	16	54	26	.5	263	260	.13	.05	.5	66
274	Sections without membranes	1 cup	86	90	2	Trace	—	—	—	22	74	36	.7	360	360	.18	.07	.7	90
	Orange juice:																		
275	Raw, all varieties	1 cup	88	110	2	Trace	—	—	—	26	27	42	.5	496	500	.22	.07	1.0	124
276	Canned, unsweetened	1 cup	87	120	2	Trace	—	—	—	28	25	45	1.0	496	500	.17	.05	.7	100
	Frozen concentrate:																		
277	Undiluted, 6-fl oz can	1 can	55	360	5	Trace	—	—	—	87	75	126	.9	1,500	1,620	.68	.11	2.8	360
278	Diluted with 3 parts water by volume.	1 cup	87	120	2	Trace	—	—	—	29	25	42	.2	503	540	.23	.03	.9	120
279	Dehydrated crystals, prepared with water (1 lb yields about 1 gal).	1 cup	88	115	1	Trace	—	—	—	27	25	40	.5	518	500	.20	.07	1.0	109
	Orange and grapefruit juice:																		
	Frozen concentrate:																		
280	Undiluted, 6-fl oz can	1 can	59	330	4	1	—	—	—	78	61	99	.8	1,308	800	.48	.06	2.3	302
281	Diluted with 3 parts water by volume.	1 cup	88	110	1	Trace	—	—	—	26	20	32	.2	439	270	.15	.02	.7	102
282	Papayas, raw, 1/2-in cubes	1 cup	89	55	1	Trace	—	—	—	14	28	22	.4	328	2,450	.06	.06	.4	78
	Peaches:																		
	Raw:																		
283	Whole, 2 1/2-in diam., peeled, pitted (about 4 per lb with peels and pits).	1 peach	89	40	1	Trace	—	—	—	10	9	19	.5	202	[34]1,330	.02	.05	1.0	7
284	Sliced	1 cup	89	65	1	Trace	—	—	—	16	15	32	.9	343	[34]2,260	.03	.09	1.7	12
	Canned, yellow-fleshed, solids and liquid (halves or slices):																		
285	Syrup pack	1 cup	79	200	1	Trace	—	—	—	51	10	31	.8	333	1,100	.03	.05	1.5	8
286	Water pack	1 cup	91	75	1	Trace	—	—	—	20	10	32	.7	334	1,100	.02	.07	1.5	7
	Dried:																		
287	Uncooked	1 cup	25	420	5	1	—	—	—	109	77	187	9.6	1,520	6,240	.02	.30	8.5	29
288	Cooked, unsweetened, halves and juice.	1 cup	77	205	3	1	—	—	—	54	38	93	4.8	743	3,050	.01	.15	3.8	5

(A)	(B)	Measure	Weight (g)	(C)	(D)	(E)	(F)	(G)	(H)	(I)	(J)	(K)	(L)	(M)	(N)	(O)	(P)	(Q)	(R)	(S)
	Frozen, sliced, sweetened:																			
289	10-oz container	1 container	284	77	250	1	Trace	—	—	—	64	11	37	1.4	352	1,850	0.03	0.11	2.0	[35]116
290	Cup	1 cup	250	77	220	1	Trace	—	—	—	57	10	33	1.3	310	1,630	.03	.10	1.8	[35]103
	Pears:																			
291	Raw, with skin, cored: Bartlett, 2 1/2-in diam. (about 2 1/2 per lb with cores and stems).	1 pear	164	83	100	1	1	—	—	—	25	13	18	.5	213	30	.03	.07	.2	7
292	Bosc, 2 1/2-in diam. (about 3 per lb with cores and stems).	1 pear	141	83	85	1	1	—	—	—	22	11	16	.4	83	30	.03	.06	.1	6
293	D'Anjou, 3-in diam. (about 2 per lb with cores and stems).	1 pear	200	83	120	1	1	—	—	—	31	16	22	.6	260	40	.04	.08	.2	8
294	Canned, solids and liquid, sirup pack, heavy (halves or slices).	1 cup	255	80	195	1	1	—	—	—	50	13	18	.5	214	10	.03	.05	.3	3
	Pineapple:																			
295	Raw, diced	1 cup	155	85	80	1	Trace	—	—	—	21	26	12	.8	226	110	.14	.05	.3	26
	Canned, heavy sirup pack, solids and liquid:																			
296	Crushed, chunks, tidbits	1 cup	255	80	190	1	Trace	—	—	—	49	28	13	.8	245	130	.20	.05	.5	18
	Slices and liquid:																			
297	Large	1 slice; 2 1/4 tbsp liquid.	105	80	80	Trace	Trace	—	—	—	20	12	5	.3	101	50	.08	.02	.2	7
298	Medium	1 slice; 1 1/4 tbsp liquid.	58	80	45	Trace	Trace	—	—	—	11	6	3	.2	56	30	.05	.01	.1	4
299	Pineapple juice, unsweetened, canned.	1 cup	250	86	140	1	Trace	—	—	—	34	38	23	.8	373	130	.13	.05	.5	[27]80
	Plums:																			
	Raw, without pits:																			
300	Japanese and hybrid (2 1/8-in diam., about 6 1/2 per lb with pits).	1 plum	66	87	30	Trace	Trace	—	—	—	8	8	12	.3	112	160	.02	.02	.3	4
301	Prune-type (1 1/2-in diam, about 15 per lb with pits).	1 plum	28	79	20	Trace	Trace	—	—	—	6	3	5	.1	48	80	.01	.01	.1	1
	Canned, heavy sirup pack (Italian prunes), with pits and liquid:																			
302	Cup[36]	1 cup[36]	272	77	215	1	Trace	—	—	—	56	23	26	2.3	367	3,130	.05	.05	1.0	5
303	Portion[36]	3 plums; 2 3/4 tbsp liquid.[36]	140	77	110	1	Trace	—	—	—	29	12	13	1.2	189	1,610	.03	.03	.5	3
	Prunes, dried, "softenized," with pits:																			
304	Uncooked	4 extra large or 5 large prunes.[36]	49	28	110	1	Trace	—	—	—	29	22	34	1.7	298	690	.04	.07	.7	1
305	Cooked, unsweetened, all sizes, fruit and liquid.	1 cup[36]	250	66	255	2	1	—	—	—	67	51	79	3.8	695	1,590	.07	.15	1.5	2
306	Prune juice, canned or bottled	1 cup	256	80	195	1	Trace	—	—	—	49	36	51	1.8	602	—	.03	.03	1.0	5
	Raisins, seedless:																			
307	Cup, not pressed down	1 cup	145	18	420	4	Trace	—	—	—	112	90	146	5.1	1,106	30	.16	.12	.7	1
308	Packet, 1/2 oz (1 1/2 tbsp)	1 packet	14	18	40	Trace	Trace	—	—	—	11	9	14	.5	107	Trace	.02	.01	.1	Trace
	Raspberries, red:																			
309	Raw, capped, whole	1 cup	123	84	70	1	1	—	—	—	17	27	27	1.1	207	160	.04	.11	1.1	31
310	Frozen, sweetened, 10-oz container	1 container	284	74	280	2	1	—	—	—	70	37	48	1.7	284	200	.06	.17	1.7	60
	Rhubarb, cooked, added sugar:																			
311	From raw	1 cup	270	63	380	1	Trace	—	—	—	97	211	41	1.6	548	220	.05	.14	.8	16
312	From frozen, sweetened	1 cup	270	63	385	1	Trace	—	—	—	93	211	32	1.9	475	190	.05	.11	.5	16

[27]Based on product with label claim of 100% of U.S. RDA in 6 fl oz.

[28]Weight includes rind. Without rind, the weight of the edible portion is 272 g for item 271 and 149 g for item 272.

[35]Represents yellow-fleshed varieties. For white-fleshed varieties, value is 50 International Units (I.U.) for 1 peach, 90 I.U. for 1 cup of slices.

[35]Value represents products without added ascorbic acid. For products with added ascorbic acid, value in milligrams is 116 for a 10-oz container, 103 for 1 cup.

[36]Weight includes pits. After removal of the pits, the weight of the edible portion is 258 g for item 302, 133 g for item 303, 43 g for item 304, and 213 g for item 305.

A–13

NUTRITIVE VALUES OF THE EDIBLE PART OF FOODS - Continued

(Dashes (—) denote lack of reliable data for a constituent believed to be present in measurable amount)

Item No. (A)	Foods, approximate measures, units, and weight (edible part unless footnotes indicate otherwise) (B)		Grams	Water (C) Percent	Food energy (D) Calories	Protein (E) Grams	Fat (F) Grams	Fatty Acids Saturated (total) (G) Grams	Unsaturated Oleic (H) Grams	Unsaturated Linoleic (I) Grams	Carbohydrate (J) Grams	Calcium (K) Milligrams	Phosphorus (L) Milligrams	Iron (M) Milligrams	Potassium (N) Milligrams	Vitamin A value (O) International units	Thiamin (P) Milligrams	Riboflavin (Q) Milligrams	Niacin (R) Milligrams	Ascorbic acid (S) Milligrams
	FRUITS AND FRUIT PRODUCTS—Con.																			
	Strawberries:																			
313	Raw, whole berries, capped	1 cup	149	90	55	1	1	—	—	—	13	31	31	1.5	244	90	0.04	0.10	0.9	88
	Frozen, sweetened:																			
314	Sliced, 10-oz container	1 container	284	71	310	1	1	—	—	—	79	40	48	2.0	318	90	.06	.17	1.4	151
315	Whole, 1-lb container (about 1 3/4 cups).	1 container	454	76	415	2	1	—	—	—	107	59	73	2.7	472	140	.09	.27	2.3	249
316	Tangerine, raw, 2 3/8-in diam., size 176, without peel (about 4 per lb with peels and seeds).	1 tangerine	86	87	40	1	Trace	—	—	—	10	34	15	.3	108	360	.05	.02	.1	27
317	Tangerine juice, canned, sweetened.	1 cup	249	87	125	1	Trace	—	—	—	30	44	35	.5	440	1,040	.15	.05	.2	54
318	Watermelon, raw, 4 by 8 in wedge with rind and seeds (1/16 of 32 2/3-lb melon, 10 by 16 in).	1 wedge with rind and seeds[17]	926	93	110	2	1	—	—	—	27	30	43	2.1	426	2,510	.13	.13	.9	30
	GRAIN PRODUCTS																			
	Bagel, 3-in diam.:																			
319	Egg	1 bagel	55	32	165	6	2	0.5	0.9	0.8	28	9	43	1.2	41	30	.14	.10	1.2	0
320	Water	1 bagel	55	29	165	6	1	.2	.4	.6	30	8	41	1.2	42	0	.15	.11	1.4	0
321	Barley, pearled, light, uncooked	1 cup	200	11	700	16	2	.3	.2	.8	158	32	378	4.0	320	0	.24	.10	6.2	0
	Biscuits, baking powder, 2-in diam. (enriched flour, vegetable shortening):																			
322	From home recipe	1 biscuit	28	27	105	2	5	1.2	2.0	1.2	13	34	49	.4	33	Trace	.08	.08	.7	Trace
323	From mix	1 biscuit	28	29	90	2	3	.6	1.1	.7	15	19	65	.6	32	Trace	.09	.08	.8	Trace
324	Breadcrumbs (enriched):[38] Dry, grated	1 cup (items 349–350).	100	7	390	13	5	1.0	1.6	1.4	73	122	141	3.6	152	Trace	.35	.35	4.8	Trace
	Breads: Soft. See White bread (items 349–350).																			
325	Boston brown bread, canned, slice, 3 1/4 by 1/2 in.[38]	1 slice	45	45	95	2	1	.1	.2	.2	21	41	72	.9	131	[39]0	.06	.04	.7	0
	Cracked-wheat bread (3/4 enriched wheat flour, 1/4 cracked wheat):[38]																			
326	Loaf, 1 lb	1 loaf	454	35	1,195	39	10	2.2	3.0	3.9	236	399	581	9.5	608	Trace	1.52	1.13	14.4	Trace
327	Slice (18 per loaf)	1 slice	25	35	65	2	1	.1	.2	.2	13	22	32	.5	34	Trace	.08	.06	.8	Trace
	French or vienna bread, enriched:[38]																			
328	Loaf, 1 lb	1 loaf	454	31	1,315	41	14	3.2	4.7	4.6	251	195	386	10.0	408	Trace	1.80	1.10	15.0	Trace
	Slice:																			
329	French (5 by 2 1/2 by 1 in)	1 slice	35	31	100	3	1	.2	.4	.4	19	15	30	.8	32	Trace	.14	.08	1.2	Trace
330	Vienna (4 3/4 by 4 by 1/2 in).	1 slice	25	31	75	2	1	.1	.3	.3	14	11	21	.6	23	Trace	.10	.06	.8	Trace
	Italian bread, enriched:																			
331	Loaf, 1 lb	1 loaf	454	32	1,250	41	4	.6	Trace	1.5	256	77	349	10.0	336	0	1.80	1.10	15.0	0
332	Slice, 4 1/2 by 3 1/4 by 3/4 in.	1 slice	30	32	85	3	Trace	Trace	Trace	.1	17	5	23	.7	22	0	.12	.07	1.0	0
	Raisin bread, enriched:[38]																			
333	Loaf, 1 lb	1 loaf	454	35	1,190	30	13	3.0	4.7	3.9	243	322	395	10.0	1,057	Trace	1.70	1.07	10.7	Trace
334	Slice (18 per loaf)	1 slice	25	35	65	2	1	.2	.3	.2	13	18	22	.6	58	Trace	.09	.06	.6	Trace

(A)	(B)	(C)	(D)	(E)	(F)	(G)	(H)	(I)	(J)	(K)	(L)	(M)	(N)	(O)	(P)	(Q)	(R)	(S)
	Rye Bread:																	
	American, light (2/3 enriched wheat flour, 1/3 rye flour):																		
335	Loaf, 1 lb ---------------- 1 loaf	454	1,100	41	5	0.7	0.5	2.2	236	340	667	9.1	658	0	1.35	0.98	12.9	0
336	Slice (4 3/4 by 3 3/4 by 7/16 in) --- 1 slice	25	60	2	Trace	Trace	Trace	.1	13	19	37	.5	36	0	.07	.05	.7	0
	Pumpernickel (2/3 rye flour, 1/3 enriched wheat flour):																		
337	Loaf, 1 lb ---------------- 1 loaf	454	1,115	41	5	.7	.5	2.4	241	381	1,039	11.8	2,059	0	1.30	.93	8.5	0
338	Slice (5 by 4 by 3/8 in) --- 1 slice	32	80	3	Trace	.1	Trace	.2	17	27	73	.8	145	0	.09	.07	.6	0
	White bread, enriched:[38]																		
	Soft-crumb type:																		
339	Loaf, 1 lb ---------------- 1 loaf	454	1,225	39	15	3.4	5.3	4.6	229	381	440	11.3	476	Trace	1.80	1.10	15.0	Trace
340	Slice (18 per loaf) ------- 1 slice	25	70	2	1	.2	.3	.3	13	21	24	.6	26	Trace	.10	.06	.8	Trace
341	Slice, toasted ----------- 1 slice	22	70	2	1	.2	.3	.3	13	21	24	.6	26	Trace	.08	.06	.8	Trace
342	Slice (22 per loaf) ------- 1 slice	20	55	2	1	.2	.2	.2	10	17	19	.5	21	Trace	.08	.05	.7	Trace
343	Slice, toasted ----------- 1 slice	17	55	2	1	.2	.2	.2	10	17	19	.5	21	Trace	.06	.05	.7	Trace
344	Loaf, 1 1/2 lb ----------- 1 loaf	680	1,835	59	22	5.2	7.9	6.9	343	571	660	17.0	714	Trace	2.70	1.65	22.5	Trace
345	Slice (24 per loaf) ------- 1 slice	28	75	2	1	.2	.3	.3	14	24	27	.7	29	Trace	.11	.07	.9	Trace
346	Slice, toasted ----------- 1 slice	24	75	2	1	.2	.3	.3	14	24	27	.7	29	Trace	.09	.07	.9	Trace
347	Slice (28 per loaf) ------- 1 slice	24	65	2	1	.2	.2	.2	12	20	23	.6	25	Trace	.10	.06	.8	Trace
348	Slice, toasted ----------- 1 slice	21	65	2	1	.2	.2	.2	12	20	23	.6	25	Trace	.08	.06	.8	Trace
349	Cubes -------------------- 1 cup	30	80	3	1	.2	.3	.3	15	25	29	.8	32	Trace	.12	.07	1.0	Trace
350	Crumbs ------------------- 1 cup	45	120	4	1	.3	.5	.5	23	38	44	1.1	47	Trace	.18	.11	1.5	Trace
	Firm-crumb type:																		
351	Loaf, 1 lb ---------------- 1 loaf	454	1,245	41	17	3.9	5.9	5.2	228	435	463	11.3	549	Trace	1.80	1.10	15.0	Trace
352	Slice (20 per loaf) ------- 1 slice	23	65	2	1	.2	.3	.3	12	22	23	.6	28	Trace	.09	.06	.8	Trace
353	Slice, toasted ----------- 1 slice	20	65	2	1	.2	.3	.3	12	22	23	.6	28	Trace	.07	.06	.8	Trace
354	Loaf, 2 lb --------------- 1 loaf	907	2,495	82	34	7.7	11.8	10.4	455	871	925	22.7	1,097	Trace	3.60	2.20	30.0	Trace
355	Slice (34 per loaf) ------- 1 slice	27	75	2	1	.2	.3	.3	14	26	28	.7	33	Trace	.11	.06	.9	Trace
356	Slice, toasted ----------- 1 slice	23	75	2	1	.2	.3	.3	14	26	28	.7	33	Trace	.09	.06	.9	Trace
	Whole-wheat bread:																		
	Soft-crumb type:[38]																		
357	Loaf, 1 lb ---------------- 1 loaf	454	1,095	41	12	2.2	2.9	4.2	224	381	1,152	13.6	1,161	Trace	1.37	.45	12.7	Trace
358	Slice (16 per loaf) ------- 1 slice	28	65	3	1	.1	.2	.2	14	24	71	.8	72	Trace	.09	.03	.8	Trace
359	Slice, toasted ----------- 1 slice	24	65	3	1	.1	.2	.2	14	24	71	.8	72	Trace	.07	.03	.8	Trace
	Firm-crumb type:[38]																		
360	Loaf, 1 lb ---------------- 1 loaf	454	1,100	48	14	2.5	3.3	4.9	216	449	1,034	13.6	1,238	Trace	1.17	.54	12.7	Trace
361	Slice (18 per loaf) ------- 1 slice	25	60	3	1	.1	.2	.3	12	25	57	.8	68	Trace	.06	.03	.7	Trace
362	Slice, toasted ----------- 1 slice	21	60	3	1	.1	.2	.3	12	25	57	.8	68	Trace	.05	.03	.7	Trace
	Breakfast cereals:																		
	Hot type, cooked:																		
	Corn (hominy) grits, degermed:																			
363	Enriched ----------------- 1 cup	245	125	3	Trace	Trace	Trace	.1	27	2	25	.7	27	[40]Trace	.10	.07	1.0	0
364	Unenriched --------------- 1 cup	245	125	3	Trace	Trace	Trace	.1	27	2	25	.2	27	[40]Trace	.05	.02	.5	0
365	Farina, quick-cooking, enriched --- 1 cup	245	105	3	Trace	Trace	Trace		22	147	[41]113	([42])	25	0	.12	.07	1.0	0
366	Oatmeal or rolled oats --- 1 cup	240	130	5	2	.4	.8	.9	23	22	137	1.4	146	0	.19	.05	.2	0
367	Wheat, rolled ----------- 1 cup	240	180	5	1	—	—	—	41	19	182	1.7	202	0	.17	.07	2.2	0
368	Wheat, whole-meal -------- 1 cup	245	110	4	1	—	—	—	23	17	127	1.2	118	0	.15	.05	1.5	0
	Ready-to-eat:																		
369	Bran flakes (40% bran), added sugar, salt, iron, vitamins --- 1 cup	35	105	4	1	—	—	—	28	19	125	12.4	137	1,650	.41	.49	4.1	12
370	Bran flakes with raisins, added sugar, salt, iron, vitamins --- 1 cup	50	145	4	1	—	—	—	40	28	146	17.7	154	2,350	.58	.71	5.8	18

[37] Weight includes rind and seeds. Without rind and seeds, weight of the edible portion is 426 g.

[38] Made with vegetable shortening.

[39] Applies to product made with white cornmeal. With yellow cornmeal, value is 30 International Units (I.U.).

[40] Applies to white varieties. For yellow varieties, value is 150 International Units (I.U.).

[41] Applies to products that do not contain di-sodium phosphate. If di-sodium phosphate is an ingredient, value is 162 mg.

[42] Value may range from less than 1 mg to about 8 mg depending on the brand. Consult the label.

(Dashes (—) denote lack of reliable data for a constituent believed to be present in measurable amount)

NUTRIENTS IN INDICATED QUANTITY

Item No. (A)	Foods, approximate measures, units, and weight (edible part unless footnotes indicate otherwise) (B)	(Grams)	Water (C) Per cent	Food energy (D) Calories	Protein (E) Grams	Fat (F) Grams	Fatty Acids Saturated (total) (G) Grams	Unsaturated Oleic (H) Grams	Unsaturated Linoleic (I) Grams	Carbohydrate (J) Grams	Calcium (K) Milligrams	Phosphorus (L) Milligrams	Iron (M) Milligrams	Potassium (N) Milligrams	Vitamin A value (O) International units	Thiamin (P) Milligrams	Riboflavin (Q) Milligrams	Niacin (R) Milligrams	Ascorbic acid (S) Milligrams
	GRAIN PRODUCTS—Con.																		
	Breakfast cereals—Continued																		
	Ready-to-eat—Continued																		
	Corn flakes:																		
371	Plain, added sugar, salt, iron, vitamins. 1 cup	25	4	95	2	Trace	—	—	—	21	(⁴³)	9	0.6	30	1,180	0.29	0.35	2.9	9
372	Sugar-coated, added salt, iron, vitamins. 1 cup	40	2	155	2	Trace	—	—	—	37	1	10	1.0	27	1,880	.46	.56	4.6	14
373	Corn, puffed, plain, added sugar, salt, iron, vita-mins. 1 cup	20	4	80	2	1	—	—	—	16	4	18	2.3	—	940	.23	.28	2.3	7
374	Corn, shredded, added sugar, salt, iron, thiamin, niacin. 1 cup	25	3	95	2	Trace	—	—	—	22	1	10	.6	—	0	.11	.05	.5	0
375	Oats, puffed, added sugar, salt, minerals, vitamins. 1 cup	25	3	100	3	1	—	—	—	19	44	102	2.9	—	1,180	.29	.35	2.9	9
	Rice, puffed:																		
376	Plain, added iron, thiamin, niacin. 1 cup	15	4	60	1	Trace	—	—	—	13	3	14	.3	15	0	.07	.01	.7	0
377	Presweetened, added salt, iron, vitamins. 1 cup	28	3	115	1	0	—	—	—	26	3	14	⁴⁴1.1	43	1,250	.38	.43	5.0	⁴⁵515
378	Wheat flakes, added sugar, salt, iron, vitamins. 1 cup	30	4	105	3	Trace	—	—	—	24	12	83	(⁴³)	81	1,410	.35	.42	3.5	11
	Wheat, puffed:																		
379	Plain, added iron, thiamin, niacin. 1 cup	15	3	55	2	Trace	—	—	—	12	4	48	.6	51	0	.08	.03	1.2	0
380	Presweetened, added salt, iron, vitamins. 1 cup	38	3	140	3	Trace	—	—	—	33	7	52	⁴³1.6	63	1,680	.50	.57	6.7	⁴⁵520
381	Wheat, shredded, plain. 1 oblong biscuit or 1/2 cup spoon-size biscuits.	25	7	90	2	1	—	—	—	20	11	97	.9	87	0	.06	.03	1.1	0
382	Wheat germ, without salt and sugar, toasted. 1 tbsp	6	4	25	2	1	—	—	—	3	3	70	.5	57	10	.11	.05	.3	1
383	Buckwheat flour, light, sifted. 1 cup	98	12	340	6	1	—	—	—	78	11	86	1.0	314	0	.08	.04	.4	0
384	Bulgur, canned, seasoned. 1 cup	135	56	245	8	4	0.2	0.4	0.4	44	27	263	1.9	151	0	.08	.05	4.1	0
	Cake icings. See Sugars and Sweets (items 532-536).																		
	Cakes made from cake mixes with enriched flour:⁴⁶																		
	Angelfood:																		
385	Whole cake (9 3/4-in diam. tube cake). 1 cake	635	34	1,645	36	1	—	—	—	377	603	756	2.5	381	0	.37	.95	3.6	0
386	Piece, 1/12 of cake. 1 piece	53	34	135	3	Trace	—	—	—	32	50	63	.2	32	0	.03	.08	.3	0
	Coffeecake:																		
387	Whole cake (7 3/4 by 5 5/8 by 1 1/4 in). 1 cake	430	30	1,385	27	41	11.7	16.3	8.8	225	262	748	6.9	469	690	.82	.91	7.7	1
388	Piece, 1/6 of cake. 1 piece	72	30	230	5	7	2.0	2.7	1.5	38	44	125	1.2	78	120	.14	.15	1.3	Trace
	Cupcakes, made with egg, milk, 2 1/2-in diam.:																		
389	Without icing. 1 cupcake	25	26	90	1	3	.8	1.2	.7	14	40	59	.3	21	40	.05	.05	.4	Trace
390	With chocolate icing. 1 cupcake	36	22	130	2	5	2.0	1.6	.6	21	47	71	.4	42	60	.05	.06	.4	Trace
	Devil's food with chocolate icing:																		
391	Whole, 2 layer cake (8- or 9-in diam.). 1 cake	1,107	24	3,755	49	136	50.0	44.9	17.0	645	653	1,162	16.6	1,439	1,660	1.06	1.65	10.1	1
392	Piece, 1/16 of cake. 1 piece	69	24	235	3	8	3.1	2.8	1.1	40	41	72	1.0	90	100	.07	.10	.6	Trace
393	Cupcake, 2 1/2-in diam. 1 cupcake	35	24	120	2	4	1.6	1.4	.5	20	21	37	.5	46	50	.03	.05	.3	Trace

(A)	(B)	(C)	(D)	(E)	(F)	(G)	(H)	(I)	(J)	(K)	(L)	(M)	(N)	(O)	(P)	(Q)	(R)	(S)
	Gingerbread:																	
394	Whole cake (8-in square)------- 1 cake	570	1,575	18	39	9.7	16.6	10.0	291	513	570	8.6	1,562	Trace	0.84	1.00	7.4	Trace
395	Piece, 1/9 of cake------------ 1 piece	63	175	2	4	1.1	1.8	1.1	32	57	63	.9	173	Trace	.09	.11	.8	Trace
	White, 2 layer with chocolate icing:[47]																	
396	Whole cake (8- or 9-in diam.)-- 1 cake	1,140	4,000	44	122	48.2	46.4	20.0	716	1,129	2,041	11.4	1,322	680	1.50	1.77	12.5	2
397	Piece, 1/16 of cake----------- 1 piece	71	250	3	8	3.0	2.9	1.2	45	70	127	.7	82	40	.09	.11	.8	Trace
	Yellow, 2 layer with chocolate icing:[47]																	
398	Whole cake (8- or 9-in diam.)-- 1 cake	1,108	3,735	45	125	47.8	47.8	20.3	638	1,008	2,017	12.2	1,208	1,550	1.24	1.67	10.6	2
399	Piece, 1/16 of cake----------- 1 piece	69	235	3	8	3.0	3.0	1.3	40	63	126	.8	75	100	.08	.10	.7	Trace
	Cakes made from home recipes using enriched flour:[48]																	
	Boston cream pie with custard filling:																	
400	Whole cake (8-in diam.)------- 1 cake	825	2,490	41	78	23.0	30.1	15.2	412	553	833	8.2	[49]734	1,730	1.04	1.27	9.6	2
401	Piece, 1/12 of cake----------- 1 piece	69	210	3	6	1.9	2.5	1.3	34	46	70	.7	[49]61	140	.09	.11	.8	Trace
402	Fruitcake, dark: Loaf, 1-lb (7 1/2 by 2 by 1 1/2 in)---- 1 loaf	454	1,720	22	69	14.4	33.5	14.8	271	327	513	11.8	2,250	540	.72	.73	4.9	2
403	Plain, sheet cake: Slice, 1/30 of loaf-------- 1 slice	15	55	1	2	.5	1.1	.5	9	11	17	.4	74	20	.02	.02	.2	Trace
	Plain, sheet cake: Without icing:																	
404	Whole cake (9-in square)------ 1 cake	777	2,830	35	108	29.5	44.4	23.9	434	497	793	8.5	[49]614	1,320	1.21	1.40	10.2	2
405	Piece, 1/9 of cake------------ 1 piece	86	315	4	12	3.3	4.9	2.6	48	55	88	.9	[49]68	150	.13	.15	1.1	Trace
	With uncooked white icing:																	
406	Whole cake (9-in square)------ 1 cake	1,096	4,020	37	129	42.2	49.5	24.4	694	548	822	8.2	[49]869	2,190	1.22	1.47	10.2	2
407	Piece, 1/9 of cake------------ 1 piece	121	445	4	14	4.7	5.5	2.7	77	61	91	.8	[49]74	240	.14	.16	1.1	Trace
	Pound:[50]																	
408	Loaf, 8 1/2 by 3 1/2 by 3 1/4 in.---- 1 loaf	565	2,725	31	170	42.9	73.1	39.6	273	107	418	7.9	345	1,410	.90	.99	7.3	0
409	Slice, 1/17 of loaf---------- 1 slice	33	160	2	10	2.5	4.3	2.3	16	6	24	.5	20	80	.05	.06	.4	0
410	Spongecake: Whole cake (9 3/4-in diam. tube cake)---- 1 cake	790	2,345	60	45	13.1	15.8	5.7	427	237	885	13.4	687	3,560	1.10	1.64	7.4	Trace
411	Piece, 1/12 of cake---------- 1 piece	66	195	5	4	1.1	1.3	.5	36	20	74	1.1	57	300	.09	.14	.6	Trace
	Cookies made with enriched flour:[50][51]																	
	Brownies with nuts:																	
	Home-prepared, 1 3/4 by 1 3/4 by 7/8 in:																	
412	From home recipe----------- 1 brownie	20	95	1	6	1.5	3.0	1.2	10	8	30	.4	38	40	.04	.03	.2	Trace
413	From commercial recipe----- 1 brownie	20	85	1	4	.9	1.4	1.3	13	9	27	.4	34	20	.03	.02	.2	Trace
414	Frozen, with chocolate icing,[52] 1 1/2 by 1 3/4 by 7/8 in.---- 1 brownie	25	105	1	5	2.0	2.2	.7	15	10	31	.4	44	50	.03	.03	.2	Trace
	Chocolate chip:																	
415	Commercial, 2 1/4-in diam., 3/8 in thick.---- 4 cookies	42	200	2	9	2.8	2.9	2.2	29	16	48	1.0	56	50	.10	.17	.9	Trace
416	From home recipe, 2 1/3-in diam., 3/8 in thick.---- 4 cookies	40	205	2	12	3.5	4.5	2.9	24	14	40	.8	47	40	.06	.06	.5	Trace
417	Fig bars, square (1 5/8 by 1 5/8 by 3/8 in) or rectangular (1 1/2 by 1 3/4 by 1/2 in).---- 4 cookies	56	200	2	3	.8	1.2	.7	42	44	34	1.0	111	60	.04	.14	.9	Trace
418	Gingersnaps, 2-in diam., 1/4 in thick.---- 4 cookies	28	90	2	2	.7	1.0	.6	22	20	13	.7	129	20	.08	.06	.7	0
419	Macaroons, 2 3/4-in diam., 1/4 in thick.---- 2 cookies	38	180	2	9	—	—	—	25	10	32	.3	176	0	.02	.06	.2	0
420	Oatmeal with raisins, 2 5/8-in diam., 1/4 in thick.---- 4 cookies	52	235	3	8	2.0	3.3	2.0	38	11	53	1.4	192	30	.15	.10	1.0	Trace

[44] Value varies with the brand. Consult the label.
[45] Value varies with the brand. Consult the label.
[46] Applies to product with added ascorbic acid. Without added ascorbic acid, value is trace.
[47] Excepting angelfood cake, cakes were made from mixes containing vegetable shortening; icings, with butter.
[48] Excepting spongecake, vegetable shortening used for cake portion; butter, for icing. If butter or margarine used for cake portion, vitamin A values would be higher.
[49] Applies to product made with a sodium aluminum-sulfate type baking powder. With a low-sodium type baking powder containing potassium, value would be about twice the amount shown.
[50] Equal weights of flour, sugar, eggs, and vegetable shortening.
[51] Products are commercial unless otherwise specified.
[52] Made with enriched flour and vegetable shortening except for macaroons which do not contain flour or shortening.
[53] Icing made with butter.

NUTRITIVE VALUES OF THE EDIBLE PART OF FOODS - Continued

(Dashes (—) denote lack of reliable data for a constituent believed to be present in measurable amount)

Item No.	Foods, approximate measures, units, and weight (edible part unless footnotes indicate otherwise)		Water	Food energy	Protein	Fat	Fatty Acids Saturated (total)	Fatty Acids Unsaturated Oleic	Fatty Acids Unsaturated Linoleic	Carbohydrate	Calcium	Phosphorus	Iron	Potassium	Vitamin A value	Thiamin	Riboflavin	Niacin	Ascorbic acid
(A)	(B)	Grams	(C) Percent	(D) Calories	(E) Grams	(F) Grams	(G) Grams	(H) Grams	(I) Grams	(J) Grams	(K) Milligrams	(L) Milligrams	(M) Milligrams	(N) Milligrams	(O) International units	(P) Milligrams	(Q) Milligrams	(R) Milligrams	(S) Milligrams
	GRAIN PRODUCTS—Con.																		
	Cookies made with enriched flour[50][51]—Continued																		
421	Plain, prepared from commercial chilled dough, 2 1/2-in diam., 1/4 in thick. 4 cookies	48	5	240	2	12	3.0	5.2	2.9	31	17	35	0.6	23	30	0.10	0.08	0.9	0
422	Sandwich type (chocolate or vanilla), 1 3/4-in diam., 3/8 in thick. 4 cookies	40	2	200	2	9	2.2	3.9	2.2	28	10	96	.7	15	0	.06	.10	.7	0
423	Vanilla wafers, 1 3/4-in diam., 1/4 in thick. 10 cookies	40	3	185	2	6	—	—	—	30	16	25	.6	29	50	.10	.09	.8	0
424	Cornmeal: Whole-ground, unbolted, dry form. 1 cup	122	12	435	11	5	.5	1.0	2.5	90	24	312	2.9	346	[53]620	.46	.13	2.4	0
425	Bolted (nearly whole-grain), dry form. 1 cup	122	12	440	11	4	.5	.9	2.1	91	21	272	2.2	303	[53]590	.37	.10	2.3	0
426	Degermed, enriched: Dry form 1 cup	138	12	500	11	2	.2	.4	.9	108	8	137	4.0	166	[53]610	.61	.36	4.8	0
427	Cooked 1 cup	240	88	120	3	Trace	Trace	.1	.2	26	2	34	1.0	38	[53]140	.14	.10	1.2	0
428	Degermed, unenriched: Dry form 1 cup	138	12	500	11	2	.2	.4	.9	108	8	137	1.5	166	[53]610	.19	.07	1.4	0
429	Cooked 1 cup	240	88	120	3	Trace	Trace	.1	.2	26	2	34	.5	38	[53]140	.05	.02	.2	0
430	Crackers:[38] Graham, plain, 2 1/2-in square 2 crackers	14	6	55	1	1	.3	.5	.3	10	6	21	.5	55	0	.02	.08	.5	0
431	Rye wafers, whole-grain, 1 7/8 by 3 1/2 in. 2 wafers	13	6	45	2	Trace	—	—	—	10	7	50	.5	78	0	.04	.03	.2	0
432	Saltines, made with enriched flour. 4 crackers or 1 packet	11	4	50	1	1	.3	.5	.4	8	2	10	.5	13	0	.05	.05	.4	0
433	Danish pastry (enriched flour), plain without fruit or nuts:[54] Packaged ring, 12 oz 1 ring	340	22	1,435	25	80	24.3	31.7	16.5	155	170	371	6.1	381	1,050	.97	1.01	8.6	Trace
434	Round piece, about 4 1/4-in diam. by 1 in. 1 pastry	65	22	275	5	15	4.7	6.1	3.2	30	33	71	1.2	73	200	.18	.19	1.7	Trace
435	Ounce 1 oz	28	22	120	2	7	2.0	2.7	1.4	13	14	31	.5	32	90	.08	.08	.7	Trace
436	Doughnuts, made with enriched flour:[38] Cake type, plain, 2 1/2-in diam., 1 in high. 1 doughnut	25	24	100	1	5	1.2	2.0	1.1	13	10	48	.4	23	20	.05	.05	.4	Trace
437	Yeast-leavened, glazed, 3 3/4-in diam., 1 1/4 in high. 1 doughnut	50	26	205	3	11	3.3	5.8	3.3	22	16	33	.6	34	25	.10	.10	.8	0
438	Macaroni, enriched, cooked (cut lengths, elbows, shells): Firm stage (hot): 1 cup	130	64	190	7	1	—	—	—	39	14	85	1.4	103	0	.23	.13	1.8	0
439	Tender stage: Cold macaroni 1 cup	105	73	115	4	Trace	—	—	—	24	8	53	.9	64	0	.15	.08	1.2	0
440	Hot macaroni 1 cup	140	73	155	5	1	—	—	—	32	11	70	1.3	85	0	.20	.11	1.5	0
441	Macaroni (enriched) and cheese: Canned[55] 1 cup	240	80	230	9	10	4.2	3.1	1.4	26	199	182	1.0	139	260	.12	.24	1.0	Trace
442	From home recipe (served hot)[56] 1 cup	200	58	430	17	22	8.9	8.8	2.9	40	362	322	1.8	240	860	.20	.40	1.8	Trace
443	Muffins made with enriched flour:[38] From home recipe: Blueberry, 2 3/8-in diam., 1 1/2 in high. 1 muffin	40	39	110	3	4	1.1	1.4	.7	17	34	53	.6	46	90	.09	.10	.7	Trace
444	Bran 1 muffin	40	35	105	3	4	1.2	1.4	.8	17	57	162	1.5	172	90	.07	.10	1.7	Trace
445	Corn (enriched degermed cornmeal and flour), 2 3/8-in diam., 1 1/2 in high. 1 muffin	40	33	125	3	4	1.2	1.6	.9	19	42	68	.7	54	[57]120	.10	.10	.7	Trace

(A)	(B)	(grams)	(C)	(D)	(E)	(F)	(G)	(H)	(I)	(J)	(K)	(L)	(M)	(N)	(O)	(P)	(Q)	(R)	(S)
446	Plain, 3-in diam., 1 1/2 in high — 1 muffin	40	38	120	3	4	1.0	1.7	1.0	17	42	60	0.6	50	40	0.09	0.12	0.9	Trace
447	From mix, egg, milk: Corn, 2 3/8-in diam., 1 1/2 in high.[58] — 1 muffin	40	30	130	3	4	1.2	1.7	.9	20	96	152	.6	44	[57]100	.08	.09	.7	Trace
448	Noodles (egg noodles), enriched,[59] cooked — 1 cup	160	71	200	7	2	—	—	—	37	16	94	1.4	70	110	.22	.13	1.9	0
449	Noodles, chow mein, canned — 1 cup	45	1	220	6	11	—	—	—	26	—	—	—	—	—	—	—	—	—
450	Pancakes, (4-in diam.):[38] Buckwheat, made from mix (with buckwheat and enriched flours), egg and milk added — 1 cake	27	58	55	2	2	.8	.9	.4	6	59	91	—	66	60	.04	.05	.2	Trace
451	Plain: Made from home recipe using enriched flour — 1 cake	27	50	60	2	2	.5	.8	.5	9	27	38	.4	33	30	.06	.07	.5	Trace
452	Made from mix with enriched flour, egg and milk added — 1 cake	27	51	60	2	2	.7	.7	.3	9	58	70	.3	42	70	.04	.06	.2	Trace
453	Pies, piecrust made with enriched flour, vegetable shortening (9-in diam.): Apple: Whole — 1 pie	945	48	2,420	21	105	27.0	44.5	25.2	360	76	208	6.6	756	280	1.06	.79	9.3	9
454	Sector, 1/7 of pie — 1 sector	135	48	345	3	15	3.9	6.4	3.6	51	11	30	.9	108	40	.15	.11	1.3	2
455	Banana cream: Whole — 1 pie	910	54	2,010	41	85	26.7	33.2	16.2	279	601	746	7.3	1,847	2,280	.77	1.51	7.0	9
456	Sector, 1/7 of pie — 1 sector	130	54	285	6	12	3.8	4.7	2.3	40	86	107	1.0	264	330	.11	.22	1.0	1
457	Blueberry: Whole — 1 pie	945	51	2,285	23	102	24.8	43.7	25.1	330	104	217	9.5	614	280	1.03	.80	10.0	28
458	Sector, 1/7 of pie — 1 sector	135	51	325	3	15	3.5	6.2	3.6	47	15	31	1.4	88	40	.15	.11	1.4	4
459	Cherry: Whole — 1 pie	945	47	2,465	25	107	28.2	45.0	25.3	363	132	236	6.6	992	4,160	1.09	.84	9.8	Trace
460	Sector, 1/7 of pie — 1 sector	135	47	350	4	15	4.0	6.4	3.6	52	19	34	.9	142	590	.16	.12	1.4	Trace
461	Custard: Whole — 1 pie	910	58	1,985	56	101	33.9	38.5	17.5	213	874	1,028	8.2	1,247	2,090	.79	1.92	5.6	0
462	Sector, 1/7 of pie — 1 sector	130	58	285	8	14	4.8	5.5	2.5	30	125	147	1.2	178	300	.11	.27	.8	0
463	Lemon meringue: Whole — 1 pie	840	47	2,140	31	86	26.1	33.8	16.4	317	118	412	6.7	420	1,430	.61	.84	5.2	25
464	Sector, 1/7 of pie — 1 sector	120	47	305	4	12	3.7	4.8	2.3	45	17	59	1.0	60	200	.09	.12	.7	4
465	Mince: Whole — 1 pie	945	43	2,560	24	109	28.0	45.9	25.2	389	265	359	13.3	1,682	20	.96	.86	9.8	9
466	Sector, 1/7 of pie — 1 sector	135	43	365	3	16	4.0	6.6	3.6	56	38	51	1.9	240	Trace	.14	.12	1.4	1
467	Peach: Whole — 1 pie	945	48	2,410	24	101	24.8	43.7	25.1	361	95	274	8.5	1,400	6,900	1.04	.97	14.0	28
468	Sector, 1/7 of pie — 1 sector	135	48	345	3	14	3.5	6.2	3.6	52	14	39	1.2	201	990	.15	.14	2.0	4
469	Pecan: Whole — 1 pie	825	20	3,450	42	189	27.8	101.0	44.2	423	388	850	25.6	1,015	1,320	1.80	.95	6.9	Trace
470	Sector, 1/7 of pie — 1 sector	118	20	495	6	27	4.0	14.4	6.3	61	55	122	3.7	145	190	.26	.14	1.0	Trace
471	Pumpkin: Whole — 1 pie	910	59	1,920	36	102	37.4	37.5	16.6	223	464	628	7.3	1,456	22,480	.78	1.27	7.0	Trace
472	Sector, 1/7 of pie — 1 sector	130	59	275	5	15	5.4	5.4	2.4	32	66	90	1.0	208	3,210	.11	.18	1.0	Trace
473	Piecrust (home recipe) made with enriched flour and vegetable shortening, baked — 1 pie shell, 9-in diam.	180	15	900	11	60	14.8	26.1	14.9	79	25	90	3.1	89	0	.47	.40	5.0	0
474	Piecrust mix with enriched flour and vegetable shortening, 10-oz pkg. prepared and baked — Piecrust for 2-crust pie, 9-in diam.	320	19	1,485	20	93	22.7	39.7	23.4	141	131	272	6.1	179	0	1.07	.79	9.9	0

[38] Made with vegetable shortening.
[50] Products are commercial unless otherwise specified.
[51] Made with enriched flour and vegetable shortening except for macaroons which do not contain flour or shortening.
[53] Applies to yellow varieties; white varieties contain only a trace.
[54] Made with corn oil.
[55] Contains vegetable shortening and butter.
[56] Made with regular margarine.
[57] Applies to product made with yellow cornmeal.
[58] Made with enriched degermed cornmeal and enriched flour.
[59] Made with enriched flour.

NUTRITIVE VALUES OF THE EDIBLE PART OF FOODS - Continued

(Dashes (—) denote lack of reliable data for a constituent believed to be present in measurable amount)

NUTRIENTS IN INDICATED QUANTITY

Item No. (A)	Foods, approximate measures, units, and weight (edible part unless footnotes indicate otherwise) (B)		Grams	Water (C) Percent	Food energy (D) Calories	Protein (E) Grams	Fat (F) Grams	Fatty Acids Saturated (total) (G) Grams	Unsaturated Oleic (H) Grams	Linoleic (I) Grams	Carbohydrate (J) Grams	Calcium (K) Milligrams	Phosphorus (L) Milligrams	Iron (M) Milligrams	Potassium (N) Milligrams	Vitamin A value (O) International units	Thiamin (P) Milligrams	Riboflavin (Q) Milligrams	Niacin (R) Milligrams	Ascorbic acid (S) Milligrams
	GRAIN PRODUCTS—Con.																			
475	Pizza (cheese) baked, 4 3/4-in sector; 1/8 of 12-in diam. pie.[13]	1 sector	60	45	145	6	4	1.7	1.5	0.6	22	86	89	1.1	67	230	0.16	0.18	1.6	4
	Popcorn, popped:																			
476	Plain, large kernel	1 cup	6	4	25	1	Trace	Trace	.1	.2	5	1	17	.2	—	—	—	.01	.1	0
477	With oil (coconut) and salt added; large kernel.	1 cup	9	3	40	1	2	1.5	.2	.2	5	1	19	.2	—	—	—	.01	.2	0
478	Sugar coated	1 cup	35	4	135	2	1	.5	.2	.4	30	2	47	.5	—	—	—	.02	.4	0
	Pretzels, made with enriched flour:																			
479	Dutch, twisted, 2 3/4 by 2 5/8 in.	1 pretzel	16	5	60	2	1	—	—	—	12	4	21	.2	21	0	.05	.04	.7	0
480	Thin, twisted, 3 1/4 by 2 1/4 by 1/4 in.	10 pretzels	60	5	235	6	3	—	—	—	46	13	79	.9	78	0	.20	.15	2.5	0
481	Stick, 2 1/4 in long	10 pretzels	3	5	10	Trace	Trace	—	—	—	2	1	4	Trace	4	0	.01	.01	.1	0
	Rice, white, enriched:																			
482	Instant, ready-to-serve, hot	1 cup	165	73	180	4	Trace	Trace	Trace	Trace	40	5	31	1.3	—	0	.21	([58])	1.7	0
	Long grain:																			
483	Raw	1 cup	185	12	670	12	1	.2	.2	.2	149	44	174	5.4	170	0	.81	.06	6.5	0
484	Cooked, served hot	1 cup	205	73	225	4	Trace	.1	.1	.1	50	21	57	1.8	57	0	.23	.02	2.1	0
	Parboiled:																			
485	Raw	1 cup	195	10	685	14	1	.2	.1	.2	150	111	370	5.4	278	0	.81	.07	6.5	0
486	Cooked, served hot	1 cup	175	73	185	4	Trace	.1	.1	.1	41	33	100	1.4	75	0	.19	.02	2.1	0
	Rolls, enriched:[38]																			
	Commercial:																			
487	Brown-and-serve (12 per 12-oz pkg.), browned.	1 roll	26	27	85	2	2	.4	.7	.5	14	20	23	.5	25	Trace	.10	.06	.9	Trace
488	Cloverleaf or pan, 2 1/2-in diam., 2 in high.	1 roll	28	31	85	2	2	.4	.6	.4	15	21	24	.5	27	Trace	.11	.07	.9	Trace
489	Frankfurter and hamburger (8 per 11 1/2-oz pkg.).	1 roll	40	31	120	3	2	.5	.8	.6	21	30	34	.8	38	Trace	.16	.10	1.3	Trace
490	Hard, 3 3/4-in diam., 2 in high.	1 roll	50	25	155	5	2	.4	.6	.5	30	24	46	1.2	49	Trace	.20	.12	1.7	Trace
491	Hoagie or submarine, 11 1/2 by 3 by 2 1/2 in.	1 roll	135	31	390	12	4	.9	1.4	1.4	75	58	115	3.0	122	Trace	.54	.32	4.5	Trace
	From home recipe:																			
492	Cloverleaf, 2 1/2-in diam., 2 in high.	1 roll	35	26	120	3	3	.8	1.1	.7	20	16	36	.7	41	30	.12	.12	1.2	Trace
	Spaghetti, enriched, cooked:																			
493	Firm stage, "al dente," served hot.	1 cup	130	64	190	7	1	—	—	—	39	14	85	1.4	103	0	.23	.13	1.8	0
494	Tender stage, served hot	1 cup	140	73	155	5	1	—	—	—	32	11	70	1.3	85	0	.20	.11	1.5	0
	Spaghetti (enriched) in tomato sauce with cheese:																			
495	From home recipe	1 cup	250	77	260	9	9	2.0	5.4	.7	37	80	135	2.3	408	1,080	.25	.18	2.3	13
496	Canned	1 cup	250	80	190	6	2	.5	.3	.4	39	40	88	2.8	303	930	.35	.28	4.5	10
	Spaghetti (enriched) with meat balls and tomato sauce:																			
497	From home recipe	1 cup	248	70	330	19	12	3.3	6.3	3.9	39	124	236	3.7	665	1,590	.25	.30	4.0	22
498	Canned	1 cup	250	78	260	12	10	2.2	3.3	3.9	29	53	113	3.3	245	1,000	.15	.18	2.3	5
499	Toaster pastries	1 pastry	50	12	200	3	6	—	—	—	36	[6]54	[6]67	1.9	[6]74	500	.16	.17	2.1	([60])
	Waffles, made with enriched flour, 7-in diam.:[39]																			
500	From home recipe	1 waffle	75	41	210	7	7	2.3	2.8	1.4	28	85	130	1.3	109	250	.17	.23	1.4	Trace
501	From mix, egg and milk added	1 waffle	75	42	205	7	8	2.8	2.9	1.2	27	179	257	1.0	146	170	.14	.22	.9	Trace

(A)	(B)		(C)	(D)	(E)	(F)	(G)	(H)	(I)	(J)	(K)	(L)	(M)	(N)	(O)	(P)	(Q)	(R)	(S)
	Wheat flours:																		
	All-purpose or family flour, enriched:																		
502	Sifted, spooned	1 cup	115	12	420	12	1	0.2	0.1	0.5	88	18	100	3.3	109	0	0.74	0.46	6.1	0
503	Unsifted, spooned	1 cup	125	12	455	13	1	.2	.1	.5	95	20	109	3.6	119	0	.80	.50	6.6	0
504	Cake or pastry flour, enriched, sifted, spooned.	1 cup	96	12	350	7	1	.1	.1	.3	76	16	70	2.8	91	0	.61	.38	5.1	0
505	Self-rising, enriched, unsifted, spooned.	1 cup	125	12	440	12	1	.2	.1	.5	93	331	583	3.6	—	0	.80	.50	6.6	0
506	Whole-wheat, from hard wheats, stirred.	1 cup	120	12	400	16	2	.4	.2	1.0	85	49	446	4.0	444	0	.66	.14	5.2	0
	LEGUMES (DRY), NUTS, SEEDS; RELATED PRODUCTS																			
	Almonds, shelled:																			
507	Chopped (about 130 almonds)	1 cup	130	5	775	24	70	5.6	47.7	12.8	25	304	655	6.1	1,005	0	.31	1.20	4.6	Trace
508	Slivered, not pressed down (about 115 almonds).	1 cup	115	5	690	21	62	5.0	42.2	11.3	22	269	580	5.4	889	0	.28	1.06	4.0	Trace
	Beans, dry:																			
	Common varieties as Great Northern, navy, and others:																			
	Cooked, drained:																			
509	Great Northern	1 cup	180	69	210	14	1	—	—	—	38	90	266	4.9	749	0	.25	.13	1.3	0
510	Pea (navy)	1 cup	190	69	225	15	1	—	—	—	40	95	281	5.1	790	0	.27	.13	1.3	0
	Canned, solids and liquid:																			
	White with—																			
511	Frankfurters (sliced)	1 cup	255	71	365	19	18	2.4	2.8	.6	32	94	303	4.8	668	330	.18	.15	3.3	Trace
512	Pork and tomato sauce	1 cup	255	71	310	16	7	4.3	5.0	1.1	48	138	235	4.6	536	330	.20	.08	1.5	5
513	Pork and sweet sauce	1 cup	255	66	385	16	12	—	—	—	54	161	291	5.9	—	—	.15	.10	1.3	—
514	Red kidney	1 cup	255	76	230	15	1	—	—	—	42	74	278	4.6	673	10	.13	.10	1.5	—
515	Lima, cooked, drained	1 cup	190	64	260	16	1	—	—	—	49	55	293	5.9	1,163	—	.25	.11	1.3	—
516	Blackeye peas, dry, cooked (with residual cooking liquid).	1 cup	250	80	190	13	1	—	—	—	35	43	238	3.3	573	30	.40	.10	1.0	—
517	Brazil nuts, shelled (6-8 large kernels).	1 oz	28	5	185	4	19	4.8	6.2	7.1	3	53	196	1.0	203	Trace	.27	.03	.5	—
518	Cashew nuts, roasted in oil	1 cup	140	5	785	24	64	12.9	36.8	10.2	41	53	522	5.3	650	140	.60	.35	2.5	—
	Coconut meat, fresh:																			
519	Piece, about 2 by 2 by 1/2 in	1 piece	45	51	155	2	16	14.0	.9	.3	4	6	43	.8	115	0	.02	.01	.2	1
520	Shredded or grated, not pressed down.	1 cup	80	51	275	3	28	24.8	1.6	.5	8	10	76	1.4	205	0	.04	.02	.4	2
521	Filberts (hazelnuts), chopped (about 80 kernels).	1 cup	115	6	730	14	72	5.1	55.2	7.3	19	240	388	3.9	810	—	.53	—	1.0	Trace
522	Lentils, whole, cooked	1 cup	200	72	210	16	Trace	—	—	—	39	50	238	4.2	498	40	.14	.12	1.2	0
523	Peanuts, roasted in oil, salted (whole, halves, chopped).	1 cup	144	2	840	37	72	13.7	33.0	20.7	27	107	577	3.0	971	0	.46	.19	24.8	0
524	Peanut butter	1 tbsp	16	2	95	4	8	1.5	3.7	2.3	3	9	61	.3	100	—	.02	.02	2.4	0
525	Peas, split, dry, cooked	1 cup	200	70	230	16	1	—	—	—	42	22	178	3.4	592	80	.30	.18	1.8	—
526	Pecans, chopped or pieces (about 120 large halves).	1 cup	118	3	810	11	84	7.2	50.5	20.0	17	86	341	2.8	712	150	1.01	.15	1.1	2
527	Pumpkin and squash kernels, dry, hulled.	1 cup	140	4	775	41	65	11.8	23.5	27.5	21	71	1,602	15.7	1,386	100	.34	.27	3.4	—
528	Sunflower seeds, dry, hulled	1 cup	145	5	810	35	69	8.2	13.7	43.2	29	174	1,214	10.3	1,334	70	2.84	.33	7.8	—
	Walnuts:																			
	Black:																			
529	Chopped or broken kernels	1 cup	125	3	785	26	74	6.3	13.3	45.7	19	Trace	713	7.5	575	380	.28	.14	.9	—
530	Ground (finely)	1 cup	80	3	500	16	47	4.0	8.5	29.2	12	Trace	456	4.8	368	240	.18	.09	.6	—
531	Persian or English, chopped (about 60 halves).	1 cup	120	4	780	18	77	8.4	11.8	42.2	19	119	456	3.7	540	40	.40	.16	1.1	2

[13]Crust made with vegetable shortening and enriched flour. Consult the label.
[38]Made with vegetable shortening.
[59]Product may or may not be enriched with riboflavin. Consult the label.
[60]Value varies with the brand. Consult the label.

NUTRITIVE VALUES OF THE EDIBLE PART OF FOODS - Continued

(Dashes (—) denote lack of reliable data for a constituent believed to be present in measurable amount)

SUGARS AND SWEETS

Item No. (A)	Foods, approximate measures, units, and weight (B)	Grams	Water % (C)	Food energy Cal. (D)	Protein g (E)	Fat g (F)	Saturated (total) g (G)	Oleic g (H)	Linoleic g (I)	Carbohydrate g (J)	Calcium mg (K)	Phosphorus mg (L)	Iron mg (M)	Potassium mg (N)	Vitamin A value IU (O)	Thiamin mg (P)	Riboflavin mg (Q)	Niacin mg (R)	Ascorbic acid mg (S)
	Cake icings:																		
	Boiled, white:																		
532	Plain------------- 1 cup	94	18	295	1	0	0	0	0	75	2	2	Trace	17	0	Trace	0.03	Trace	0
533	With coconut------ 1 cup	166	15	605	3	13	11.0	.9	Trace	124	10	50	0.8	277	0	0.02	.07	0.3	0
	Uncooked:																		
534	Chocolate made with milk and butter------ 1 cup	275	14	1,035	9	38	23.4	11.7	1.0	185	165	305	3.3	536	580	.06	.28	.6	1
535	Creamy fudge from mix and water------ 1 cup	245	15	830	7	16	5.1	6.7	3.1	183	96	218	2.7	238	Trace	.05	.20	.7	Trace
536	White------------- 1 cup	319	11	1,200	2	21	12.7	5.1	.5	260	48	38	Trace	57	860	Trace	.06	Trace	Trace
	Candy:																		
537	Caramels, plain or chocolate--- 1 oz	28	8	115	1	3	1.6	1.1	.1	22	42	35	.4	54	Trace	.01	.05	.1	Trace
	Chocolate:																		
538	Milk, plain------- 1 oz	28	1	145	2	9	5.5	3.0	.3	16	65	65	.3	109	80	.02	.10	.1	Trace
539	Semisweet, small pieces (60 per oz)--- 1 cup or 6-oz pkg	170	1	860	7	61	36.2	19.8	1.7	97	51	255	4.4	553	30	.02	.14	.9	0
540	Chocolate-coated peanuts--- 1 oz	28	1	160	5	12	4.0	4.7	2.1	11	33	84	.4	143	Trace	.10	.05	2.1	Trace
541	Fondant, uncoated (mints, candy corn, other)--- 1 oz	28	8	105	Trace	1	—	—	—	25	4	2	.3	1	0	Trace	Trace	Trace	0
542	Fudge, chocolate, plain--- 1 oz	28	8	115	Trace	3	1.3	1.4	.6	21	22	24	.3	42	Trace	.01	.03	.1	Trace
543	Gum drops--------- 1 oz	28	12	100	Trace	Trace	—	—	—	25	2	Trace	.1	1	0	0	Trace	0	0
544	Hard-------------- 1 oz	28	1	110	0	Trace	—	—	—	28	6	2	.5	1	0	0	0	0	0
545	Marshmallows------ 1 oz	28	17	90	1	Trace	—	—	—	23	5	2	.5	2	0	0	Trace	Trace	0
	Chocolate-flavored beverage powders (about 4 heaping tsp per oz):																		
546	With nonfat dry milk--- 1 oz	28	2	100	5	1	.5	.3	Trace	20	167	155	.5	227	10	.04	.21	.2	1
547	Without milk------ 1 oz	28	1	100	1	1	.4	.2	Trace	25	9	48	.6	142	0	.01	.03	.1	0
548	Honey, strained or extracted--- 1 tbsp	21	17	65	Trace	0	0	0	0	17	1	1	.1	11	0	Trace	.01	.1	Trace
549	Jams and preserves--- 1 tbsp	20	29	55	Trace	Trace	—	—	—	14	4	2	.2	18	Trace	Trace	.01	Trace	Trace
550	--- 1 packet	14	29	40	Trace	Trace	—	—	—	10	3	1	.1	12	Trace	Trace	.01	Trace	Trace
551	Jellies----------- 1 tbsp	18	29	50	Trace	Trace	—	—	—	13	4	1	.3	14	Trace	Trace	.01	Trace	1
552	--- 1 packet	14	29	40	Trace	Trace	—	—	—	10	3	1	.2	11	Trace	Trace	Trace	Trace	1
	Sirups:																		
	Chocolate-flavored sirup or topping:																		
553	Thin type------- 1 fl oz or 2 tbsp	38	32	90	1	1	.5	.3	Trace	24	6	35	.6	106	Trace	.01	.03	.2	0
554	Fudge type------ 1 fl oz or 2 tbsp	38	25	125	2	5	3.1	1.6	.1	20	48	60	.5	107	60	.02	.08	.2	Trace
	Molasses, cane:																		
555	Light (first extraction)--- 1 tbsp	20	24	50	—	—	—	—	—	13	33	9	.9	183	—	.01	.01	Trace	—
556	Blackstrap (third extraction)--- 1 tbsp	20	24	45	—	—	—	—	—	11	137	17	3.2	585	—	.02	.04	.4	—
557	Sorghum---------- 1 tbsp	21	23	55	—	—	—	—	—	14	35	5	2.6	—	—	—	.02	Trace	—
558	Table blends, chiefly corn, light and dark--- 1 tbsp	21	24	60	0	0	0	0	0	15	9	3	.8	1	0	0	0	0	0
	Sugars:																		
559	Brown, pressed down--- 1 cup	220	2	820	0	0	0	0	0	212	187	42	7.5	757	0	.02	.07	.4	0
	White:																		
560	Granulated------- 1 cup	200	1	770	0	0	0	0	0	199	0	0	.2	6	0	0	0	0	0
561	--- 1 tbsp	12	1	45	0	0	0	0	0	12	0	0	Trace	Trace	0	0	0	0	0
562	--- 1 packet	6	1	23	0	0	0	0	0	6	0	0	Trace	Trace	0	0	0	0	0
563	Powdered, sifted, spooned into cup--- 1 cup	100	1	385	0	0	0	0	0	100	0	0	.1	3	0	0	0	0	0

VEGETABLE AND VEGETABLE PRODUCTS

(A)	(B)	(C)	(D)	(E)	(F)	(G)	(H)	(I)	(J)	(K)	(L)	(M)	(N)	(O)	(P)	(Q)	(R)	(S)
	Asparagus, green:																	
	Cooked, drained:																	
	Cuts and tips, 1 1/2- to 2-in lengths:																	
564	From raw---------- 1 cup	94	30	3	Trace	---	---	---	5	30	73	0.9	265	1,310	0.23	0.26	2.0	38
565	From frozen------- 1 cup	93	40	6	Trace	---	---	---	6	40	115	2.2	396	1,530	.25	.23	1.8	41
	Spears, 1/2-in diam. at base:																	
566	From raw---------- 4 spears	94	10	1	Trace	---	---	---	2	13	30	.4	110	540	.10	.11	.8	16
567	From frozen------- 4 spears	92	15	2	Trace	---	---	---	2	10	40	.7	143	470	.10	.08	.7	16
568	Canned, spears, 1/2-in diam. at base. 4 spears	93	15	2	Trace	---	---	---	3	15	42	1.5	133	640	.05	.08	.6	12
	Beans:																	
	Lima, immature seeds, frozen, cooked, drained:																	
569	Thick-seeded types (Fordhooks) 1 cup	74	170	10	Trace	---	---	---	32	34	153	2.9	724	390	.12	.09	1.7	29
570	Thin-seeded types (baby limas) 1 cup	69	210	13	Trace	---	---	---	40	63	227	4.7	709	400	.16	.09	2.2	22
	Snap:																	
	Green:																	
571	From raw (cuts and French style). 1 cup	92	30	2	Trace	---	---	---	7	63	46	.8	189	680	.09	.11	.6	15
	From frozen:																	
572	Cuts--------- 1 cup	92	35	2	Trace	---	---	---	8	54	43	.9	205	780	.09	.12	.5	7
573	French style------- 1 cup	92	35	2	Trace	---	---	---	9	49	39	1.2	177	690	.08	.10	.4	9
574	Canned, drained solids (cuts). 1 cup	92	30	2	Trace	---	---	---	7	61	34	2.0	128	630	.04	.07	.4	5
	Yellow or wax:																	
	Cooked, drained:																	
575	From raw (cuts and French style). 1 cup	93	30	2	Trace	---	---	---	6	63	46	.8	189	290	.09	.11	.6	16
576	From frozen (cuts)------ 1 cup	92	35	2	Trace	---	---	---	8	47	42	.9	221	140	.09	.11	.5	8
577	Canned, drained solids (cuts). 1 cup	92	30	2	Trace	---	---	---	7	61	34	2.0	128	140	.04	.07	.4	7
	Beans, mature. See Beans, dry (items 509-515) and Blackeye peas, dry (item 516).																	
	Bean sprouts (mung):																	
578	Raw----------- 1 cup	89	35	4	Trace	---	---	---	7	20	67	1.4	234	20	.14	.14	.8	20
579	Cooked, drained------- 1 cup	91	35	4	Trace	---	---	---	7	21	60	1.1	195	30	.11	.13	.9	8
	Beets:																	
	Cooked, drained, peeled:																	
580	Whole beets, 2-in diam.------ 2 beets	91	30	1	1	---	---	---	7	14	23	.5	208	20	.03	.04	.3	6
581	Diced or sliced------ 1 cup	91	55	2	1	---	---	---	12	24	39	.9	354	30	.05	.07	.5	10
	Canned, drained solids:																	
582	Whole beets, small----- 1 cup	89	60	2	Trace	---	---	---	14	30	29	1.1	267	30	.02	.05	.2	5
583	Diced or sliced------ 1 cup	89	65	2	Trace	---	---	---	15	32	31	1.2	284	30	.02	.05	.2	5
584	Beet greens, leaves and stems, cooked, drained. 1 cup	94	25	2	Trace	---	---	---	5	144	36	2.8	481	7,400	.10	.22	.4	22
	Blackeye peas, immature seeds, cooked and drained:																	
585	From raw----------- 1 cup	72	180	13	1	---	---	---	30	40	241	3.5	625	580	.50	.18	2.3	28
586	From frozen---------- 1 cup	66	220	15	1	---	---	---	40	43	286	4.8	573	290	.68	.19	2.4	15
	Broccoli, cooked, drained:																	
	From raw:																	
587	Stalk, medium size------ 1 stalk	91	45	6	1	---	---	---	8	158	112	1.4	481	4,500	.16	.36	1.4	162
588	Stalks cut into 1/2-in pieces- 1 cup	91	40	5	Trace	---	---	---	7	136	96	1.2	414	3,880	.14	.31	1.2	140
	From frozen:																	
589	Stalk, 4 1/2 to 5 in long----- 1 stalk	91	10	1	Trace	---	---	---	1	12	17	.2	66	570	.02	.03	.2	22
590	Chopped----------- 1 cup	92	50	5	1	---	---	---	9	100	104	1.3	392	4,810	.11	.22	.9	105
591	Brussels sprouts, cooked, drained: From raw, 7-8 sprouts (1 1/4- to 1 1/2-in diam.). 1 cup	88	55	7	1	---	---	---	10	50	112	1.7	423	810	.12	.22	1.2	135
592	From frozen--------- 1 cup	89	50	5	Trace	---	---	---	10	33	95	1.2	457	880	.12	.16	.9	126

NUTRITIVE VALUES OF THE EDIBLE PART OF FOODS - Continued

[Dashes (—) denote lack of reliable data for a constituent believed to be present in measurable amount]

VEGETABLE AND VEGETABLE PRODUCTS—Con.

Item No. (A)	Foods, approximate measures, units, and weight (edible part unless footnotes indicate otherwise) (B)	Grams	Water (C) Percent	Food energy (D) Calories	Protein (E) Grams	Fat (F) Grams	Fatty Acids Saturated (total) (G) Grams	Unsaturated Oleic (H) Grams	Unsaturated Linoleic (I) Grams	Carbohydrate (J) Grams	Calcium (K) Milligrams	Phosphorus (L) Milligrams	Iron (M) Milligrams	Potassium (N) Milligrams	Vitamin A value (O) International units	Thiamin (P) Milligrams	Riboflavin (Q) Milligrams	Niacin (R) Milligrams	Ascorbic acid (S) Milligrams
	Cabbage:																		
	Common varieties:																		
	Raw:																		
593	Coarsely shredded or sliced—1 cup	70	92	15	1	Trace	—	—	—	4	34	20	0.3	163	90	0.04	0.04	0.2	33
594	Finely shredded or chopped—1 cup	90	92	20	1	Trace	—	—	—	5	44	26	.4	210	120	.05	.05	.3	42
595	Cooked, drained—1 cup	145	94	30	2	Trace	—	—	—	6	64	29	.4	236	190	.06	.06	.4	48
596	Red, raw, coarsely shredded or sliced—1 cup	70	90	20	1	Trace	—	—	—	5	29	25	.6	188	30	.06	.04	.3	43
597	Savoy, raw, coarsely shredded or sliced—1 cup	70	92	15	2	Trace	—	—	—	3	47	38	.6	188	140	.04	.06	.2	39
598	Cabbage, celery (also called pe-tsai or wongbok), raw, 1-in pieces—1 cup	75	95	10	1	—	—	—	—	2	32	30	.5	190	110	.04	.03	.5	19
599	Cabbage, white mustard (also called bokchoy or pakchoy), cooked, drained—1 cup	170	95	25	2	Trace	—	—	—	4	252	56	1.0	364	5,270	.07	.14	1.2	26
	Carrots:																		
	Raw, without crowns and tips, scraped:																		
600	Whole, 7 1/2 by 1 1/8 in, or strips, 2 1/2 to 3 in. long—1 carrot or 18 strips	72	88	30	1	Trace	—	—	—	7	27	26	.5	246	7,930	.04	.04	.4	6
601	Grated—1 cup	110	88	45	1	Trace	—	—	—	11	41	40	.8	375	12,100	.07	.06	.7	9
602	Cooked (crosswise cuts), drained—1 cup	155	91	50	1	Trace	—	—	—	11	51	48	.9	344	16,280	.08	.08	.8	9
	Canned:																		
603	Sliced, drained solids—1 cup	155	91	45	1	Trace	—	—	—	10	47	34	1.1	186	23,250	.03	.05	.6	3
604	Strained or junior (baby food)—1 oz (1 3/4 to 2 tbsp)	28	92	10	Trace	Trace	—	—	—	2	7	6	.1	51	3,690	.01	.01	.1	1
	Cauliflower:																		
605	Raw, chopped—1 cup	115	91	31	3	Trace	—	—	—	6	29	64	1.3	339	70	.13	.12	.8	90
	Cooked, drained:																		
606	From raw (flower buds)—1 cup	125	93	30	3	Trace	—	—	—	5	26	53	.9	258	80	.11	.10	.8	69
607	From frozen (flowerets)—1 cup	180	94	30	3	Trace	—	—	—	6	31	68	.9	373	50	.07	.09	.7	74
608	Celery, Pascal type, raw: Stalk, large outer, 8 by 1 1/2 in, at root end—1 stalk	40	94	5	Trace	Trace	—	—	—	2	16	11	.1	136	110	.01	.01	.1	4
609	Pieces, diced—1 cup	120	94	20	1	Trace	—	—	—	5	47	34	.4	409	320	.04	.04	.4	11
	Collards, cooked, drained:																		
610	From raw (leaves without stems)—1 cup	190	90	65	7	1	—	—	—	10	357	99	1.5	498	14,820	.21	.38	2.3	144
611	From frozen (chopped)—1 cup	170	90	50	5	1	—	—	—	10	299	87	1.7	401	11,560	.10	.24	1.0	56
	Corn, sweet:																		
612	Cooked, drained: From raw, ear 5 by 1 3/4 in—1 ear[61]	140	74	70	2	1	—	—	—	16	2	69	.5	151	310	.09	.08	1.1	7
	From frozen:																		
613	Ear, 5 in long—1 ear[61]	229	73	120	4	1	—	—	—	27	4	121	1.0	291	[62]440	.18	.10	2.1	9
614	Kernels—1 cup	165	77	130	5	1	—	—	—	31	5	120	1.3	304	[62]580	.15	.10	2.5	8
	Canned:																		
615	Cream style—1 cup	256	76	210	5	2	—	—	—	51	8	143	1.5	248	[62]840	.08	.13	2.6	13
	Whole kernel:																		
616	Vacuum pack—1 cup	210	76	175	5	1	—	—	—	43	6	153	1.1	204	[62]740	.06	.13	2.3	11
617	Wet pack, drained solids—1 cup	165	76	140	4	1	—	—	—	33	8	81	.8	160	[62]580	.05	.08	1.5	7
	Cowpeas. See Blackeye peas. (Items 585-586).																		
	Cucumber slices, 1/8 in thick (large, 2 1/8-in diam.; small, 1 3/4-in diam.):																		
618	With peel—6 large or 8 small slices	28	95	5	Trace	Trace	—	—	—	1	7	8	.3	45	70	.01	.01	.1	3

(A)	(B)		(C)	(D)	(E)	(F)	(G)	(H)	(I)	(J)	(K)	(L)	(M)	(N)	(O)	(P)	(Q)	(R)	(S)
619	Without peel---- 6 1/2 large or 9 small pieces.	28	96	5	Trace	Trace	—	—	—	1	1	5	0.1	45	Trace	0.01	0.01	0.1	3
620	Dandelion greens, cooked, drained---- 1 cup----	105	90	35	2	1	—	—	—	7	147	44	1.9	244	12,290	.14	.17		19
621	Endive, curly (including escarole), raw, small pieces---- 1 cup----	50	93	10	1	Trace	—	—	—	2	41	27	.9	147	1,650	.04	.07	.3	5
	Kale, cooked, drained:																		
622	From raw (leaves without stems and midribs)---- 1 cup----	110	88	45	5	1	—	—	—	7	206	64	1.8	243	9,130	.11	.20	1.8	102
623	From frozen (leaf style)---- 1 cup----	130	91	40	4	1	—	—	—	7	157	62	1.3	251	10,660	.08	.20	.9	49
	Lettuce, raw: Butterhead, as Boston types:																		
624	Head, 5-in diam[63]---- 1 head[63]----	220	95	25	2	Trace	—	—	—	4	57	42	3.3	430	1,580	.10	.10	.5	13
625	Leaves---- 1 outer or 2 inner or 3 heart leaves.	15	95	Trace	Trace	Trace	—	—	—	Trace	5	4	.3	40	150	.01	.01	Trace	1
	Crisphead, as Iceberg:																		
626	Head, 6-in diam[64]---- 1 head[64]----	567	96	70	5	1	—	—	—	16	108	118	2.7	943	1,780	.32	.32	1.6	32
627	Wedge, 1/4 of head---- 1 wedge----	135	96	20	1	Trace	—	—	—	4	27	30	.7	236	450	.08	.08	.4	8
628	Pieces, chopped or shredded---- 1 cup----	55	96	5	Trace	Trace	—	—	—	2	11	12	.3	96	180	.03	.03	.2	3
629	Looseleaf (bunching varieties including romaine or cos), chopped or shredded pieces---- 1 cup----	55	94	10	1	Trace	—	—	—	2	37	14	.8	145	1,050	.03	.04	.2	10
630	Mushrooms, raw, sliced or chopped---- 1 cup----	70	90	20	2	Trace	—	—	—	3	4	81	.6	290	Trace	.07	.32	2.9	2
631	Mustard greens, without stems and midribs, cooked, drained---- 1 cup----	140	93	30	3	1	—	—	—	6	193	45	2.5	308	8,120	.11	.20	.8	67
632	Okra pods, 3 by 5/8 in, cooked---- 10 pods----	106	91	30	2	Trace	—	—	—	6	98	43	.5	184	520	.14	.19	1.0	21
	Onions: Mature: Raw:																		
633	Chopped---- 1 cup----	170	89	65	3	Trace	—	—	—	15	46	61	.9	267	[65]Trace	.05	.05	.3	17
634	Sliced---- 1 cup----	115	89	45	2	Trace	—	—	—	10	31	41	.6	181	[65]Trace	.03	.05	.2	12
635	Cooked (whole or sliced), drained---- 1 cup----	210	92	60	3	Trace	—	—	—	14	50	61	.8	231	[65]Trace	.06	.06	.4	15
636	Young green, bulb (3/8 in diam.) and white portion of top---- 6 onions----	30	88	15	Trace	Trace	—	—	—	3	12	12	.2	69	Trace	.02	.01	.1	8
637	Parsley, raw, chopped---- 1 tbsp----	4	85	Trace	Trace	Trace	—	—	—	Trace	7	2	.2	25	300	Trace	.01	Trace	6
638	Parsnips, cooked (diced or 2-in lengths)---- 1 cup----	155	82	100	2	1	—	—	—	23	70	96	.9	587	50	.11	.12	.2	16
	Peas, green: Canned:																		
639	Whole, drained solids---- 1 cup----	170	77	150	8	1	—	—	—	29	44	129	3.2	163	1,170	.15	.10	1.4	14
640	Strained (baby food)---- 1 oz (1 3/4 to 2 tbsp)----	28	86	15	1	Trace	—	—	—	3	3	18	.3	28	140	.02	.03	.3	3
641	Frozen, cooked, drained---- 1 cup----	160	82	110	8	Trace	—	—	—	19	30	138	3.0	216	960	.43	.14	2.7	21
642	Peppers, hot, red, without seeds, dried (ground chili powder, added seasonings)---- 1 tsp----	2	9	5	Trace	Trace	—	—	—	1	5	4	.3	20	1,300	Trace	.02	.2	Trace
	Peppers, sweet (about 5 per lb, whole), stem and seeds removed:																		
643	Raw---- 1 pod----	74	93	15	1	Trace	—	—	—	4	7	16	.5	157	310	.06	.06	.4	94
644	Cooked, boiled, drained---- 1 pod----	73	95	15	1	Trace	—	—	—	3	7	12	.4	109	310	.05	.05	.4	70
	Potatoes, cooked:																		
645	Baked, peeled after baking (about 2 per lb, raw)---- 1 potato----	156	75	145	4	Trace	—	—	—	33	14	101	1.1	782	Trace	.15	.07	2.7	31
	Boiled (about 3 per lb, raw):																		
646	Peeled after boiling---- 1 potato----	137	80	105	3	Trace	—	—	—	23	10	72	.8	556	Trace	.12	.05	2.0	22
647	Peeled before boiling---- 1 potato----	135	83	90	3	Trace	—	—	—	20	8	57	.7	385	Trace	.12	.05	1.6	22
	French-fried, strip, 2 to 3 1/2 in long:																		
648	Prepared from raw---- 10 strips----	50	45	135	2	7	1.7	1.2	3.3	18	8	56	.7	427	Trace	.07	.04	1.6	11
649	Frozen, oven heated---- 10 strips----	50	53	110	2	4	1.1	.8	2.1	17	5	43	.9	326	Trace	.07	.01	1.3	11
650	Hashed brown, prepared from frozen---- 1 cup----	155	56	345	3	18	4.6	3.2	9.0	45	28	78	1.9	439	Trace	.11	.03	1.6	12
	Mashed, prepared from— Raw:																		
651	Milk added---- 1 cup----	210	83	135	4	2	.7	.4	Trace	27	50	103	.8	548	40	.17	.11	2.1	21

[61] Weight includes cob. Without cob, weight is 77 g for item 612, 126 g for item 613.
[62] Based on yellow varieties. For white varieties, value is trace.
[63] Weight includes refuse of outer leaves and core. Without these parts, weight is 163 g.
[64] Weight includes core. Without core, weight is 539 g.
[65] Value based on white-fleshed varieties. For yellow-fleshed varieties, value in International Units (I.U.) is 70 for item 633, 50 for item 634, and 80 for item 635.

NUTRITIVE VALUES OF THE EDIBLE PART OF FOODS - Continued

(Dashes (—) denote lack of reliable data for a constituent believed to be present in measurable amount)

Item No. (A)	Foods, approximate measures, units, and weight (edible part unless footnotes indicate otherwise) (B)	Grams	Water (C) Percent	Food energy (D) Calories	Protein (E) Grams	Fat (F) Grams	Fatty Acids Saturated (total) (G) Grams	Unsaturated Oleic (H) Grams	Unsaturated Linoleic (I) Grams	Carbohydrate (J) Grams	Calcium (K) Milligrams	Phosphorus (L) Milligrams	Iron (M) Milligrams	Potassium (N) Milligrams	Vitamin A value (O) International units	Thiamin (P) Milligrams	Riboflavin (Q) Milligrams	Niacin (R) Milligrams	Ascorbic acid (S) Milligrams
	VEGETABLE AND VEGETABLE PRODUCTS—Con.																		
	Potatoes, cooked—Continued																		
	Mashed, prepared from—Continued																		
652	Milk and butter added----- 1 cup	210	80	195	4	9	5.6	2.3	0.2	26	50	101	0.8	525	360	0.17	0.11	2.1	19
653	Dehydrated flakes (without milk), water, milk, butter, and salt added. 1 cup	210	79	195	4	7	3.6	2.1	.2	30	65	99	.6	601	270	.08	.08	1.9	11
654	Potato chips, 1 3/4 by 2 1/2 in oval cross section. 10 chips	20	2	115	1	8	2.1	1.4	4.0	10	8	28	.4	226	Trace	.04	.01	1.0	3
655	Potato salad, made with cooked salad dressing. 1 cup	250	76	250	7	7	2.0	2.7	1.3	41	80	160	1.5	798	350	.20	.18	2.8	28
656	Pumpkin, canned--------- 1 cup	245	90	80	2	1	—	—	—	19	61	64	1.0	588	15,680	.07	.12	1.5	12
657	Radishes, raw (prepackaged) stem ends, rootlets cut off. 4 radishes	18	95	5	Trace	Trace	—	—	—	1	5	6	.2	58	Trace	.01	.01	.1	5
658	Sauerkraut, canned, solids and liquid. 1 cup	235	93	40	2	Trace	—	—	—	9	85	42	1.2	329	120	.07	.09	.5	33
	Southern peas. See Blackeye peas (items 585-586).																		
	Spinach:																		
659	Raw, chopped-------- 1 cup	55	91	15	2	Trace	—	—	—	2	51	28	1.7	259	4,460	.06	.11	.3	28
	Cooked, drained:																		
660	From raw--------- 1 cup	180	92	40	5	1	—	—	—	6	167	68	4.0	583	14,580	.13	.25	.9	50
	From frozen:																		
661	Chopped-------- 1 cup	205	92	45	6	1	—	—	—	8	232	90	4.3	683	16,200	.14	.31	.8	39
662	Leaf-------- 1 cup	190	92	45	6	1	—	—	—	7	200	84	4.8	688	15,390	.15	.27	1.0	53
663	Canned, drained solids-------- 1 cup	205	91	50	6	1	—	—	—	7	242	53	5.3	513	16,400	.04	.25	.6	29
	Squash, cooked:																		
664	Summer (all varieties), diced, drained. 1 cup	210	96	30	2	Trace	—	—	—	7	53	53	.8	296	820	.11	.17	1.7	21
665	Winter (all varieties), baked, mashed. 1 cup	205	81	130	4	1	—	—	—	32	57	98	1.6	945	8,610	.10	.27	1.4	27
	Sweetpotatoes:																		
	Cooked (raw, 5 by 2 in; about 2 1/2 per lb):																		
666	Baked in skin, peeled------- 1 potato	114	64	160	2	1	—	—	—	37	46	66	1.0	342	9,230	.10	.08	.8	25
667	Boiled in skin, peeled------- 1 potato	151	71	170	3	1	—	—	—	40	48	71	1.1	367	11,940	.14	.09	.9	26
668	Candied, 2 1/2 by 2-in piece------- 1 piece	105	60	175	1	3	2.0	.8	.1	36	39	45	.9	200	6,620	.06	.04	.4	11
	Canned:																		
669	Solid pack (mashed)------- 1 cup	255	72	275	5	1	—	—	—	63	64	105	2.0	510	19,890	.13	.10	1.5	36
670	Vacuum pack, piece 2 3/4 by 1 in. 1 piece	40	72	45	1	Trace	—	—	—	10	10	16	.3	80	3,120	.02	.02	.2	6
	Tomatoes:																		
671	Raw, 2 3/5-in diam. (3 per 12 oz pkg.). 1 tomato[66]	135	94	25	1	Trace	—	—	—	6	16	33	.6	300	1,110	.07	.05	.9	[6,7]28
672	Canned, solids and liquid------- 1 cup	241	94	50	2	Trace	—	—	—	10	[6,8]14	46	1.2	523	2,170	.12	.07	1.7	41
673	Tomato catsup------- 1 cup	273	69	290	5	1	—	—	—	69	60	137	2.2	991	3,820	.25	.19	4.4	41
674	------- 1 tbsp	15	69	15	Trace	Trace	—	—	—	4	3	8	.1	54	210	.01	.01	.2	2
	Tomato juice, canned:																		
675	Cup------- 1 cup	243	94	45	2	Trace	—	—	—	10	17	44	2.2	552	1,940	.12	.07	1.9	39
676	Glass (6 fl oz)------- 1 glass	182	94	35	2	Trace	—	—	—	8	13	33	1.6	413	1,460	.09	.05	1.5	29
677	Turnips, cooked, diced------- 1 cup	155	94	35	1	Trace	—	—	—	8	54	37	.6	291	Trace	.06	.08	.5	34
	Turnip greens, cooked, drained:																		
678	From raw (leaves and stems)------- 1 cup	145	94	30	3	Trace	—	—	—	5	252	49	1.5	—	8,270	.15	.33	.7	68
679	From frozen (chopped)------- 1 cup	165	93	40	4	Trace	—	—	—	6	195	64	2.6	246	11,390	.08	.15	.7	31
680	Vegetables, mixed, frozen, cooked------- 1 cup	182	83	115	6	1	—	—	—	24	46	115	2.4	348	9,010	.22	.13	2.0	15

MISCELLANEOUS ITEMS

(A)	(B)	(C)	(D)	(E)	(F)	(G)	(H)	(I)	(J)	(K)	(L)	(M)	(N)	(O)	(P)	(Q)	(R)	(S)
	Baking powders for home use:																	
	Sodium aluminum sulfate:																	
681	With monocalcium phosphate monohydrate. — 1 tsp — 3.0	2	5	Trace	Trace	0	0	0	0	58	87	—	5	0	0	0	0	0
682	With monocalcium phosphate monohydrate, calcium sulfate. — 1 tsp — 2.9	1	5	Trace	Trace	0	0	0	1	183	45	—	—	0	0	0	0	0
683	Straight phosphate — 1 tsp — 3.8	2	5	Trace	Trace	0	0	0	1	239	359	—	6	0	0	0	0	0
684	Low sodium — 1 tsp — 4.3	2	5	Trace	Trace	0	0	0	2	207	314	—	471	0	0	0	0	0
685	Barbecue sauce — 1 cup — 250	81	230	4	17	2.2	4.3	10.0	20	53	50	2.0	435	900	.03	.03	.8	13
	Beverages, alcoholic:																	
686	Beer — 12 fl oz — 360	92	150	1	0	0	0	0	14	18	108	Trace	90	—	.01	.11	2.2	—
	Gin, rum, vodka, whisky:																	
687	80-proof — 1 1/2-fl oz jigger — 42	67	95	—	—	0	0	0	Trace	—	—	—	—	—	—	—	—	—
688	86-proof — 1 1/2-fl oz jigger — 42	64	105	—	—	0	0	0	Trace	—	—	—	—	—	—	—	—	—
689	90-proof — 1 1/2-fl oz jigger — 42	62	110	—	—	0	0	0	Trace	—	—	—	—	—	—	—	—	—
	Wines:																	
690	Dessert — 3 1/2-fl oz glass — 103	77	140	Trace	0	0	0	0	8	8	—	—	77	—	.01	.02	.2	—
691	Table — 3 1/2-fl oz glass — 102	86	85	Trace	0	0	0	0	4	9	10	.4	94	—	Trace	.01	.1	—
	Beverages, carbonated, sweetened, nonalcoholic:																	
692	Carbonated water — 12 fl oz — 366	92	115	0	0	0	0	0	29	—	—	—	—	0	0	0	0	0
693	Cola type — 12 fl oz — 369	90	145	0	0	0	0	0	37	—	—	—	—	0	0	0	0	0
694	Fruit-flavored sodas and Tom Collins mixer. — 12 fl oz — 372	88	170	0	0	0	0	0	45	—	—	—	—	0	0	0	0	0
695	Ginger ale — 12 fl oz — 366	92	115	0	0	0	0	0	29	—	—	—	0	0	0	0	0	0
696	Root beer — 12 fl oz — 370	90	150	0	0	0	0	0	39	—	—	—	0	0	0	0	0	0
	Chili powder. See Peppers, hot, red (item 642).																	
	Chocolate:																	
697	Bitter or baking — 1 oz — 28	2	145	3	15	8.9	4.9	.4	8	22	109	1.9	235	20	.01	.07	.4	0
	Semisweet, see Candy, chocolate (item 539).																	
698	Gelatin, dry — 1 7-g envelope — 7	13	25	6	Trace	0	0	0	0	—	—	—	—	—	—	—	—	—
699	Gelatin dessert prepared with gelatin dessert powder and water. — 1 cup — 240	84	140	4	0	0	0	0	34	—	—	—	—	—	—	—	—	—
700	Mustard, prepared, yellow — 1 tsp or individual serving pouch or cup. — 5	80	5	Trace	Trace	—	—	Trace	Trace	4	4	.1	7	—	Trace	Trace	—	—
	Olives, pickled, canned:																	
701	Green — 4 medium or 3 extra large or 2 giant.[69] — 16	78	15	Trace	2	.2	1.2	.1	Trace	8	2	.2	7	40	—	—	—	—
702	Ripe, Mission — 3 small or 2 large[69] — 10	73	15	Trace	2	.2	1.2	.1	Trace	9	1	.1	2	10	Trace	Trace	—	—
	Pickles, cucumber:																	
703	Dill, medium, whole, 3 3/4 in long, 1 1/4-in diam. — 1 pickle — 65	93	5	Trace	Trace	—	—	Trace	1	17	14	.7	130	70	Trace	.01	Trace	4
704	Fresh-pack, slices 1 1/2-in diam. 1/4 in thick. — 2 slices — 15	79	10	Trace	Trace	—	—	—	3	5	4	.3	—	20	Trace	Trace	Trace	1
705	Sweet, gherkin, small, whole, about 2 1/2 in long, 3/4-in diam. — 1 pickle — 15	61	20	Trace	Trace	—	—	—	5	2	2	.2	—	10	Trace	Trace	Trace	1
706	Relish, finely chopped, sweet — 1 tbsp — 15	63	20	Trace	Trace	—	—	—	5	3	2	.1	—	—	—	—	—	—
	Popcorn. See items 476-478.																	
707	Popsicle, 3-fl oz size — 1 popsicle — 95	80	70	0	0	0	0	0	18	0	—	Trace	—	0	0	0	0	0

[66] Weight includes cores and stem ends. Without these parts, weight is 123 g.
[67] Based on year-round average. For tomatoes marketed from November through May, value is about 12 mg; from June through October, 32 mg.
[68] Applies to product without calcium salts added. Value for products with calcium salts added may be as much as 63 mg for whole tomatoes, 241 mg for cut forms.
[69] Weight includes pits. Without pits, weight is 13 g for item 701, 9 g for item 702.

TABLE 2.— NUTRITIVE VALUES OF THE EDIBLE PART OF FOODS - Continued

(Dashes (—) denote lack of reliable data for a constituent believed to be present in measurable amount)

(A) Item No.	(B) Foods, approximate measures, units, and weight (edible part unless footnotes indicate otherwise)		Grams	(C) Water Percent	(D) Food energy Calories	(E) Protein Grams	(F) Fat Grams	(G) Saturated (total) Grams	(H) Oleic Grams	(I) Linoleic Grams	(I) Carbohydrate Grams	(K) Calcium Milligrams	(L) Phosphorus Milligrams	(M) Iron Milligrams	(N) Potassium Milligrams	(O) Vitamin A value International units	(P) Thiamin Milligrams	(Q) Riboflavin Milligrams	(R) Niacin Milligrams	(S) Ascorbic acid Milligrams
	MISCELLANEOUS ITEMS—Con.																			
	Soups:																			
	Canned, condensed:																			
	Prepared with equal volume of milk:																			
708	Cream of chicken	1 cup	245	85	180	7	10	4.2	3.6	1.3	15	172	152	0.5	260	610	0.05	0.27	0.7	2
709	Cream of mushroom	1 cup	245	83	215	7	14	5.4	2.9	4.6	16	191	169	.5	279	250	.05	.34	.7	1
710	Tomato	1 cup	250	84	175	7	7	3.4	1.7	1.0	23	168	155	.8	418	1,200	.10	.25	1.3	15
	Prepared with equal volume of water:																			
711	Bean with pork	1 cup	250	84	170	8	6	1.2	1.8	2.4	22	63	128	2.3	395	650	.13	.08	1.0	3
712	Beef broth, bouillon, consomme.	1 cup	240	96	30	5	0	0	0	0	3	Trace	31	.5	130	Trace	Trace	.02	1.2	—
713	Beef noodle	1 cup	240	93	65	4	3	.6	.7	.8	7	7	48	1.0	77	50	.05	.07	1.0	Trace
714	Clam chowder, Manhattan type (with tomatoes, without milk).	1 cup	245	92	80	2	3	.5	.4	1.3	12	34	47	1.0	184	880	.02	.02	1.0	—
715	Cream of chicken	1 cup	240	92	95	3	6	1.6	2.3	1.1	8	24	34	.5	79	410	.02	.05	.5	Trace
716	Cream of mushroom	1 cup	240	90	135	2	10	2.6	1.7	4.5	10	41	50	.5	98	70	.02	.12	.7	Trace
717	Minestrone	1 cup	245	90	105	5	3	1.1	.9	1.3	14	37	59	1.0	314	2,350	.07	.05	1.0	—
718	Split pea	1 cup	245	85	145	9	3	1.1	1.2	.4	21	29	149	1.5	270	440	.25	.15	1.5	1
719	Tomato	1 cup	245	91	90	2	3	.5	.5	1.0	16	15	34	.7	230	1,000	.05	.05	1.2	12
720	Vegetable beef	1 cup	245	92	80	5	2	—	—	—	10	12	49	.7	162	2,700	.05	.05	1.0	—
721	Vegetarian	1 cup	245	92	80	2	2	—	—	—	13	20	39	1.0	172	2,940	.05	.05	1.0	—
	Dehydrated:																			
722	Bouillon cube, 1/2 in	1 cube	4	4	5	1	Trace	—	—	—	Trace	—	—	—	4	—	—	—	—	—
	Mixes:																			
	Unprepared:																			
723	Onion	1 1/2-oz pkg	43	3	150	6	5	1.1	2.3	1.0	23	42	49	.6	238	30	.05	.03	.3	6
	Prepared with water:																			
724	Chicken noodle	1 cup	240	95	55	2	1	—	—	—	8	7	19	.2	19	50	.07	.05	.5	Trace
725	Onion	1 cup	240	96	35	1	1	—	—	—	6	10	12	.2	58	Trace	Trace	Trace	Trace	2
726	Tomato vegetable with noodles.	1 cup	240	93	65	1	1	—	—	—	12	7	19	.2	29	480	.05	.02	.5	5
727	Vinegar, cider	1 tbsp	15	94	Trace	Trace	0	0	0	0	1	1	1	.1	15	—	—	—	—	—
728	White sauce, medium, with enriched flour.	1 cup	250	73	405	10	31	19.3	7.8	.8	22	288	233	.5	348	1,150	.12	.43	.7	2
	Yeast:																			
729	Baker's, dry, active	1 pkg	7	5	20	3	Trace	—	—	—	3	3	90	1.1	140	Trace	.16	.38	2.6	Trace
730	Brewer's, dry	1 tbsp	8	5	25	3	Trace	—	—	—	3	[70]17	140	1.4	152	Trace	1.25	.34	3.0	Trace

[70]Value may vary from 6 to 60 mg.

APPENDIX B

Teaching Ideas

The purpose of this appendix is to suggest various learning experiences for both teacher and student in the areas of nutrition and weight control. The material is mainly geared for teaching on the secondary level, but many of the ideas are flexible and allow for modification and adaptation to individual curricula and needs.

Also provided is a list of agencies and associations which are potential sources of nutrition education information and materials to aid you in teaching and in stimulating student interest.

The appendix is in no way meant to be the last word in nutrition education. Build on it, modify it to meet your individual needs, but by all means, be innovative in your approach to this very contemporary subject!

LESSON PLANS

Objective: The student will be able to identify the major nutrients and their roles in the body, and be able to choose foods for an individualized, sound diet.

NECESSARY NUTRIENTS

Concept: The substances in food which provide nourishment and perform certain functions in the body are called nutrients.

Learning Activity. Flash cards with each nutrient's name on one side and its function on the reverse side. These can be used for competition games, individual study, test review and learning in pairs.

Concept: An individual must consider several factors in making food selections.

Learning Activity. Special project and report
Assign several students to visit a local market and discover the comparative costs of protein-rich foods available. Have them calculate the cost per serving of each food and decide which foods are the best buys. Have one student report findings to the class, and provide written copies of results to all.

Concept: The healthy person makes wise choices in selecting foods for meals and snacks.

Learning Activity. Current Status of the Teenage Diet: A Survey
Select several students to conduct a survey among their classmates to determine common excesses and deficiencies of carbohydrates, fats, proteins, vitamins and

minerals in the teenage diet. Results of the survey may be reported in a panel discussion with the student surveyors acting as the panel of experts. Suggestions should be made as to how to vary caloric and nutrient intake for a sound diet and weight control.

Learning Activity. Present three menus to the class and encourage discussion on such questions as: a) Is the U.S. RDA met in every case? b) Is more food energy needed? If so, what foods would you supply? c) If more food or nutrients are needed, from what food groups would you select? d) Any changes or substitutions in snacks? e) How could you modify the menu if you were overweight? If you were on a very limited budget?

Concept: Each nutrient has specific functions in the body, but the amounts needed by an individual vary according to age, size, sex, activity, and health status.

Learning Activity. Students are divided into several committees to report on specific nutritional needs and hazards in such groups as: a) pregnant women, b) diabetics, c) alcoholics, d) teenagers, e) the elderly (over sixty-five), f) children, g) athletes, and h) heart disease patients.

Special Learning Activity. Experimental Tests for Determining Presence of Starch and Minerals in Various Foods.

Starch Test. 1) Make test solution by adding 10 ml tincture of iodine to 500 ml cold water and stirring until mixed.
2) Select several different foods and test for presence of starch by dropping a small amount of the solution on the food with a medicine dropper. Presence of starch is indicated by a purple color.
3) Experiment may be conducted as a demonstration by the instructor, or as a project by the students, who mark an answer sheet as they proceed to indicate the foods that contain starch.

(Note to teacher: Starch is a carbohydrate found in some foods, but some carbohydrate foods do not contain it.)

Mineral Test. 1) Materials needed: several different foods, aluminum foil, hot plate.
2) Place each food piece on its own section of foil and place in a pan on the hot plate. Allow to burn until only ashes remain.
3) Minerals do not burn, so if ashes are left the food contains minerals.
4) This experiment may be either a demonstration by the teacher or a project by the students themselves.

Objective: The student will understand the importance of vitamins in proper nutrition and will identify how each vitamin and mineral contributes to the particular health needs of his/her age group.

Concept: Vitamins and minerals are a necessary part of a balanced diet.

Learning Activity. Assign special reports on individual vitamins and minerals and how they contribute to health. Reports may be presented briefly in class with a worksheet for each student to complete as an aid in taking notes. An example of a worksheet follows:

Vitamin (or Mineral):
Fat or Water Soluble:
Function in the Body:
Effect on body when deficient:
Any harmful effects of overdose or excess:
Excellent food sources of the nutrient:
Good food sources of the nutrient:
RDA:

Learning Activity. For younger groups, role play the major vitamin and mineral deficiency diseases. A student describes symptoms and presumed diet (which would be deficient or inadequate in the specific nutrient). The remaining students guess what the particular disease is and how to correct or prevent it. This can be conducted with the class divided into teams.

Learning Activity. "Fact or Misconception?" Exercise
Each student identifies a popular belief or idea about a particular nutrient such as vitamin C or protein. Assign each student to use library research to either validate or invalidate the claim according to recent studies. The instructor may wish to compile a list of common misconceptions from the results of the students' study.

Concept: Fluoride, a necessary trace element, can be supplied in the diet through drinking fluoridated water.

Learning Activity. Debate the pros and cons of fluoridation of the public water supply, following study and preparation by the student panel members. After the debate, summarize recent scientific findings and common fallacies and misconceptions.

Objective: Each student will evaluate his or her diet for a week by recording intake and comparing it to that recommended for the particular age group.

Learning Activity. Each student records complete dietary intake for a full 24-hour period on the following sheet (see Table B-1). He or she then calculates the nutritional value of each item, recording it in the columns provided for the various nutrients. They may be done with the aid of labeling information on food packages and additional charts and information provided by the teacher.

The student then evaluates his or her diet for a week according to the Basic Four Food Groups summary chart, as shown in Table B-2.

Objective: Each student will evaluate the nutritional value of four different cereal products according to the nutritional information provided on the package or label.

Learning Activity. Each student chooses four different cereal products and completes a nutritional information sheet (similar to the one detailed below) for each of the four products.

NUTRITION INFORMATION

Name and brand of food _____
Number of servings per container _____
Serving size _____

calories _____ protein _____

carbohydrate _____ fat _____

Percentages of U.S. RDA provided: _____

Protein _____ Riboflavin (B_2) _____

Vitamin A _____ Niacin _____

Vitamin C _____ Calcium _____

Thiamine (B_1) _____ Iron _____

FIBER *Objective:* The student will recognize the need for sufficient fiber in his/her diet and know how to obtain it.

Concept: Adequate dietary fiber is essential for maintenance of optimal health.

Learning Activity. Instructor researches the latest scientific findings on the relationship between certain disorders or diseases, such as colonic cancer, diverticulosis, and hemorrhoids, and consumption of dietary fiber, and then presents a lecture and discussion with the use of overhead transparencies or a slide-cassette recorder.

Concept: Various foods are good sources of dietary fiber.

Learning Activity. As an at-home assignment, have each student list as many commonly eaten foods as possible that are at least good sources of fiber in the diet. In class request each student to name one food on his/her list, alternating until all have been mentioned. (This exercise could be used particularly as an introduction to the section on fiber, possibly as a preassessment technique.) The instructor then compiles a list of the foods, ranking the foods in order from fair to excellent sources of fiber.

Table B-1. 24-Hour Food and Drink Record Calculation Sheet

Meal B=breakfast S=snack L=lunch D=dinner	Food	Size Serving S=small M=medium L=large	Calories	Protein gm	Fat gm	Fatty Acids Saturated gm	Fatty Acids Linoleic gm	Carbo-hydrate gm	Calcium mg	Iron mg	Vitamin A IU	Thiamine mg	Riboflavin mg	Niacin mg	Vitamin C mg
Day's Total															
RDAs															
Difference (+ or −)															

B–5

Name _____

Date _____

Table B-2. Summary Evaluation of Basic Four Food Groups

Day	Food	Protein	Milk & Dairy Products	Fruits & Vegetables	Breads & Cereals	Snacks Desserts & Other
1						
2						
3						
4						
5						
6						
7						

Objective: The student will recognize both some advantages and some potential hazards of a vegetarian diet.

Concept: A nutritionally balanced vegetarian diet requires considerable planning and evaluation.

Learning Activity. Discuss the specific dietary needs of vegetarians and how these needs can be economically met. This discussion should include emphasis on the need for various protein sources and vitamin B_{12} for strict vegetarians. Ask the class to contribute as many advantages and disadvantages of vegetarianism as they can observe.

Learning Activity. Divide the class into three groups. The first group plans a balanced diet for an adult for one day (three meals), omitting all meats and animal products except eggs, but allowing for consumption of poultry and fish. The second group does the same, but omits poultry and fish while allowing for milk, milk products, and eggs. The third group plans a strict vegetarian diet, omitting all animal flesh and animal products, poultry, fish, and eggs. This exercise can be done in buzz groups under a time limit with a discussion following.

Objective: The student will be able to explain how various controls and safeguards help make our food supply safe for our use.

Concept: Modern methods of food processing and preparation provide us with a wide selection of foods and help safeguard our health.

Learning Activity. Plan a field trip to a restaurant, school cafeteria, milk or food processing plant, and observe all sanitary methods used in preparation, serving, cleanup and/or storage.

Learning Activity. Invite a representative from the County Extension Service, local FDA, or Department of Agriculture or a college professor to present a discussion, film, or other program on governmental controls in food production, e.g., animal diets, use of pesticides, soil conservation and preparation, seed preparation, etc. Invite the representative to also address the issue of organic vs. chemical fertilizers and pest control. Students may also submit questions in advance.

Objective: The student will recognize the role of any food-handler in preventing foodborne disease.

Concept: Improper food handling and/or preparation can cause disease.

Learning Activity. Invite a local health department representative for a discussion on foodborne diseases. After the discussion, provide a brief case history of several common types of food poisonings. Have the students determine (in groups) how the cases in point could have been prevented by proper food-handling techniques. Examples of particular foodborne diseases: (a) Salmonella (from eggs or improperly cooked poultry), (b) Staphylococcus (from improperly prepared or stored potato salad, chicken salad, cream pie, etc., (c) Trichinosis (from improperly cooked pork), (d) Botulism (from improper home canning).

FATS   *Objective:* The student will be able to determine from a variety of commonly eaten fats which are saturated and which are unsaturated.

Concept: A convenient way of evaluating whether a fat is saturated or unsaturated is to remember that saturated fats tend to be more solid at room temperature while unsaturated fats are more liquid.

Learning Activity. A display of the various commonly used fats (i.e. lard, vegetable oils, butter, margarine, etc.) available and a question-answer discussion with the students could be used as a preassessment technique for this concept. The discussion should also involve an explanation (very basic) of the chemical structure of fats and the difference between saturated and unsaturated and why that is important.

Concept: Consumption of less saturated fats and cholesterol may reduce one's risk of heart and circulatory disease.

Learning Activity. Prepare a bulletin board using models or diagrams of commonly eaten foods, comparing the relative amounts of cholesterol and saturated fats they contain. (Amounts per serving can be identified from the labels in most cases.)

Learning Activity. Prepare a copy of a typical high-saturated-fat, high-cholesterol diet for each student. Assign them to substitute foods of lower cholesterol value without changing the nutritional value or eliminating fat from the diet. Discuss possible advantages of reducing saturated fat in the diet.

BREAKFAST   *Objective:* The student will recognize the common excuses for failure to eat an adequate breakfast, and will replace them with reasons in favor of starting the day with breakfast.

Concept: An adequate breakfast is a necessary part of a good family nutrition program.

Learning Activity. Role play involving several students (10–12) divided into two groups. The first group role plays a typical morning scene of the "Breakfast Bandits," a non-breakfast-eating family. Emphasize excuses for not eating breakfast, and possible consequences. The second group then role plays the "Breakfast

Beneficiaries," a family of breakfast eaters. Emphasis should be placed on all types of benefits of eating breakfast—psychological, social, nutritional, familial, etc. Following the role play, class discussion can center on alternative plans and suggestions for changing a non-breakfast-eating family into one that enjoys breakfast together.

Objective: The student will learn to recognize the proper role of sugar in the diet.   ***SUGAR***

Concept: Sugar is not an essential "nutrient" and can actually be detrimental to health when consumed in excess.

Learning Activity. Debate, with each team consisting of four to five students. One team defends the statement "Sugar is necessary in the diet," while the other team defends "Sugar is a poison." Following the debate, summarize the facts presented and identify any misconceptions, emphasizing that neither of the statements is entirely correct.

Learning Activity. Through use of a bulletin board presentation, compare the nutritional value, calories, and cost per serving of white table sugar, brown sugar, and honey.

Objective: The student will be able to evaluate a diet as to its probable validity and safety for weight reduction.   ***DIETING AND WEIGHT CONTROL***

Concept: Careful evaluation is necessary in order to discriminate between a sound reduction program and a fad diet.

Learning Activity. Students collect newspaper/magazine advertisements on crash diets, reducing fads, machines, pills, etc. Discuss the most popular ones and analyze, during class discussion, nutritional deficits, values, potential harmful effects, and fraudulent or misleading claims.

Learning Activity. Brainstorm a checklist of concepts to consider when evaluating any diet as to probable effectiveness and safety. Compile a list for each student. Some examples of items on the checklist should include:

- Does it cause or claim more than a 2 lb/week weight loss?
- Does it contain food choices from all four food groups?
- Does it rely on unusual or unpleasant products in order to be successful?
- Does it cause or promote a change in eating behavior?
- Does it discourage or ignore physical activity?

Concept: A sound weight control or weight reducing program can help improve health status and alleviate some physiological problems.

Learning Activity. Assign two or three students to visit a reputable weight reducing clinic and interview the physician or other professional in charge. Help students plan the questions to ask and the information to obtain for later evaluation. Have the students report their findings to the class.

Concept: Obesity is a growing problem in the United States among all age groups.

Learning Activity. Discuss the physiological conditions or disorders which can be aggravated by obesity. Examples include: arthritis, diabetes, heart disease, high blood pressure, hernia, respiratory difficulty.

Learning Activity. Competition Game
Divide the class into two groups. One student from each team goes to the chalkboard and writes down a disadvantage of obesity. The disadvantages may be psychological, emotional, physiological, or sociological in nature. The team with the most disadvantages (without repetition) at the end of a set time period wins.

SPECIAL TERM PROJECTS

1. Rat experiment in which one group of rats is fed a nutritionally balanced diet, and the other group receives a diet deficient in one or more nutrients. Students are responsible for all care and feeding of the animals. A paper explaining the experiment, observations, and results of the study is required.

2. Several students work together in designing and conducting a public awareness campaign in one of a number of aspects of nutrition and/or weight control. Examples of possible campaigns:
   How to recognize nutritional quackery
   The importance of a good breakfast—a family affair
   The role of fiber
   Dollars and "sense" in meal planning OR How to eat well on a limited budget
   Why fluoridation?
   The project could include selecting an appropriate target population, surveys, posters, radio announcements, displays, fact sheets for distribution, etc.

3. Arrangements may be made with an elementary school principal for interested students to present an assembly for younger children on food, eating, and nutrition. Charts or displays geared to young children's interests and comprehension may be substituted for the assembly.

4. Well-researched, well-documented written reports on specific areas, such as:
   Recent findings on the relationship between cardiovascular disease and trace minerals

Nutrition and brain development
Facts and fallacies about food additives
Why do we eat?
Cultural and/or familial influences and obesity
The use of drugs in weight control: pro and con
Bypass surgery as a means of weight control
Recent findings on vitamin E or vitamin C and their relationship to the
     cure or prevention of disease

5. Students design and conduct a special "quiz show" assembly or meeting
   in which panels of students compete in responding to questions on
   nutrition and weight control. Students make up the questions and
   conduct the assembly and scoring of the contestants.

CROSSWORD PUZZLE

Across:

1. High serum levels of this sterol are often associated with atherosclerosis and heart attack.
4. An excellent source of dietary iron.
6. A major protein source, not consumed by vegetarians.
8. A measurement of energy.
9. Added to salt to prevent goiter.
10. A major source of vitamin D (in the environment).
11. Recommended Daily Allowance (abbr.).
14. An element required in relatively large amounts in the diet (more than 100 mg per day), such as calcium, sodium, or potassium.
15. A term indicating that nutrients have been added beyond the level present before processing.
17. Dietary roughage.
18. The average American adult consumes over 100 lb yearly of this substance—which contributes nothing in the way of nutrients for the body.

Down:

1. Major mineral found in milk
2. A term meaning that the four nutrients niacin, thiamine, riboflavin, and iron have been added to a food.
3. Excessive overweight due to a surplus of body fat.
5. Ascorbic acid, Calciferol, and Tocopherol all belong to this important group of nutrients.
7. Insufficient iodine in the diet may cause simple _____.
12. Its building blocks are amino acids.
13. Consumption of this nutrient provides a concentrated source of energy, and helps in the transport and absorption of certain vitamins in the body.
15. To ensure a balanced diet, we should choose foods daily from the _____ Basic Food Groups.
16. The federal agency (abbr.) that determines the Recommended Daily Allowance and helps ensure the purity of our food supply.

Answers: (Across) 1. cholesterol; 4. liver; 6. meat, 8. calorie, 9. iodine; 10. sun; 11. RDA; 14. macromineral; 15. fortified; 17. fiber; 18. sugar. (Down) 1. calcium; 2. enriched; 3. obesity; 5. vitamin; 7. goiter; 12. protein; 13. fat; 15. four; 16. FDA.

SAMPLE TEST QUESTIONS

(These questions may be used for preassessment, pre-test or post-test.)

1. Many Americans suffer from poor nutrition because
   a. we have so many poor people who don't have the money to buy proper food
   b. our soil is being depleted of the necessary nutrients; therefore, a lot of our food stuff is poor quality
   c. we eat too much of the wrong kinds of food and not enough of the right
   d. our bodies don't handle the breakdown and metabolism of food properly
2. The best way to get the different nutrients we need for body processes is
   a. to eat a wide variety of foods
   b. to take vitamin and mineral supplements
   c. to eat only organically grown foods
   d. to eat large amounts of a limited variety of foods
3. A main function of protein is to provide
   a. quick energy to the body systems
   b. materials for building and maintaining body tissues
   c. subcutaneous fat to protect the inner organs
   d. warmth
4. The building blocks of protein are
   a. vitamins and minerals
   b. carbohydrates and water
   c. polyunsaturates
   d. amino acids
5. Jim, a football player, was surprised to learn that
   a. he needed an increase in protein to maintain his physical activity
   b. he did not need an increase in protein to maintain his physical activity
   c. his energy supply came from protein
   d. vitamin and mineral supplements were necessary to keep him in top shape
6. The best source of high-quality protein is
   a. vegetable products
   b. powdered protein supplements
   c. shellfish
   d. animal products
7. The best way to obtain sufficient amounts of protein for daily use is to eat
   a. a combination of animal and vegetable protein
   b. only animal protein
   c. cereal and bread
   d. diet supplements
8. Carbohydrates are those foods that are made up of
   a. amino acids
   b. fatty acids
   c. muscle tissue
   d. sugars and starches

9. A main function of carbohydrates is
   a. to build and repair the body
   b. to supply the body with energy
   c. to regulate body temperature
   d. to manufacture hormones and enzymes

10. An excess intake of carbohydrates can cause
    a. constipation
    b. a person to become overweight
    c. excess energy and hyperactivity
    d. diarrhea

11. A carbohydrate that is a source of calories only (no other nutrients) is
    a. refined sugar
    b. glucose
    c. human milk
    d. there is no such food

12. Which of the following is true about fats?
    a. as a nutrient, fats are essential and good for the body
    b. they are a concentrated source of energy
    c. they aid in the absorption of fat-soluble vitamins
    d. all of the above

13. A main difference between saturated and unsaturated fats is
    a. saturated fats are missing nitrogen atoms, and unsaturated fats tend to be liquid at room temperature
    b. saturated fats tend to be solid at room temperature, while unsaturated fats tend to be liquid at room temperature
    c. animal fats are more liquid, and vegetable fats tend to be unsaturated
    d. saturated fats are liquid at room temperature, and unsaturated fats are solid at room temperature

14. The main nutritional problem in our country is
    a. overweight
    b. lack of adequate protein
    c. lack of adequate vitamins and minerals
    d. too much protein

15. Many processed foods, such as bread, baked goods, noodles, and dried fruit, are rich in:
    a. fats
    b. proteins
    c. cholesterol
    d. carbohydrates

16. Which of the following may increase blood cholesterol?
    a. a diet high in polyunsaturated fats
    b. a diet low in saturated fats
    c. unsaturated fat
    d. a diet high in saturated fats

17. This vitamin helps in the absorption of calcium and phosphorus in bone formation:
    a. vitamin B_2
    b. vitamin B_{12}
    c. vitamin D
    d. vitamin E

18. This vitamin is found only in the animal kingdom and strict vegetarians often suffer a deficiency of it:
    a. vitamin B_2 —riboflavin
    b. vitamin B_{12} —cyanocabalamin
    c. vitamin D—calciferol
    d. vitamin E—tocopherol

19. Natural vitamins are better than synthesized vitamins because
    a. they do not contain any additives
    b. they are much cheaper
    c. the body can digest them much better due to their chemical makeup
    d. none of the above

20. The function of minerals is to
    a. act as a catalyst to allow chemical reactions to take place
    b. provide the body with fuel and energy
    c. allow the breakdown and use of vitamins
    d. build and regulate body functions

21. Stems of salad greens, celery, and apple skins are rich sources of:
    a. sugars
    b. calcium
    c. B_{12}
    d. fiber

22. If a person is having trouble with hemorrhoids, colitis, or constipation, the doctor may tell the person to
    a. decrease the bulk and roughage in her diet
    b. go on an all-liquid diet
    c. include more bulk and roughage in her diet
    d. increase foods higher in cholesterol

23. Good replacements for meat in the diet are
    a. meat analogs
    b. nuts
    c. legumes
    d. all of the above

24. An excess consumption of fats has been found to be associated with
    a. obesity
    b. high level of blood cholesterol
    c. high incidence of coronary heart disease
    d. all of the above

25. Athletes do not necessarily need increased protein when they are engaged in sports because
    a. too much protein causes sluggishness
    b. athletes should restrict their food intake
    c. energy needs are best met by carbohydrates and fats
    d. proteins form antibodies

26. You can reduce the intake of saturated fats by switching to
    a. lard
    b. liquid vegetable oils
    c. hydrogenated shortenings
    d. margarines

27. Susan followed a high-protein diet for a month and was disgusted to discover she gained five pounds instead of losing weight. How could this have happened?
    a. extra protein is used for calories or converted to body fat
    b. excess protein causes an uncontrollable desire for sweets
    c. excess protein causes weight gain from extra muscle growth
    d. Susan has a slow metabolism, slowed even more by excess protein

28. Which of the following groups would have the least amount of fat?
    a. baked potato, beans, consomme
    b. broiled round steak, olives, apple pie
    c. walnuts, bacon, baking chocolate
    d. broiled cod, milk, creamed soups

29. Which is the best source of vitamin A?
    a. nuts
    b. melon
    c. yellow vegetables and fruits
    d. dark green leafy vegetables

30. Which of the following is the best source of vitamin C?
    a. berries, tomatoes, potatoes
    b. squash
    c. milk, grains, eggs
    d. peas, kumquats, carrots

31. Neglecting iodine-rich foods may cause
    a. gout
    b. goiter
    c. gall bladder infection
    d. gangrene

32. From what sources do we get roughage or fiber?
    a. plant sources
    b. vitamins
    c. animal sources
    d. beverages

33. Certain vitamins taken in excess of the RDA will protect an individual against
    a. miscarriage
    b. colds
    c. heart disease
    d. multiple sclerosis
    e. none of the above

34. Which of the following vitamins would be most likely to cause problems when taken in large amounts above the RDA during pregnancy?
    a. vitamin B_{12}
    b. vitamin B_6
    c. vitamin D
    d. vitamin A
    e. vitamins are not harmful in large doses

35. Trace elements can be maintained in adequate quantity in the diet by
    a. emphasizing the dairy products food group
    b. taking vitamin and mineral supplements
    c. taking mineral supplements only
    d. eating a well-balanced diet from the four food groups
    e. sprouting alfalfa and eating the uncooked sprouts

36. The quantity of fiber in the diet will be adequate if an individual consumes
    a. plenty of meat and white bread
    b. recommended servings from the dairy group of the basic four food groups
    c. a fiber supplement such as raisins
    d. a diet made up of selections from all of the basic food groups

37. The most reliable source of calcium is
    a. turnip greens
    b. milk
    c. collards
    d. mustard greens

38. Pick out the true statement:
    a. proteins are made up of 10 different amino acids
    b. dietary protein cannot contribute to fat weight gain
    c. muscle growth is stimulated by consumption of large quantities of protein
    d. protein cannot be stored for growth and repair as fats and sugars can be for energy

39. The main danger of a strict vegetarian diet is
    a. lack of essential amino acids
    b. too much bulk and fiber content
    c. lack of vitamin B_{12}
    d. heart attack

40. One advantage of whole-wheat flour over refined flour is
    a. it offers more roughage because of the bran
    b. it is much more nutritious
    c. it is a "natural" food
    d. there isn't any advantage of one over the other

41. The word "fortified" on a box of cereal means
    a. nutrients lost in the milling process have been replaced
    b. nutrients have been added beyond the natural level
    c. it is a "health" food
    d. it is high in cholesterol

42. The nutrients added to enriched bread are
    a. iron, thiamine, riboflavin, and niacin
    b. proteins
    c. fiber
    d. calcium and vitamin C

43. In regard to sucrose, it has been found that
    a. the body does not require it
    b. it promotes tooth decay and gum disease
    c. it is less damaging to the teeth when taken in liquid form
    d. too much may play a part in coronary artery disease
    e. all of the above

44. The main reason additives and preservatives are used in foods is
    a. to prevent spoilage
    b. to replace lost nutrients
    c. to make food taste better
    d. to give the public a wide variety of foods
    e. all of the above

45. A diet high in saturated fats tends to
    a. have little effect on serum cholesterol
    b. lower serum cholesterol
    c. raise serum cholesterol
    d. be better for health reasons than one high in polyunsaturates

46. The best way to reduce serum cholesterol is to
    a. stop eating polyunsaturates
    b. there is no way to reduce serum cholesterol, since the body manufactures it
    c. stop exercising
    d. reduce the amount of dietary saturated fat consumed

47. Food processing is necessary for
    a. feeding the populace of the world
    b. helping to improve texture, flavor, and appearance in some foods
    c. killing some bacteria and enzymes which destroy food over a period of time
    d. all of the above

48. During cooking, some vitamins
    a. are destroyed
    b. are chemically broken down
    c. pass out of the food into the cooking water

49. One of the problems encountered with quickie restaurant food is
    a. spread of germs and bacteria from so many people handling the food
    b. too high in fat content
    c. too expensive
    d. none of the above

50. The major difference between "organic" and "inorganic" food is:
    a. inorganic is more likely to be infected with parasites
    b. organic is far superior in quality of nutrients
    c. plants treated with organic fertilizer are healthier and produce more food
    d. organic is more costly

51. What essential nutrients does refined sugar contain?
    a. no nutrients; it is a source of calories only
    b. B vitamins
    c. trace minerals
    d. fats

52. Why are whole-grain products superior to highly refined products?
    a. whole-grain products contain the nutrient-rich bran and wheat germ, as well as the starchy endosperm portion from which processed cereal products are made
    b. processed cereal products void of sugars contain more nutrients
    c. processed cereal products are harder to digest
    d. enriched flour contains all the nutrients of whole grains

53. Indicate the misleading nutrition statement among the following:
    a. whether food is bought fresh, canned, or frozen has less influence on its nutritional value than how it is prepared
    b. in a general sense, food processing decreases the overall nutrient content of foods
    c. breastfeeding is superior nutritionally to bottle-feeding
    d. sugar, honey, sweets, and other high-energy foods taken immediately before short-term competitive sports events will enhance performance
    e. certain foods such as carrots and spinach are more nutritious cooked than raw

54. Which of the following is not a method for determining total body fat?
    a. measurement of basal metabolic rate
    b. measurement of body density
    c. measurement of body water content
    d. total body radiopotassium content

55. Which one of the following affects feelings of hunger?
    a. the pituitary gland
    b. the glucose level in the blood
    c. the thyroid gland
    d. the adrenal system

56. Overweight persons have a higher incidence of all the following problems except
    a. liver disease
    b. diabetes
    c. cancer
    d. high blood pressure
57. Which one of the following is not normally associated with obesity?
    a. diabetes
    b. gall bladder problems
    c. increased complications during pregnancy
    d. hernia
    e. none of the above
58. Verna has decided to change her eating habits in order to lose weight. She should do all of the following *except:*
    a. read or watch TV while eating
    b. confine her eating to the family's usual eating place
    c. eat foods that take more time to eat, such as oranges
    d. avoid lingering at the table when the meal is over
59. Hal is following a high-protein diet, eating mostly meat, cheese, eggs, and fish. What is the greatest danger of this type of diet?
    a. diverticulitis
    b. breakdown of muscle tissue
    c. hypoglycemia
    d. increased serum cholesterol
60. Which of the following cooking habits is not a good idea?
    a. broil all meat that normally would be fried
    b. remove the skin and any loose fat from chicken before cooking
    c. cook vegetables in margarine or butter instead of water
    d. learn which are the low- and no-calorie foods and serve them often
61. A person usually becomes obese because of
    a. heredity
    b. total energy input (calories) exceeding total energy output
    c. high blood cholesterol levels
    d. stress factors
    e. all of the above
62. The most accurate way to determine body fat would be
    a. weighing on bathroom scales
    b. height and weight charts
    c. skin caliper assessments
    d. looking in a mirror
63. As people grow older, even though they remain physically active, they must
    a. increase their intake of protein
    b. reduce caloric intake
    c. take thyroid pills to increase the BMR
    d. sleep more in order to decrease BMR

64. Which of the following diseases is usually not associated with obesity?
    a. premature aging
    b. angina pectoris
    c. emphysema
    d. diabetes mellitus

65. Obesity may reduce a person's life span as much as
    a. 15 years
    b. 20 years
    c. 25 years

66. A fasting diet often causes
    a. too much of a strain on the kidneys
    b. the loss of lean body mass
    c. ketosis
    d. diarrhea

67. Among the mechanical gadgets offered to help reduce weight, which of the following has been proven to be the most effective?
    a. body suits
    b. weighted waistbelts
    c. constricting bands
    d. they are all equally worthless

68. Which of the following is the best diet program?
    a. cutting back the portions of normal meals
    b. hormone shots (HCG)
    c. substituting foods with higher fat content
    d. a high-protein diet

69. Weight loss can be best accomplished by
    a. isometric exercise
    b. isotonic exercise
    c. exercise that requires a significant increase in cardiorespiratory (heart-lung) activity
    d. stretching exercises that activitate fat cells
    e. exercise that provides some type of massaging in order to facilitate the breaking up of fat pads

70. Which of the following is true concerning exercise and weight control?
    a. it takes a gargantuan effort to work off a tiny bit of weight
    b. exercise makes you hungry, so you end up eating more and gaining weight
    c. once you reach middle age, exercise suppresses the appetite and causes excessive weight loss
    d. obesity in the U.S. is more a problem of under-exercising than overeating
    e. weight loss through exercise is usually only water loss

71. If caloric restriction is being used to lose weight, a man should not restrict daily caloric intake to less than _____ calories per day without consulting a physician.
    a. 1,800
    b. 1,500
    c. 1,000
    d. 600
    e. 300

72. Which of the following makes the greatest contribution to obesity?
    a. hormonal disorders
    b. lack of physical exercise
    c. the presence of cellulite as a type of fat deposition
    d. low basal metabolic rate
    e. eating habits

73. The main nutritional problem in our country is
    a. too much protein
    b. lack of adequate protein
    c. lack of adequate vitamins
    d. obesity

Answers:

1) c	16) d	31) b	46) d	61) b
2) a	17) c	32) a	47) d	62) c
3) b	18) b	33) e	48) c	63) b
4) d	19) d	34) a	49) b	64) c
5) b	20) d	35) d	50) d	65) a
6) d	21) d	36) d	51) a	66) b
7) a	22) c	37) b	52) a	67) d
8) d	23) d	38) d	53) d	68) a
9) b	24) d	39) c	54) a	69) c
10) b	25) c	40) a	55) b	70) d
11) a	26) b	41) b	56) a	71) b
12) d	27) a	42) a	57) e	72) b
13) b	28) a	43) e	58) a	73) d
14) a	29) c	44) e	59) d	
15) d	30) a	45) c	60) c	

APPENDIX C

Sources of Nutrition Education Information

Following is a list of various agencies and organizations who are potential sources of materials and information in the field of nutrition and weight control. Some of the materials available are free of charge, others are not.

Abbott Laboratories
14th and Sheridan Road
North Chicago, Illinois 60600
materials: recipe books for the overweight or diabetic

American Alliance for Health, Physical Education and Recreation
1201 Sixteenth Street, N.W.
Washington, D.C. 20036
materials: pamphlets, films, lists

American Association for Maternal and Child Health (AAMCH)
P.O. Box 965
Los Altos, California 94022

American Cancer Society
Director of Public Education
777 Third Avenue
New York, New York 10017
materials: films, pamphlets, posters, etc.

American Dental Association
Bureau of Dental Health Education
211 E. Chicago Avenue
Chicago, Illinois 60611
materials: pamphlets, charts, posters, models

American Diabetes Association
1 West 18th Street
New York, New York 10020
"A.D.A. Forecase" bimonthly magazine reprints, pamphlets

American Dietetic Association
430 North Michigan Avenue
Chicago, Illinois 60611

American Heart Association
7320 Greenville Avenue
Dallas, Texas 75231

American Home Economics Association
2010 Massachusetts Avenue, N.W.
Washington, D.C. 20036
materials: pamphlets, reprints

American Institute of Baking
Department of Nutrition Education
400 E. Ontario Street
Chicago, Illinois 60611

American Medical Association
Bureau of Health Education
535 North Dearborn Street
Chicago, Illinois 60610

American Nurses Association
Public Relations Department
2420 Pershing Road
Kansas City, Missouri 64108

American Public Health Association
1015 18th Street, N.W.
Washington, D.C. 20036

Borden Company
Consumer Services
350 Madison Avenue
New York, New York 10000

Cereal Institute, Inc.
Educational Director
135 S. LaSalle Street
Chicago, Illinois 60603
materials: filmstrips, pamphlets

Child Study Association of America
50 Madison Avenue
New York, New York 10010

Educational Broadcasting Corporation
356 W. 58th Street
New York, New York 10019

Encyclopedia Britannica Films, Inc.
5625 Hollywood Blvd.
Hollywood, California
             OR
7250 MacArthur Blvd.
Oakland, California 94600

Evaporated Milk Association
910 17th Street, N.W.
Washington, D.C. 20006

Florida Department of Citrus
P.O. Box 148
Lakeland, Florida 33802
materials: pamphlets, posters, films

Fresh Fruit and Vegetable Association
1019 19th Street, N.W.
Washington, D.C. 20036

National Academy of Sciences
Food and Nutrition Board
Office of Information
2101 Constitution Avenue
Washington, D.C. 20418

National Better Business Bureau, Inc.
Chrysler Building
405 Lexington Avenue
New York, New York 10000

National Canners Association
Home Economics Division
1133 20th Street, N.W.
Washington, D.C. 20036

National Dairy Council
Nutrition Education
6300 N. River Road
Rosemont, Illinois 60018

National Foundation March of Dimes
Box 2000
White Plains, New York 10602
materials: charts, pamphlets concerning maternal
nutrition

National Health Council
1740 Broadway
New York, New York 10019

National Heart and Lung Institute
National Institutes of Health
9600 Rockville Pike, Bldg. 31, Rm. 5A52
Bethesda, Maryland 20014

National Livestock and Meat Board
444 N. Michigan Avenue
Chicago, Illinois 60611

National Publicity Council for Health and Welfare
Services
815 Second Avenue
New York, New York 10017

Single Service Institute (Disposables)
Public Health Committee
250 Park Avenue
New York, New York 10017
materials: periodicals on food handling and food
service sanitation

Sunkist Growers
14130 Riverside Drive
Sherman Oaks, California 91423

U.S. Department of Agriculture
Human Nutrition Research Branch
14th Street and Independence Avenue, S.W.
Washington, D.C. 20250

U.S. Public Health Service
Public Inquiries Branch
200 Independence Avenue, S.W.
Washington, D.C. 20201

Wheat Flour Institute
1776 F. Street, N.W.
Washington, D.C. 20006

World Health Organization
777 United Nations Plaza
New York, New York 10017

APPENDIX D

Suggested Nutritional References

NORMAL NUTRITION

Alfin-Slater, R., and Aftergood, L. *Nutrition for Today*. Dubuque: William C. Brown Co., 1977.

Chancey, M.S., and Ross, M. L. *Nutrition*. Boston: Houghton Mifflin Co., 1971.

Deutsch, R. *The Family Guide to Better Food and Better Health*. New York: Bantam Books, 1973.

Deutsch, R. *Realities of Nutrition*. Palo Alto: Bull Publishing Co., 1976.

Guthrie, H. *Introductory Nutrition*. Saint Louis: The C. V. Mosby Co., 1975.

Keyes, A. and M. *How to Eat Well and Stay Well the Mediterranean Way*. New York: Doubleday & Co., 1975.

Kotschevar, L. H., and McWilliams, M. *Understanding Foods*. New York: New American Library, 1975.

Labuza, T. P. *Food and Your Well Being*. St. Paul: West Publishing Co., 1977.

Martin, E., and Coolidge, A. *Nutrition in Action.* New York: Holt, Rinehart and Winston, 1978.

Mayer, J. *A Diet for Living*. Mt. Vernon, N.Y.: Consumers Union, 1975.

McWilliams, M. *Food Fundamentals,* 2nd edition. New York: Wiley, 1974.

National Academy of Sciences. *Recommended Dietary Allowances,* 8th edition. Washington, D.C.: National Academy of Sciences, 1974.

Stare, F., and McWilliams, M. *Living Nutrition*. New York: Wiley, 1977.

Stare, F., and McWilliams, M. *Nutrition for Good Health*. Redondo Beach, Ca.: Plycon Press, 1974.

U.S. Government. *Composition of Foods*. Washington, D.C.: U.S. Government Printing Office.

White, P., and Selvey, N. *Let's Talk About Food*. Boston: Publishing Sciences Group, 1974.

INFANT CARE

Fomon, S. *Infant Nutrition*. Philadelphia: W. B. Saunders Co., 1974.

Spock, B., and Lowenberg, M. *Feeding Your Baby and Child.* New York: Pocket Books, 1968.

TEENAGERS

Gilbert, S. *Fat Free: Common Sense for Young Weight Worriers.* New York: Macmillan Co., 1975.

McWilliams, M. *Nutrition for the Growing Years,* 2nd edition. New York: Wiley, 1975.

MATURE YEARS

Institute of Rehabiliation, New York University Medical Center. *Mealtime Manual for the Aged and Handicapped.* New York: Simon and Schuster, 1970.

ABOUT FOOD FADS

Barrett, S., and Knight, G. *The Health Robbers.* Philadelphia: G. F. Stickley Co., 1976.

Deutsch, R. *The New Nuts Among the Berries.* Palo Alto: Bull Publishing Co., 1976.

Whelan, E., and Stare, F. *Panic in the Pantry.* New York: Atheneum, 1977.

WEIGHT CONTROL

Ferguson, J. *Habits, Not Diets.* Palo Alto: Bull Publishing Co., 1976.

Jordan, H. A., et al. *Eating Is Okay: A Radical Approach to Successful Weight Loss.* New York: Rawson Associates Publishers, 1976.

Konishi, F. *Exercise Equivalents of Foods.* Carbondale: Southern Illinois University Press, 1974.

Mayer, J. *Overweight, Causes, Costs, Control.* Englewood Cliffs, N.J.: Prentice-Hall, 1968.

Redbook's Wise Woman's Diet and Exercise Book. *New York: McCall Publishing Co., 1970.*

Schoenberg, H. *Cookbook for Calorie Watchers.* New York: Good Housekeeping Books, 1972.

Stare, F., and Whelan, E. M. *How to Eat Crackers in Bed and Keep Slim.* North Quincy, Ma.: Christopher Publishing House, 1978.

VEGETARIANISM

Ewald, E. *Recipes for a Small Planet.* New York: Ballantine Books, 1975.

Lappe, F. M. *Diet for a Small Planet.* New York: Ballantine Books, 1975.

Lappe, F. M., and Ewald, E. *Great Meatless Meals.* New York: Ballantine Books, 1976.

HEART DISEASE

Cutler, C. *Haute Cuisine for Your Heart's Delight.* New York: Clarkson N. Potter, 1973.

Eshleman, R., and Winston, M. *The American Heart Association Cookbook.* New York: David McKay Co., Inc., 1973; New York: Ballantine Books, 1976.

Margolese, R. G. *A Doctor's Eat-Healthy Guide for Good Health and Long Life.* New York: Parker Publishing Co., 1974.

SPECIAL NUTRITIONAL INTERESTS

Bogert, L. J., Briggs, G. M., and Calloway, D. H. *Nutrition and Physical Fitness.* Philadelphia: W. B. Saunders Co., 1973.

Bradley, H., and Sundberg, C. *Keeping Food Safe.* New York: Doubleday & Co., 1975.

Cormican, A. *Controlling Diabetes with Diet.* Springfield, Il.: Charles C Thomas, 1971.

Kraus, B. *The Barbara Kraus Dictionary of Protein.* New York: Harper Magazine Press, 1975.

Kraus, B. *The Barbara Kraus Guide to Fiber in Foods.* New York: New American Library, 1975.

Roe, D. *A Plague of Corn.* Ithaca, N.Y.: Cornell University Press, 1973.

Rosenthal, S. *Live High on Low Fat.* Philadelphia: J. B. Lippincott Co., 1975.

Portions of this list suggested by Frederick J. Stare, M.D., Julia C. Witschi, M.S., and Martha R. Singer, M.P.H., Harvard School of Nutrition.

APPENDIX E

Combining Foods to Your Own Best Advantage

The menus on the following pages are from "Combining Foods to Your Own Best Advantage," by Mary Hill, *Yearbook of Agriculture 1974,* U.S. Department of Agriculture.

A Day's Food Intake for an Adult
Based on Specific Amounts as Listed in the Food Guide

EARLY MORNING
Fruit-flavored beverage—vitamin C added
Cooked whole wheat cereal with milk
Toast—jam
Coffee

MIDDAY MEAL
Cream of asparagus soup
Tuna salad sandwich   Iced tea
Ice cream

SNACK
Pear

EVENING MEAL
Broiled chicken
Parslied potatoes   Spinach
Lettuce-tomato salad   French dressing
Apricot-tapioca cream pudding
Coffee

EVENING SNACK
Toast with jam
Milk

Nutritional Foundation of This Day's Food

Milk Group 2 cups	Fruit-Veg. Group 4 servings	Meat or Alternate 2 servings	Bread-Cereal—4 servings (enriched or whole grain)
½ cup—on cereal	1 serving pear	1 serving tuna—	1 serving cooked
½ cup—in tapioca	1 serving potato	in sandwich	whole wheat cereal
1 cup—as beverage	1 serving spinach	1 serving chicken	2 servings in sandwich
	1 serving salad		1 slice toast

Foods That Provide Additional Nutrients and Food Energy to Meet Individual Needs

From the 4 Food Groups	From Other Foods
Milk and asparagus in soup	Fruit-flavored beverage—vitamin C added
Lettuce in sandwich	Jam
Apricots and other ingredients	Sugar in iced tea and coffee
in the pudding	French dressing on salad
Toast in evening snack	Butter on toast and hot vegetables

E-3 An Italian selection from the four food groups:

EARLY MORNING
Banana
Sweet sausage Scrambled egg
Italian bread (enriched)
Coffee

MIDDAY MEAL
Minestrone Italian bread
Mixed vegetable salad (lettuce, tomato, green pepper,
carrot, onion)—French dressing
Ice cream
Milk

EVENING MEAL
Veal Parmesan Spaghetti—tomato sauce
Kale Italian bread
Zabaglione (soft custard flavored with wine)
Coffee

Nutritional Foundation of This Day's Food

Milk Group 2 cups	Fruit-Veg. Group 4 servings	Meat or Alternate 2 servings	Bread-Cereal—4 servings (enriched or whole grain)
1 cup as beverage ½ cup equivalent in ice cream ½ cup in zabaglione	1 serving—banana 1 serving in salad 1 serving—kale 1 serving in minestrone	1 serving—sausage 1 serving—veal	3 servings—Italian bread 1 serving—enriched spaghetti

Foods That Provide Additional Nutrients and Food Energy to Meet Individual Needs

From the 4 Food Groups	From Other Foods
Scrambled egg Milk in coffee Remaining ingredients in minestrone Tomato sauce	Butter or margarine on bread Sugar in coffee French dressing

A day's food intake for a "snacker" might look like this:

7:30 a.m.	Instant breakfast (instant breakfast powder+1 cup milk)
10:00 a.m.	Two doughnuts (enriched) Milk
11:00 a.m.	Apple
12:30 p.m.	Hamburger (onion, relish, tomato slice), French fries, Cola
3:00 p.m.	Plain Danish (enriched) Milk
4:30 p.m.	Hard-boiled egg Saltines
6:00 p.m.	Lasagna, Coleslaw, Iced tea
8:30 p.m.	Cheese dip with assorted raw vegetables (carrot strips, tomato wedges, cauliflower flowerets, broccoli flowerets)

Nutritional Foundation of This Day's Food

Milk Group 2 cups	Fruit-Veg. Group 4 servings	Meat or Alternate 2 servings	Bread-Cereal—4 servings (enriched or whole grain)
1 cup in instant breakfast 1 cup as beverage	Apple—1 serving French fries—1 serving Coleslaw—1 serving Raw veg.—1 serving	Hamburger—1 serving Lasagna—1 serving (meat in it)	2 doughnuts—2 servings Hamburger roll—1 serving Danish—1 serving

Foods That Provide Additional Nutrients and Food Energy to Meet Individual Needs

From the 4 Food Groups	From Other Foods
Onion, relish, tomato Served on hamburger Hard-boiled egg Saltines—enriched Lasagna noodles (enriched) and sauce Cheese dip Milk in coffee	Instant breakfast powder Sugar in coffee Cola Dressing on coleslaw

EARLY MORNING MEAL
Pineapple juice
Wheat flakes with milk
Doughnut (enriched)
Coffee

MID-MORNING
Peach

MIDDAY MEAL
Hard-cooked eggs—cream sauce
Whole-wheat bread—butter or margarine
Brussels sprouts
Molasses cookies   Milk

EVENING MEAL
Vegetarian baked beans
Green pepper stuffed with rice and tomato sauce
Tossed green salad   French dressing
Raisin pie
Milk

Nutritional Foundation of This Day's Food

Milk Group 2 cups	Fruit-Veg. Group 4 servings	Meat or Alternate 2 servings	Bread-Cereal—4 servings (enriched or whole grain)
1 cup as beverage ½ cup with cereal ½ cup in cream sauce	1 serving—pine- apple juice 1 serving—peach 1 serving—brussels sprouts 1 serving—green pepper	1 serving—2 eggs 1 serving—vegetarian baked beans	1 serving wheat flakes 1 serving doughnut 1 serving whole-wheat bread 1 serving rice

Foods That Provide Additional Nutrients and Food Energy to Meet Individual Needs

From the 4 Food Groups	From Other Foods
Milk as beverage and in coffee Remaining ingredients in cream sauce Molasses cookies—enriched Tomato sauce Tossed green salad Raisin pie	Butter or margarine with bread Sugar in coffee French dressing

EARLY MORNING

Orange	1 medium
Bulgur	1 cup
with brewer's yeast	1 tablespoon
Toasted wheat-soy bread	1 slice
with honey	1 tablespoon

MID-MORNING SNACK

Shelled almonds	¼ cup

MIDDAY MEAL

Split pea soup	2 cups
Peanut butter sandwich:	
Peanut butter	2 tablespoons
Whole wheat bread	2 slices
Honey	1 tablespoon
Fruit-sunflower seed salad:	
Apple	½ medium
Banana	½ medium
Sunflower seeds	¼ cup
Lettuce	1 leaf

SNACK

Peach	1 medium

EVENING MEAL

Soybeans	1 cup
Brown rice cooked	1 cup
fried in oil	2 tablespoons
with chestnuts	2 tablespoons
with sesame seeds	2 tablespoons
Collards	1 cup
Pear	1 medium

EVENING SNACK

Raisins	¼ cup

E-7   A Jewish homemaker's plans for a day's meals:

EARLY MORNING
Orange juice

Poached egg   Bagel with butter

Coffee

MIDDAY MEAL
Chopped chicken liver sandwich—rye bread

Perfection salad (mixed vegetables in gelatine)

Watermelon

Hot tea

EVENING MEAL
Broiled halibut

Baked potato   Glazed carrots

Pickled beets   Roll and butter

Cheesecake

Skim milk

EVENING SNACK
Graham crackers   Skim milk

Nutritional Foundation of This Day's Food

Milk Group 2 cups	Fruit-Veg. Group 4 servings	Meat or Alternate 2 servings	Bread-Cereal—4 servings (enriched or whole grain)
2 cups as beverage	Orange juice Watermelon Baked potato Carrots	Chicken liver Halibut	1 bagel 2 slices bread 1 roll

Foods That Provide Additional Nutrients and Food Energy to Meet Individual Needs

From the 4 Food Groups	From Other Foods
Poached egg Hard-cooked egg and onion in chicken liver spread Perfection salad Pickled beets Cheesecake—enriched Graham crackers—enriched	Butter on roll and bagel Sugar for coffee and tea Dressing on salad

Glossary

ABSORPTION—In physiology, the uptake of nutrients, water, or other substances by the stomach or intestinal walls following digestion of food.

ADIPOCYTE—A fat cell.

ADIPOSE—Animal fat; adipose tissue is the part of the body where fat is stored.

AEROBIC—Living or functioning in the presence of air or free oxygen.

AFLATOXIN—A liver carcinogen, produced by some types of molds.

AMINO ACID—An organic compound of carbon, hydrogen, oxygen, and nitrogen; when amino acids are linked together in a specific pattern they form a molecule of protein.

ANAEROBIC—Living or functioning in the absence of air or free oxygen.

ANALEPTIC—A drug that stimulates the central nervous system; an example is caffeine.

ANALGESIC—A drug that relieves pain.

ANEMIA—A blood deficiency, either qualitative or quantitative in nature.

ANGINA PECTORIS—Acute chest pain due to interference with the oxygen supply to the heart.

ANOREXIA—Loss of appetite for food.

ANTIOXIDANT—A substance capable of protecting another substance against oxidation.

APOPLEXY—Stroke; a condition in which blood supply is impaired to the brain.

ARRYTHMIA—Variation from the normal heartbeat rhythm.

ASCORBIC ACID—Vitamin C.

ATHEROSCLEROSIS—A process in which fatty materials, including cholesterol, are deposited along the lining of the walls of blood vessels, sometimes impairing blood flow.

ATROPHY—Wasting away of a normally developed tissue or organ.

BRAN—The outer coarse coat of grains.

CALCIUM—A mineral element which is a vital constituent of bone and is essential for proper muscle tone, nerve function, and blood clotting.

CALORIE—(Kilocalorie) The unit by which heat or energy is measured. It is the amount of heat needed to raise the temperature of one liter of water by one degree centigrade.

CARBOHYDRATES—A group of organic compounds containing carbon, hydrogen, and oxygen which are converted to carbon dioxide and water in the body with the release of energy.

CARCINOGEN—A cancer-causing substance.

CAROTENE—A yellow compound that is a form of vitamin A and occurs in some plants.

CELLULOSE—A carbohydrate found in the fiber part of plants.

CHOLESTEROL—A fatlike substance found in animal fat and some organs. It is manufactured in the body, and when found in high levels in the blood, it is associated with increased risk of coronary heart disease.

CIRRHOSIS—An inflammation of the liver or other organ.

COFACTOR—An element whose presence is required for the proper function of another.

COLLAGEN—The protein that forms the major constituent of connective tissue, cartilage, tendon, bone, and skin.

COLLATERAL CIRCULATION—A side branch of a blood vessel.

CORONARY—Refers to the arteries that supply the heart.

DEHYDRATION—The loss of water.

DERMATITIS—Inflammation of the skin.

DIABETES MELLITUS—A disorder due to low or insufficient production of the pancreatic enzyme insulin. Insulin is necessary for oxidation of sugar in the tissues. The disorder is usually accompanied by high water requirements and excretion of large quantities of urine.

DIGESTION—The breaking down of food into simpler components in the digestive tract.

DUODENUM—The portion of the small intestine that first receives the stomach contents; the pancreatic and common bile ducts also empty into the duodenum, making it very important in digestion.

DYSPEPSIA—Indigestion.

DYSPNEA—Difficult or labored breathing.

EDEMA—An accumulation of or an excess of water in a part of the body causing swelling.

EMBOLUS—A material transported in the vascular system that obstructs blood flow.

ENDEMIC—Refers to a disease that occurs constantly but in low incidence in a given population.

ENDOCRINE—Glands that secrete internally.

ENDOSPERM—The starchy portion within the kernel of grain.

ENZYME—One of a class of substances formed in living cells which act as catalysts in chemical reactions within the body.

EPINEPHRINE—Also known as adrenalin; a hormone produced by the adrenal medulla.

ETIOLOGY—The causes(s) of a disease or disorder.

EXACERBATION—An increase in severity.

EXOGENOUS—Has its origin outside cells or tissues.

FAT—A glyceryl ester of fatty acids, generally of plant and animal origin.

FAT-SOLUBLE—Refers generally to substances that cannot be dissolved in water, but can be dissolved in fats and oils or in fat solvents. The fat-soluble vitamins are A, D, E, and K.

FIBER—Polymers of carbohydrates found in plant sources which are undigestible by humans, and thus supply no calories, but only roughage for the digestive tract.

FOLIC ACID—One of the vitamins in the B-complex, deficiency of which causes poor growth and blood disorders.

FORTIFY—to add nutrients to a foodstuff beyond the level present before processing.

GASTRITIS—Inflammation of the stomach lining.

GLUCOSE—A simple carbohydrate containing six carbon atoms; it is the principal simple sugar in blood and body fluids.

GLUTEN—The tough substance formed when the proteins in flour absorb water; it gives dough its elasticity.

GLYCEROL—The same as glycerin; one of the products of the hydrolysis of ingested fats.

GLYCOGEN—The main storage form of carbohydrate in the body, mostly in the liver.

GOITER—Enlargement of the thyroid gland; simple goiter is caused by a deficiency of iodine in the diet.

HCG—Human Chorionic Gonadotropin, a hormone secreted by the placenta, found in considerable amounts in the urine of pregnant women. Injections of this hormone are part of the HCG diet.

HEMOGLOBIN—The pigment component of the blood which carries oxygen.

HEMORRHAGE—Blood loss.

HYDROGENATION—The process of adding hydrogen.

HYPER—Prefix meaning increased or in excess or normal.

HYPERKINESIS—Abnormally increased activity.

HYPERPHAGIA—Increase in appetite.

HYPERPLASIA—Increase in cell numbers.

HYPERTENSION—High blood pressure.

HYPERTROPHY—Increase in volume of a tissue by enlargement of the cells.

HYPO-—Prefix meaning decreased.

HYPOGLYCEMIA—Condition in which glucose levels in the blood are abnormally decreased.

HYPOTENSION—Decreased blood pressure.

HYPOTHALAMUS—The portion of the brain lying under the thalamus; the hypothalamus regulates the activity of the posterior lobe of the pituitary, therefore indirectly influencing fat and carbohydrate metabolism among other things.

IMMUNE—Lack of susceptibility to a certain disease.

INFARCTION—A localized area of dead or dying tissue produced by obstruction of blood supply to that area.

INSULIN—The hormone secreted by the pancreas which regulates the rate of carbohydrate utilization in the body.

ISCHEMIC HEART DISEASE—Disorder caused by a deficiency of blood supply to a part of the heart, due to obstruction or constriction of a blood vessel.

IU—International Units, the measurement of potency of a vitamin.

KETOSIS—Condition that occurs as a result of improper utilization of carbohydrates in the body, causing an accumulation of ketone bodies which are the products of incomplete fatty acid combustion.

LACTOSE—Milk sugar.

LEGUMES—Peas and beans.

LESION—A sore, ulcer, or any other damage to a tissue.

LINOLEICACID—A polyunsaturated fatty acid that the body cannot manufacture; it must be supplied in the diet.

LIPECTOMY—Removal of fatty tissue.

LIPID—A fat or fatlike substance.

LIPOLYSIS—The breaking up of fat.

MALNUTRITION—Poor nourishment due to improper diet or a defect in the metabolism of food.

METABOLISM—The sum of the chemical changes occurring in the body as food is converted to body tissue, energy is produced, and body tissue is broken down.

MORBIDITY—Sickness or illness.

MORPHOMETRIC—The measurement of form or shape.

MYELINATION—The formation of a fatlike substance, myelin, around the nerve axon.

MYOCARDIAL—Having to do with the heart muscle.

NATAL—Having to do with birth.

NECROSIS—Death of cells due to injury or disease.

NUTRIENT—A chemical compound with a specific function(s) in the nourishment of the body.

OBESITY—Excessive overweight due to a surplus of body fat.

OLEIC ACID—A colorless, oily liquid prepared from fats, the salts of which are oleates. The formula for oleic acid is $C_8H_{34}O_2$.

OSMOSIS—The transfer of materials through a semipermeable membrane such as the wall of a living cell.

OTC DRUG—A drug obtainable without a physician's prescription; over-the-counter drug.

OVERWEIGHT—An increase in weight of the total body compartments, including essential vital tissue (muscle, liver, kidney, blood, glands, joints), water, and fat.

PATHOLOGY—The study of the effects of disease.

PERISTALSIS—The wavelike movement of the esophagus and intestines which propels the contents along the digestive tract.

PHAGOCYTE—A cell found in blood, lymph fluid, and certain organs that can engulf particles that are harmful or foreign to the body.

PHOSPHOLIPID—Fatlike substance which contains phosphorus and nitrogen along with cholesterol and fatty acids; they are abundant in nervous tissue.

PLACEBO—An inactive substance which resembles a drug or medication given experimentally or for the psychological effects it may induce.

PLAQUE—Patches or unnatural formations on tissues such as inner arterial walls or tooth surfaces.

POLYUNSATURATED FATTY ACID—A fatty acid having more than one unsaturated linkage in the carbon chain, each lacking two hydrogen atoms.

POSTPRANDIAL—Following a meal.

PREDISPOSE—To indicate a special tendency toward a particular disease or other situation.

PROCESSING—Subjecting foodstuffs to various manufacturing procedures such as canning, freezing, or dehydrating, to alter their characteristics.

PROTEIN—A complex organic compound containing nitrogen, carbon, oxygen, and hydrogen, formed by various combinations of amino acids.

PYRUVIC ACID—A substance formed during aerobic carbohydrate metabolism.

RDA—Recommended Daily Allowance.

RNA—Ribonucleic acid; essential for cellular protein synthesis.

SALMONELLA—A large group of heat-sensitive bacteria, some of which are associated with food poisoning.

SATIETY—A feeling of fulness.

SATURATED FATTY ACID—Fatty acids having all the hydrogens the carbon chain can accommodate.

SICKLE CELL DISEASE—A blood disorder in which the red blood cells are shaped like sickles due to varying proportions of hemoglobin.

SOLUBLE—Capable of being dissolved or entering into solution.

STARCH—The storage form of carbohydrates in plants.

STASIS—A stoppage of the flow of blood or other body fluid.

STENOSIS—A narrowing of a body opening or passage such as a blood vessel.

STONE GROUND—The grinding of grains by old-fashioned millstones, generally resulting in a higher extraction rate.

SUBCUTANEOUS—Underneath the skin layers.

SYNCOPE—Fainting.

SYNDROME—A medical term meaning a group of symptoms that occur together.

SYNTHESIS—The coming together of two or more substances to form a new material.

THERAPEUTIC—Refers to curing a disease or disorder.

THROMBOSIS—A blood clot or mass.

TOXIC—Poisonous.

TRABECULATION—The formation of fibrous bands as a supporting structure in some organs such as the heart.

TRIGLYCERIDE—The storage form of fat in the body.

VASCULAR—In physiology, having to do with the blood and lymph vessels of the body.

VITAMINS—A group of substances that in relatively small amounts are necessary for life and proper growth.

WHEAT GERM—The heart or kernel of the wheat; the embryo, from which a new plant may develop.

Glossary References:

Encyclopedia and Dictionary of Medicine and Nursing. Benjamin F. Miller and Claire Brackman Keane. Philadelphia: J. B. Lippincott Company, 1972.

Food and Your Well-Being. Theodore P. Labuza. St. Paul, Minn.: West Publishing Co., 1977.

Food: The Yearbook of Agriculture 1959. U.S. Department of Agriculture, Washington, D.C.

"Grain Glossary," *Family Health/Today's Health,* May 1976, p. 68.

Health Foods Facts and Fakes. Sidney Margolius. New York: David McKay, Inc., 1973.

Index